Handbook of Communication in Anaesthesia and Critical Care

Handbook of Communication in Anaesthesia and Critical Care

A practical guide to exploring the art

Edited by

Allan M Cyna

Marion I Andrew

Suyin GM Tan

Andrew F Smith

OXFORD
UNIVERSITY PRESS

OXFORD
UNIVERSITY PRESS

Great Clarendon Street, Oxford OX2 6DP

Oxford University Press is a department of the University of Oxford.
It furthers the University's objective of excellence in research, scholarship,
and education by publishing worldwide in

Oxford New York

Auckland Cape Town Dar es Salaam Hong Kong Karachi Kuala Lumpur
Madrid Melbourne Mexico City Nairobi New Delhi Shanghai Taipei Toronto

With offices in

Argentina Austria Brazil Chile Czech Republic France Greece Guatemala Hungary Italy
Japan Poland Portugal Singapore South Korea Switzerland Thailand Turkey Ukraine Vietnam

Oxford is a registered trade mark of Oxford University Press
in the UK and in certain other countries

Published in the United States
by Oxford University Press Inc., New York

First published 2011

British Library Cataloguing in Publication Data
Data available

Library of Congress Cataloging in Publication Data

Handbook of communication in anaesthesia and critical care : a practical
guide to exploring the art / edited by Allan M. Cyna ... [et. al.].
p. ; cm.
Includes bibliographical references and index.
ISBN 978-0-19-957728-6 (alk. paper)
1. Anesthesiology—Handbooks, manuals, etc. 2. Communication in
medicine—Handbooks, manuals, etc. 3. Critical care medicine—Handbooks,
manuals, etc. I. Cyna, Allan M.
[DNLM: 1. Anesthesia—psychology. 2. Professional-Patient Relations. 3.
Communication. 4. Critical Care—psychology. WO 62]
RD82.2.H357 2011
617.9'6—dc22 2010029051

Typeset in Minion by Glyph International Bangalore, India
Printed in Great Britain on acid-free paper by CPI Antony Rowe

ISBN 978–0–19–957728–6

10 9 8 7 6 5 4 3 2 1

Dedicated to

Ayesha, Sophia, Benjamin
Hen, Doris, Mary, Louise
Kevin, Oban, Lewis, Arran, Todd, Ailsa
Adele, Martha and Naomi

Preface

'Whether you think you can or whether you think you can't—you are probably right!'
Adapted from Henry Ford

Communications with patients and colleagues frequently go well, yet few anaesthetists consciously appreciate how they achieve this, or how to teach what they do. Such intuitive skills are usually gained through many years of experience, rather than developing a structure of specific skills. We encourage readers to continue with their current modes of communication where these are working well. This book is primarily concerned with providing anaesthetists with a resource that offers ways of improving communication when the usual strategies are not working, or where the situation in which clinicians find themselves is unfamiliar. Strategies are suggested that can allow the anaesthetist to gain some understanding of the language structures involved, and facilitate the teaching of such skills. The concepts and tools used in this book draw on a wide range of ideas and, as such, constitute a blend of practice, teaching and research.

Unlike other books concerned with developing medical communication skills, this one discusses aspects of anaesthetic practice that can greatly enhance patients' well-being that are frequently not considered. The first of these is to optimize patients' perceptions of control over what is happening to them. Secondly, to appreciate that the way we communicate can increase the choices available to both patients and anaesthetists. Thirdly, to recognize that patients have both the ability and desire to assist and cooperate with their care wherever possible. To achieve this end, hospital experiences should be perceived by both patient and anaesthetist in the most positive mindset possible in any particular situation or context.

Although written with a view to be of interest primarily to anaesthetists, much of what is proposed would easily benefit other professional groups. We hope that paramedical, nursing and midwifery professional groups benefit from reading it, as many of the concepts could be readily adapted to these disciplines. We also envisage that this book will complement the development of comprehensive resources for communication skills teaching within postgraduate training in anaesthesia, and possibly other professional groups with whom anaesthetists work.

Finally, the reviewers of our original proposal universally recognized the need for a book on communication in anaesthesia. We are grateful for the considerable feedback from colleagues that we have received during its development and writing.

In the process, we have all learned a lot, and enjoyed ourselves along the way. The structure of the book is self-explanatory and, as a group, anaesthetists are impatient. We have therefore cut a rather wordy draft preface so that you can just get on with it ...

We would greatly value any feedback you have on this book. Please email any comments to medicine.books.uk@oup.com.

AMC
MIA
SGMT
AFS

Acknowledgements

We thank:
Evelyn M Hood for her invaluable assistance copyediting and proofreading the draft manuscript
Helen Beasley and Belinda Smith for secretarial support
&
Stavros Prineas for cartoon illustrations

Contents

Contributors

Dr Marion I Andrew
Department of Women's Anaesthesia,
Women's and Children's Hospital,
Adelaide, SA 5006, Australia

Dr Christel J Bejenke
Anesthesiologist,
Santa Barbara,
California, USA

Dr Allan M Cyna
Department of Women's Anaesthesia,
Women's and Children's Hospital,
Adelaide, SA 5006, Australia

Professor Marie-Elisabeth Faymonville
Department of Algology
and Palliative Care, Domaine
Universitaire du Sart Tilman, CHU
Liège-B 35, Belgium

Professor Ernil Hansen
Department of Anesthesiology,
University Regensburg Medical Center,
D-93042 Regensburg, Germany

Dr Gillian M Hood
Southern Group of Anaesthetic
Specialists, Flinders Private Hospital,
Bedford Park, South Australia, Australia

Dr Vincent J Kopp
Associate Professor,
Department of Anesthesiology,
School of Medicine, University of
North Carolina at Chapel Hill,
Chapel Hill, NC 27599, USA

Dr Elvira V Lang
Department of Radiology,
Beth Israel Deaconess Medical Center,
Harvard Medical School,
330 Brookline Ave, Boston,
MA 02115, USA

Dr Andrew McWilliam
Department of Anaesthesia,
Royal Lancaster Infirmary,
Lancaster LA1 4RP, UK

Professor Alan F Merry
Department of Anaesthesiology,
University of Auckland,
Private Bag 92019, Auckland,
New Zealand

Dr Sally N Merry
Werry Centre for Child and
Adolescent Mental Health,
Department of Psychological Medicine,
Faculty of Medical and Health Sciences,
University of Auckland,
Private Bag 92019, Auckland,
New Zealand

Dr Daniel Nethercott
Adult Intensive Care Unit,
Wythenshawe Hospital,
Southmoor Road,
Manchester M23 9LT, UK

Dr Stavros Prineas
Bathurst Base Hospital,
NSW Australia, Clinical Lecturer,
Notre Dame University,
Sydney, Australia

Dr Susanna Richmond
Department of Anaesthesia,
Royal Lancaster Infirmary,
Ashton Road,
Lancaster LA1 4RP, UK

Dr David Sainsbury
Department of Children's Anaesthesia,
Women's and Children's Hospital,
72 King William Rd, Adelaide, SA 5006,
Australia

Professor Audrey Shafer
Stanford University School of Medicine, Veterans Affairs Palo Alto Health Care System, 3801 Miranda Avenue, Palo Alto, CA 94304, USA

Dr Maire Shelly
Adult Intensive Care Unit, Wythenshawe Hospital, Southmoor Road, Manchester M23 9LT, UK

Dr Scott W Simmons
Department of Anaesthesia, Mercy Hospital for Women, 163 Studley Road, Heidelberg, Victoria 3084, Australia

Dr Andrew F Smith
Department of Anaesthesia and Lancaster Patient Safety Research Unit, Royal Lancaster Infirmary, Ashton Road, Lancaster, LA1 4RP, UK

Dr Diana C Strange Khursandi
Deputy Director of Clinical Training, Medical Education Unit, Caboolture Hospital, Caboolture, Queensland 4510, Australia

Dr Suyin GM Tan
Department of Anaesthesia and Pain Management, Nepean Hospital, Penrith, NSW 2750, Australia

Section 1

Principles of communication

Chapter 1

To begin...

Stavros Prineas, Andrew F Smith,
and Suyin GM Tan

'A journey of a thousand miles begins with a single step'.
Confucius

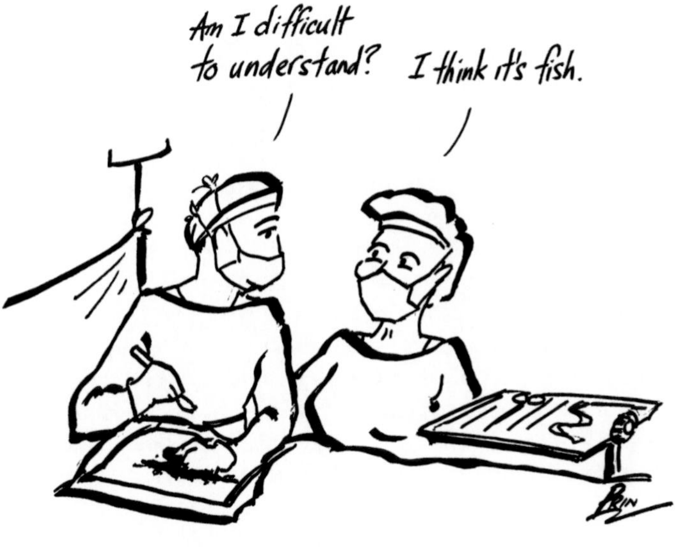

What this chapter is about

The importance of communication in anaesthetic practice

Communication is an innately fascinating and, on occasions, a somewhat mysterious topic. At its heart, it is the means of expressing, both to ourselves and to others, how we perceive the world and how we influence the world around us. It is a tool for exchanging information and meaning, but also a way to connect with others. While obviously a means to an end, it is also an end in itself—without the ability to share with others, life would be greatly impoverished. The many human dimensions of communication—the practical, the social, the linguistic, the lyrical, the subliminal, its ability to soothe and to injure, to inform, to entertain, to terrify—are what make this topic so challenging.

Anaesthesia has come a very long way since the 1840s. The advent of safer and more selective drugs, coupled with ever more sophisticated technology, has made the practice of anaesthesia safer, yet also more complicated. The patients that we treat are often older, have multiple co-morbidities, and are undergoing procedures that would have been unthinkable 20 years ago.

Yet with the increasingly complex workload have come the additional pressures of time and resource allocation. Patients are admitted on the day of surgery, leaving minimal time for anaesthetic assessment. Anaesthetists are frequently busy, isolated and unavailable when working in theatre, or find themselves working at multiple sites with little opportunity for interaction with colleagues. Similarly, theatre staff rarely work in the same operating room with the same team on a regular basis. The hospital administrators are under constant pressure as they strain to contain costs and reduce length of stay, while wards are increasingly understaffed and overworked. In the midst of all this, patients are left wondering who is actually caring for them, and if anyone is listening to their concerns.

Anaesthetists play a crucial role in multi-professional teams in a wide variety of clinical settings of which theatre is only one. There is the high dependency unit (HDU), the labour suite[1], paediatrics, the chronic pain clinic—to name but a few. In almost every aspect of anaesthetic clinical practice the ability to communicate effectively is a vital component of patient care. Many anaesthetists voice more concerns regarding communication challenges than about technical skills which they are generally well equipped to handle[2]. A recent survey of anaesthetists showed that over 90% believed poor communication caused procedural delay and that further work is required to improve communication in the stressful operating room environment, particularly at the surgeon–anaesthetist interface[3].

Anaesthetists frequently communicate using highly technical language[4]. This can be off-putting to some patients, is likely to promote misunderstandings and, in some contexts, can adversely affect patient safety.

When communication breaks down

There is growing recognition that many of the problems that beset modern healthcare stem from deficiencies in communication. Studies of adverse events show that communication failure is a root cause in about 50% of cases. Similarly a substantial proportion of patient complaints and litigation stems from communication breakdown between patients and their carers[5]. Consider the following cases …

A 'broken routine'

Induction communication is designed to reassure the patient, whilst also signalling to others that induction is taking place (see Chapter 8), thus helping to ensure that it is accomplished successfully[6]. The following interview with an anaesthetist's assistant shows what happens when the usual communication routine is absent and how the smooth, predictable sequence of events can be disrupted:

> 'There have been a couple of other cases where I've felt uneasy really. In one particular instance, the anaesthetist gave the anaesthetic without warning the patient, and the patient panicked. I felt uneasy then, I felt very uneasy because the patient sat bolt upright and started grabbing hold of her throat and I felt bad because I hadn't warned the patient. I thought the anaesthetist was going to do it … the patient was scared stiff … If that was me, I would have quite a phobia about coming into theatres now.'
>
> (Interview with anaesthetist's assistant conducted during communication research)[6].

This vignette illustrates how careful anaesthetists need to be to make sure that the patient's journey into unconsciousness is made not only in safety, but also with the appropriate psychological preparation and communication. It also underlines how closely individuals within the anaesthesia team work together. It is fortunately rare for a member of the team not to 'fill in' another member's gaps in communication.

Power relationships in complex hierarchical organizations, such as a teaching hospital, can often determine how, and whether or not, staff are willing to speak up and escalate concern—particularly in the face of a deteriorating patient or an obvious error by a colleague. The concept of 'authority gradients' and their impact is discussed in Chapter 16.

Failure of handover with fatal consequences[7]

A 68-year-old man was admitted to hospital for a craniotomy to remove a large pituitary adenoma. Immediately prior to induction of anaesthesia, the anaesthetist who was in charge of the case was called to take care of an emergency craniotomy in a trauma patient. He gave only a brief report to the anaesthetist who took over the case, and did not mention that 2 weeks previously the tumour had been partially debulked via a transnasal, trans-sphenoidal approach. Unaware of this, the second anaesthetist decided to intubate the patient via the nasal route, as was the usual custom for craniotomy patients at that facility. After induction, the anaesthetist attempted to advance the nasotracheal tube through the left nostril and, after a slight resistance, inadvertently passed the tube through the freshly granulating hole made from the previous operation and into the brainstem of the patient, leading to immediate circulatory collapse. The patient remained unconscious and died 4 days later from this devastating injury.

What was remarkable about this case report was that while much discussion (over two pages) was devoted to the technical details—that is, the anatomical course taken through the brain by the wayward tube, the incidence and outcomes of traumatic foreign bodies in the brain, etc., only one sentence was given to discussion on the lack of handover. This observation is not made to disparage the specific team in question, but rather to make a more general assertion: that frequently in the analyses of clinical events, poor communication is not examined with the same due diligence as other technical aspects of a given clinical scenario. The authors believe this to be the case around the world, and not just in this report.

Right advice, wrong manner and timing

This case is taken from the archives of a medical defence organization[8].

An anaesthetist at a private clinic gave a lumbar epidural to a patient in preparation for elective Caesarean section. The patient was in her twenties and in good health, although she was a heavy smoker. During the procedure, the patient appeared to have a satisfactory block for surgical anaesthesia. However, she did experience pain during washout of the peritoneal cavity following delivery. This was managed with epidural top up, and nitrous oxide inhalation.

The patient subsequently complained that the insertion of the intravenous cannula and the epidural catheter had been painful and that the anaesthetist had 'harassed' her during the surgery about her smoking habit. The anaesthetist, on the other hand, had been concerned that the patient's absence from the ward for a cigarette had disrupted the operating list, and that her coughing perioperatively had made the surgical procedure much more difficult. He expressed his views about smoking, '*You've seen your daughter born; if you give up smoking you might see her get married too*'.

The patient refused to discuss the case with the anaesthetist and declined his written suggestion of a meeting. She claimed the experience left her with severe postnatal depression. She began a legal claim for pain and psychological distress, alleging that the anaesthetist had failed to provide the proper pre-anaesthetic care, failed to ensure adequate surgical anaesthesia and failed to ensure that she did not suffer unnecessary pain and distress after the delivery. The claimant also alleged that the anaesthetist's manner towards the patient had contributed to the postnatal depression.

The experts consulted felt that the technical aspects of the anaesthetic had been carried out in a competent and appropriate manner. The evidence was, however, that the anaesthetist's manner and poor communication had indeed contributed to the patient's psychological condition. The case was settled for a five-figure sum.

Well-intentioned health promotion advice here led to an unsatisfactory outcome. Whilst it is without doubt correct that smoking reduces life expectancy, this was neither the time nor the manner in which to communicate this.

Benefits of improved communication

In contrast to the problems caused when communication breaks down, many benefits can be expected from improved clinical communication. The literature on patient benefits has been carefully reviewed for a number of outcomes in a variety of health-care settings[9,10]. Little of this work has been carried out within the domain of the anaesthetist, though there are some notable exceptions[11,12]. More recently, training in communication skills for the pre-operative visit was found to increase patient satisfaction[13].

The perception that clinicians are more effective can only enhance personal and professional self-esteem and work satisfaction, and the general improvement in interaction with other human beings should extend also to relationships with colleagues[13]. Further, hospitals can benefit too. If it is perceived that more effective care is being provided for patients, the reputation of the institution will be enhanced amongst patients, referring doctors and the community in general. One might also expect a decrease in litigation by patients[5].

Models of communication

The various models of conceptualizing communication differ largely in the semantics and language used to describe what are fundamentally similar, or even identical, concepts. Some of these concepts and tools may not initially appear consistent with existing models. There are many conceptual patterns of communication, such as the Calgary–Cambridge model[14] for conducting medical consultations or team communication models[15]. However, training in communication skills has focused on content and process, whereas many aspects of communication occur by implication[16].

Important aspects of how to learn and teach effective interpersonal communication skills have, until recently, been largely unrecognized and poorly understood. Explicit or conscious aspects, and implicit, tacit or subconscious aspects, all need consideration when learning and teaching effective communication (see Chapters 2 and 4). This concept underpins much of the content of this book.

There are several 'traditions' of thought regarding communication research[17], and studies of communication theory tend to reflect the agendas pursued by researchers of each tradition. Given the highly technical and scientific backgrounds of anaesthetists, it is tempting for them to be drawn to technical constructs of communication theory—theories which frame communication as packages of signals that are exchanged through organs designed to transmit, receive and interpret those signals.

There are two broad traditions that deal with this: ***semiotics*** (communication as 'signs' that convey 'meaning') and ***cybernetics*** (flow of 'quanta' of information between transmitters and receivers). These inform, among many other things, a number of tools outlined in Chapter 16, as well as much of the enormous field of medical informatics, which is not within the scope of this book.

The ***rhetorical*** tradition, which dates back to Aristotle (4th century BCE), deals with identifying the available means of persuasion in any discourse between a '*rhetor*'—the speaker—and his or her 'audience'. Rhetoric, a term that in modern times is often used pejoratively, has significant implications for a range of clinical topics such as: forming logical or emotive arguments for or against certain treatments; the power of medical anecdotes and storytelling; techniques of assertiveness; the communication responsibilities of leadership in clinical teams; medical politics; and identifying the most persuasive communication approaches with particular types of patient—for example, paediatric or needle-phobic patients (see Chapters 10 and 14). This invariably relies on subconscious processes which have traditionally been thought to be intuitive skills that could be neither learned nor taught, since being subconscious they were 'below the radar' and not reaching conscious awareness.

The ***phenomenological*** tradition is largely philosophical, conceptualizing communication as a reflection of how we experience the world and others in a broader sense: how 'vibes' affect us consciously or subconsciously; how communication relates to 'consciousness'; whether and how we are able to perceive ourselves as being able to 'walk in another's shoes'. This tradition suggests that all observations are subject to interpretation, and that we need to communicate in order to truly experience events from another person's perspective.

Although we can attempt to bridge the gap, it is impossible to truly experience events from another person's perspective. This tradition has links to clinical empathy skills, non-verbal communication and its impact on anaesthetists as clinicians and their patients, understanding the needs of patients, regarding, for instance, the disclosure of adverse events, and what our clinical environments tell us about the way we work, and in some cases 'direct' us. Some of the most illuminating examples of this tradition are 'doctor-as-patient' stories[18]. See also Chapter 5.

The ***socio-psychological*** and ***socio-cultural*** traditions, while relatively new, have grown prodigiously in the last 50 years. They focus on communication as a means of interaction between social beings, and the role of communication in forming, nurturing and disrupting relationships, communities and society as a whole. They counterpoint the rhetorical and phenomenological traditions by striving towards a more scientific approach, drawing on psychology and sociology with a focus on careful testing through social experiments, some of which have become legendary[19].

The socio-cultural tradition looks at how social and cultural norms affect and are reflected in communication trends—essentially looking at communication in society from the 'top down' as opposed to the socio-psychological tradition, which essentially views many of the same issues from the individual relationship level, and extrapolating up.

This tradition is relevant in examining specific features of organizational, professional, and other cultures which influence the way anaesthetists behave and communicate in the workplace, the reporting or non-reporting of adverse events, traditional doctor–nurse hierarchies, workplace harassment, differences in the way 'Baby Boomers' (older clinicians) and 'Gen Y' (younger clinicians) communicate, and so on. To anaesthetists, socio-psychological studies are relevant to a diverse range of topics from constructive communication styles between colleagues, the placebo and nocebo effects[20] (see Chapter 3), to using 'bedside manner' to establish a trusting doctor–patient relationship, to using communication to nurture cohesive, clinical teams.

Finally the ***critical*** tradition is an interesting hybrid of several traditions, its focus being communication as a means of reflecting upon unexamined habits, beliefs, ideologies and power relationships across the gamut of human experience. Dialectic—the art of inquiry through questioning—is at the heart of this tradition. Plato's Socratic dialogues are an archetypal example. This tradition seeks a reasoned means of conveying not just ***how*** but ***why*** we should do things. As such it is part philosophy, part science and, even in trying to distinguish itself from rhetoric, is a form of rhetoric itself. Medical practitioners must be able to reflect analytically upon their practice. Working in departments, they must be able to share and discuss their performance constructively, and be brave enough to challenge beliefs, however cherished, especially if these are based on assumptions.

A common theme that is directly and indirectly apparent within most of these traditions is that every context of communication has *conscious* or explicit, and *subconscious* or implicit/tacit aspects. One of the early representations of this idea was the 'Johari window' named after the two psychologists who formulated it (Figure 1.1)[21]. They proposed that at any given moment in time, individuals are receiving and transmitting information from four distinct sources: the 'open self', where both transmitter and receiver consciously share information; the 'hidden self', where the transmitter attempts to communicate around issues or agendas of which the receiver is unaware; the 'blind self' where the transmitter is sending verbal or non-verbal signals without being consciously aware of them; and the 'unknown self', from which signals are being sent and received without the conscious awareness of either party.

Mehrabian's classic study[22] suggests that over 90% of the emotional meaning of an interaction between any two people is carried non-verbally by body language, tone of voice, etc. The hypnosis literature is explicit in its use of conscious–subconscious

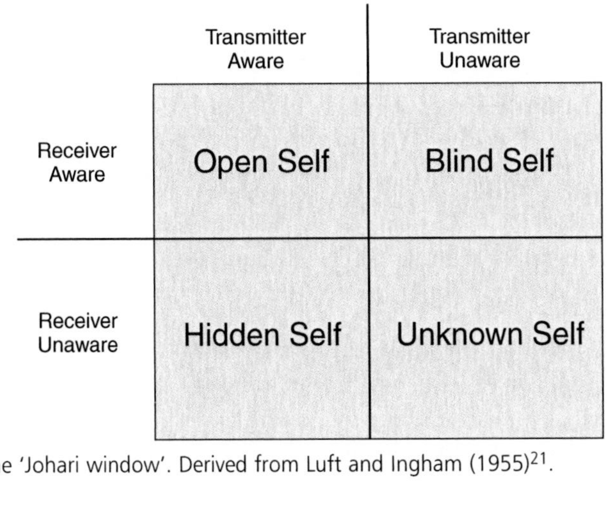

Fig. 1.1 The 'Johari window'. Derived from Luft and Ingham (1955)[21].

communication which has an established role in clinical psychology (see Chapters 2–4 and 20). We explicitly discuss suggestibility in influencing subconscious responses— in particular how this increases with increasing stress, be this of patients, anaesthetists themselves or their colleagues. This is frequently of relevance in optimizing anaesthetic care.

The practical import of this concept for anaesthetists is to emphasize that when two people, such as an anaesthetist and a patient, interact, communication is naturally occurring at several levels—verbal and non-verbal, explicit and implicit—and that all levels of communication are amenable to influence, both positive and negative. Influential communication can be learned, used therapeutically and readily taught to most people, including most anaesthetists.

A number of the communication paradigms discussed in this book may appear unfamiliar, yet they are evidence based and have structures which can be learned. It is hoped this approach will provide anaesthetists with a range of strategies to deal successfully with challenges in practice that were previously deemed almost impossible to overcome.

Communication will inevitably play an increasing role in the anaesthetist's armamentarium during clinical practice, teaching and research. Current research is designed to improve our understanding of the fundamental concepts involved including the psychophysiology of emotion, an understanding of cognition, perception, semantics and metaphor. There is a wealth of knowledge from the fields of psychology and neuroscience, safety and human factors that can enable us to better understand how we communicate, especially in the time-pressured stressful environment of the operating theatre. Unfortunately, this information has been slow to percolate into anaesthetic practice.

Communication skills training in anaesthesia

Anaesthetists are taught vast amounts of information on the molecular structure of drugs and the physical principles of the equipment they use, but few will have had any training on how to talk to a distressed patient, or to deal with an angry surgeon or a frightened child. Nevertheless, these are scenarios which confront anaesthetists daily. In addition poor communication is recognized as the root of many difficulties that anaesthetists find themselves in, including adverse events, patient dissatisfaction and medico-legal issues. Although much has been written about communication and doctors in general, there are almost no writings on useful communication skills of relevance to the anaesthetist in their various roles within and outside the theatre environment. Training in communication facilitates the addressing of these issues[16].

Much of the research and teaching to date on communication skills comes from models looking at communication with patients within the clinical context of taking a history, examining the patient, performing investigation and making diagnoses. Expert anaesthetists have a capacity for critical self-reflection that pervades all aspects of their clinical and professional practice. This includes solving problems, eliciting a highly focused anaesthetic-relevant history and examination while, at the same time, providing and obtaining critical information. The experienced anaesthetist then makes any necessary evidence-based decisions and performs only appropriate technical procedures.

Current communication skills training, is explicitly emphasised as important by the anaesthesia colleges in the UK, USA and Australia. The CanMEDS model[23] proposes some key communication competencies such as: gaining rapport and trust; eliciting relevant information; conveying relevant information and explanations; developing a common understanding with patients and families, colleagues and other professionals; and conveying effective oral and written information about a medical encounter.

Similarly key communication evidence-based strategies have been advocated by the Calgary–Cambridge group in the context of the medical consultation[14]. Although some of these are of relevance and value to anaesthetists particularly in the context of the pre-anaesthetic clinic, there are many areas of anaesthetic practice that require supplemental approaches.

Much of the knowledge required for anaesthetic practice, such as drug doses and physiological mechanisms, are taught explicitly. Such teachings are readily implemented, accessible to conscious awareness, are quantifiable and are therefore easily translated into evidence-based guidelines. The intuitive nature of many of the professional skills required of a consultant anaesthetist has led to the erroneous belief that they cannot be taught explicitly. Indeed most teaching of such skills relies on the subconscious learning obtained through the modelling of mentors or peers.

Being aware of the subconscious aspects of our lives facilitates an engagement in moment-to-moment self-monitoring that brings into conscious awareness tacit personal knowledge and deeply held values that are usually 'below the radar'[24]. These aspects of anaesthetic care are receiving increasing attention and are being recognized as an essential component of patient care[25].

Addressing patient needs

Communication is maximally effective when it is seen as a tool directed to patients' needs as well as to those of the anaesthetist. The consultation model proposed by Tate is useful here[26] (see Figure 1.2). It is based on the assumption that patients and doctors bring quite different agendas to any consultation.

These agendas may not align and may even conflict. For instance, the anaesthetist's first priority may be to gather information and collect facts, with the sharing of understanding further down the agenda. The patient, on the other hand, may be more concerned with hopes, fears and hidden or perceived problems, with the exact detail of previous anaesthetic problems being of less importance.

It is useful to keep in mind the shorter and longer term goals of the patient–anaesthetist encounter. The first two of these goals are usually foremost in every patient–anaesthetist interaction: to ensure that patient ***safety*** is maximized and, by implication, any risk minimized; and to optimize patient ***comfort*** before, during and after the procedure. The third goal is frequently neither recognized nor considered a priority—it is to allow patients to feel a sense of ***control*** in, what is frequently for them, an out-of-control situation where they become increasingly dependent on the anaesthetist's skill and care.

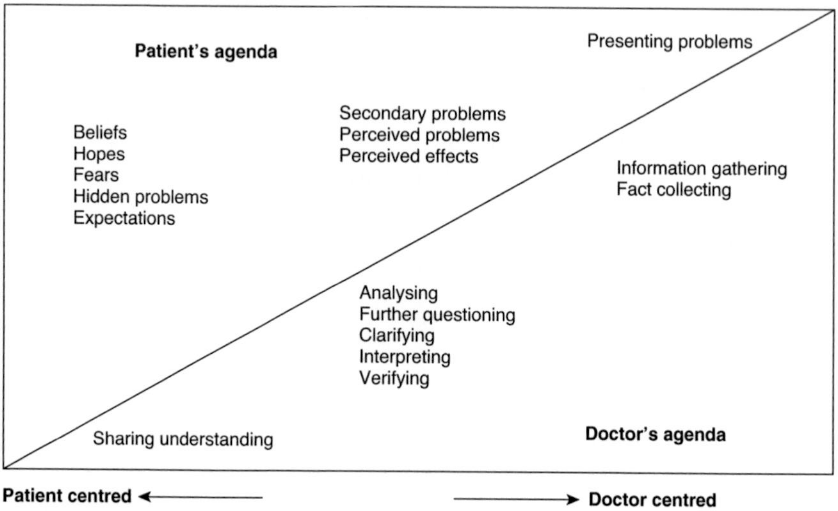

Fig. 1.2 A power-shift model of the consultation. Reproduced from Tate (1997)[26] with permission from the publishers.

Patients not infrequently consider themselves victims of their illness or helpless in the face of incomprehensible technology[27]. The way in which anaesthetists communicate can greatly change the patient's perception of being a passive bystander just having to accept whatever care is provided, rather than being allowed to participate in that care. This can be empowering for both parties. The final goal to consider is how to recognize and respect the choices available to both patient and anaesthetist in any particular context.

Exactly which path is optimal will be dependent not only on the patient's wishes but also on the anaesthetist's level of comfort and skill for any particular path. A 'one size fits all' approach to communication is frequently inappropriate as communication must be tailored to the individual needs and responses of the patient. For example, in some situations good communication will be facilitated by frequent eye contact, while in others it may be optimized by avoiding any eye contact whatsoever.

Although communication superficially is individualized, there are generic patterns such as the concepts of 'utilization', 'reframing' and the use of 'suggestion' that are an integral part of the two main communication tools used in many of the chapters that follow—the '**LAURS**' and '**GREAT**' concepts detailed in Chapter 2. They function as one possible framework from which an individualized approach can be generated. Reflective listening and observing are key aspects of a patient-centred approach to communication relevant to anaesthetists.

There is a growing body of evidence supporting the view that 'the how' and 'the way' anaesthetists communicate can affect patient experience and be therapeutic in its own right[28]. The communications of the patient allow assessments to be made, and the patient's response will determine the anaesthetist's response. Using verbal and non-verbal communications skilfully can facilitate responses that are meaningful to both parties in the interaction.

Every patient–anaesthetist interaction involves a huge degree of trust on the part of the patient and an equal burden of responsibility on the anaesthetist. The patient is giving up control of consciousness and other aspects of physiological homeostasis and handing over control to the anaesthetist. The frequently unspoken assumption is that the anaesthetist will have the skill and knowledge to bring the patient back from being completely dependent during surgery and anaesthesia to being an autonomous functioning person again. This privilege of responsibility should not be taken lightly as it has a range of important effects on patterns of communication and how anaesthetists influence patients by their interactions. These are intended to be positive, and in the clinical setting therapeutic.

However, it is not infrequent that communications inadvertently sabotage what we are trying to do (see Chapter 3). The skills of the clinician can be increased when one understands how these paradoxical effects of communications can arise and facilitate an understanding of how they can be prevented.

What can anaesthetists learn about communication from other disciplines?

Social psychology tells us that clinicians will influence patients whether communications are verbalized or not. How this occurs will be dependent on how the interaction takes place, its context and the patient's perceptions and past experiences. Advances in communication reflect the influence of the positive psychology movement as researched by Seligman[29]. This concept is a focus on what the patient does well without overemphasizing their difficulties. Noticing and amplifying what is right with the patient, rather than what is wrong, is an approach that is unfamiliar to many anaesthetists.

Recent efforts in understanding the neurobiology underpinning nocebo-induced pain and placebo analgesia emphasize the importance of expectation in affecting patient behavioural and perceptual responses. Indeed expectation may be the driver for placebo and nocebo in equal measure[30]. Current clinical research evidence suggests that warning patients of a perceptual experience using language with negative emotional content, such as '*This will hurt!*' or sympathizing in a way that refers to negative experiences, is unhelpful[31,32] (see Chapter 3).

The patient's state of consciousness will determine the type of communication that is likely to be most effective or therapeutic. The states of consciousness blend seamlessly one with another but can be categorized for the purpose of this discussion as three states. The conscious and unconscious states are familiar to all anaesthetists, reasonably well understood and usually easily recognizable. Anaesthetists are the experts in managing the unconscious state of patients when in a coma or under general anaesthesia. However it is frequently unappreciated that all patients, whether unconscious or conscious, also have the ability to function in a third state—the subconscious state. This is further elaborated in Chapters 2 and 4.

Amongst the general public, at least until a few years ago, doctors were, and still are to a degree, seen as the equivalent of the magicians and sorcerers of old. They have access to, and knowledge of, wondrous potions and magical procedures that cure leukaemia and infection, treat injuries, relieve pain, treat diabetes and effectively contain chronic disease. For doctors, however, anaesthetists are the magicians and sorcerers of today. They enable even the most debilitated patients to survive their surgical procedures. They place intravenous access or central lines when all else, and all others, have failed. They 'miraculously' manage pre-operative anxiety, relieve post-operative pain, have a detailed understanding of the mysterious anaesthetic machine and somehow effectively manage any deviation from normal physiology. Such intricacies of anaesthetic clinical practice are but some of a range of complexities that few non-anaesthetic peers, and even fewer patients, appreciate. However, true mastery is demonstrated not only through technical prowess but also through the effectiveness of anaesthetic communications with patients and colleagues.

The more that is learned about 'useful communication' the more it is realized that there are common specific processes involved that have structure, can be readily understood and therefore can be taught.

Common problems that regularly occur in communication and which need to be recognized and addressed include:

- alternative viewpoints, perceptions, misinformation and misperceptions;
- individual anxieties and concerns;
- variation in response to direction (being told what to do);
- the importance of control for many patients and colleagues;
- the anaesthetist being in a unique and powerful position;
- the patient's vulnerability.

Possible solutions that facilitate problem resolution include:

- recognizing that the way anaesthetists communicate will inevitably change perceptions, feelings and behaviour of patients, colleagues and ourselves;
- increasing or allowing patients some control over what is happening to them;
- engendering a cooperative relationship;
- avoiding power struggles between the anaesthetist, patients and other colleagues.

Anaesthetists now have the opportunity to enhance and improve their communication skills beyond learning through role modelling, or trial and error. The acquisition of enhanced communication skills will improve patient rapport and patients' perspectives of their quality of care. In addition, improved communication makes the working environment less stressful, more efficient and a much safer place. Learning more about communication is an effective strategy for improving patient safety, making teams work and resolving complaints. Perhaps most importantly, good communication skills allow the development of expertise and professionalism[33,34] in all interactions whether with patients, colleagues, trainees or even administrators!

Key points

1. Good communication brings considerable benefits to all concerned.
2. Reflective listening and observing are key aspects of a patient-centred approach to communication relevant to anaesthetists.
3. Anaesthetists and patients may bring very different expectations and agendas to their encounters.
4. A common theme within communication models is the idea that there are both conscious (explicit) and subconscious (implicit) aspects.
5. The anaesthetist needs to be aware that communication is occurring at both a conscious and subconscious level if patient care is to be optimized.

References

1 Alder J, Christen R, Zemp E, Bitzer J (2007). Communication skills training in obstetrics and gynaecology: whom should we train? A randomized controlled trial. *Arch Gynecol Obstet*, **276**(6), 605–12.

2 Smith AF, Shelly MP (1999). Communication skills for anesthesiologists. *Can J Anaesth*, **46**(11), 1082–8.

3 Elks KN, Riley RH (2009). A survey of anaesthetists' perspectives of communication in the operating suite. *Anaesth Intensive Care*, **37**(1), 108–11.

4 Babitu UQ, Cyna AM (2010). Patients' understanding of technical terms used during the pre-anaesthetic consultation. *Anaesth Intensive Care*, **38**(2), 349–53.

5 Levinson W, Chaumeton N (1999). Communication between surgeons and patients in routine office visits. *Surgery*, **125**(2), 127–34.

6 Smith AF, Pope C, Goodwin D, Mort M (2005). Communication between anesthesiologists, patients and the anesthesia team: a descriptive study of induction and emergence. *Can J Anesth*, **52**(9), 915–20.

7 Paul M, Dueck M, Kampe S, Petzke F, Ladra A (2003). Intracranial placement of a nasotracheal tube after transnasal trans-sphenoidal surgery. *Br J Anaesth*, **91**(4), 601–4.

8 Medical Protection Society (2006). *Case reports: healthy advice or harassment?* Available at: http://www.medicalprotection.org/Default.aspx?DN=ed542160-6e13-490f-9647-998d91ab63f5 (Accessed 18 March 2010).

9 Ong LML, deHaes CJM, Hoos AM, Lammes FB (1995). Doctor–patient communication: a review of the literature. *Soc Sci Med*, **40**(7), 903–18.

10 Stewart MA (1995). Effective physician–patient communication and health outcomes: a review. *CMAJ*, **152**(9), 1423–33.

11 Egbert LD, Battit GE, Welch CE, Bartlett MK (1964). Reduction of postoperative pain by encouragement and instruction of patients—a study of doctor–patient rapport. *N Engl J Med*, **270**, 825–7.

12 Anderson EA (1987). Preoperative preparation for cardiac surgery facilitates recovery, reduces psychological distress and reduces the incidence of acute postoperative hypertension. *J Consult Clin Psychol*, **55**(4), 513–20.

13 Harms C, Young JR, Amsler F, Zettler C, Scheidegger D, Kindler CH (2004). Improving anaesthetists' communication skills. *Anaesthesia*, **59**(2), 166–72.

14 Kurtz S, Silverman J, Benson J, Draper J (2003). Marrying content and process in clinical method teaching: enhancing the Calgary–Cambridge guides. *Acad Med*, **78**(8), 802–9.

15 U.S. Department of Health & Human Resources (2010). *AHRQ, TeamSTEPPS: national implementation.* Available at: http://teamstepps.ahrq.gov/ (accessed 18 March 2010).

16 Kinnersley P, Spencer J (2008). Communication skills teaching comes of age. *Med Educ*, **42**(11), 1052–3.

17 Craig RT, Muller HL (2007) *Theorizing communication: readings across traditions.* Los Angeles: Sage Publishers.

18 Bowes D (1984) The doctor as patient: an encounter with Guillain–Barre syndrome. *CMAJ*, **131**(11): 1343–8.

19 Milgram S (1963) Behavioural study of obedience. *J Abnormal Soc Psychol*, **67**(4), 371–9 Also available online at: http://library.nhsggc.org.uk/mediaAssets/Mental%20Health%20Partnership/Peper%202%2027th%20Nov%20Milgram_Study%20KT.pdf (accessed 19 Dec 2009).

20 Benedetti F, Lanotte M, Lopiano L, Colloca L (2007). When words are painful: unraveling the mechanisms of the nocebo effect. *Neuroscience*, **147**(2), 260–71.

21 Luft J, Ingham H. (1955). The Johari window, a graphic model of interpersonal awareness. *Proceedings of the Western training laboratory in group development.* Los Angeles: UCLA.

22 Mehrabian A, Ferris SR (1967). Inference of attitudes from nonverbal communication in two channels. *J Consult Psychol*, **31**(3), 248–58.

23 Frank JR (2005). *The CanMEDS 2005 physician competency framework. Better standards. Better physicians. Better care.* Ottawa: Royal College of Physicians and Surgeons of Canada.

24 Epstein RM (1999). Mindful practice. *J Am Med Assoc*, **282**(9), 833–9.

25 Hool A and Smith AF (2009). Communication between anaesthesiologists and patients: how are we doing it now and how can we improve? *Curr Opin Anaesthesiol*, **22**, 431–5.

26 Tate P (1997). *The doctor's communication handbook.* 2nd edn. Abingdon, UK: Radcliffe Medical Press.

27 Bejenke CJ. (1996). Painful medical procedures. In: Barber J (ed.) *Hypnosis and suggestion in the treatment of pain: a clinical guide.* pp. 209–61. London: WW Norton.

28 Lang EV, Hatsiopoulou O, Koch T, Berbaum K, Lutgendorf S, Kettenmann E, et al. (2005). Can words hurt? Patient–provider interactions during invasive procedures. *Pain*, **114**(1–2), 303–9.

29 Seligman M, Csikszentmihalyi M (2000). Positive psychology: an introduction. *Am Psychol*, **55**(1), 5–14.

30 Colloca L, Sigaudo M, Benedetti F (2008). The role of learning in nocebo and placebo effects. *Pain*, **136**(1–2), 211–8.

31 Varelmann D, Pancaro C, Cappiello EC, Camman WR (2010). Nocebo-induced hyperalgesia during local anesthetic injection. *Anesth Analg*, **110**(3), 868–70.

32 Dutt-Gupta J, Bown T, Cyna AM (2007). Effect of communication on pain during intravenous cannulation: a randomized controlled trial. *Br J Anaesth*, **99**(6), 871–5.

33 Smith AF, Greaves JD (2010). Beyond competence: defining and promoting excellence in anaesthesia. *Anaesthesia*, **65**(2), 184–91.

34 Larsson J, Holmström I, Rosenqvist U (2003). Professional artist, good Samaritan, servant and co-ordinator: four ways of understanding the anaesthesiologist's work. *Acta Anaesthesiol Scand*, **47**(7), 787–93.

Chapter 2

Structures

Allan M Cyna, Marion I Andrew, and
Suyin GM Tan

'Too often we underestimate the power of a touch, a smile, a kind word, a listening ear…'.
Leo Buscaglia

What this chapter is about

Communication concepts of relevance to the practice of anaesthesia

Anaesthetic culture tends to view patients as physiological specimens to which pharmacological and technical procedures are applied and utilized to optimize various measurable parameters. However, this aspect is only one small part of a patient's anaesthetic care. The medical model to which many anaesthetists still cling is very much a paternalistic one.

Although terms such as 'patient autonomy' and 'choice' are frequently used, achieving these laudable aims in clinical practice remains elusive. Promoting patient autonomy and fostering a therapeutic relationship are areas of practice that have traditionally not been of direct concern to anaesthetists. The communication skills required to achieve this are centred on listening to what patients are really saying, and accepting the patients' alternative, but sometimes radically different, view of the world. In addition, anaesthetists can use their understanding of this alternative view to communicate in a way that is likely to engender cooperation and trust. Language affects our patients, our colleagues and our own perceptions. This has profound implications in the practice of anaesthesia.

The anatomy of communication

Dissecting the anatomy of communication begins with a message between two or more people. This message can take many forms—for example, as a request for assistance or information, a command, advice, clarification, addressing a concern or the provision of reassurance. The message, superficially, is contained only in words. However, the meaning of the communication carried in the message is invariably far more complex. Spoken words are inevitably accompanied by pitch, volume and intonation, a facial expression and body posture. For example, take the six words '*He anaesthetized that patient last Tuesday*'. Box 2.1 shows six different meanings of this sentence. Each one is dependent on just one change in emphasis on how the words are said.

The example demonstrates that with just one small change of emphasis in one word the entire meaning of the phrase can change. One can begin to imagine how many hundreds of pieces of information—probably thousands—are being passed on implicitly during any particular interpersonal interaction or communication. It is, of course, impossible to dissect every last nuance, but we can begin to understand some aspects

Box 2.1 Words and their meaning

'***He*** *anaesthetized that patient last Tuesday*'.

i.e. He, not one of the other registrars, anaesthetized the patient.

'*He* ***anaesthetized*** *that patient last Tuesday*'.

i.e. He anaesthetized the patient, rather than just used sedation.

'*He anaesthetized* ***that*** *patient last Tuesday*'.

i.e. Definitely that patient, rather than another patient.

'*He anaesthetised that* ***patient*** *last Tuesday?*'

i.e. The person is unsure whether he anaesthetized that patient, or another one.

'*He anaesthetized that patient* ***last*** *Tuesday*'.

i.e. He anaesthetized that patient last Tuesday, and not the Tuesday 3 weeks ago.

'*He anaesthetized that patient last* ***Tuesday?***'

i.e. He anaesthetized that patient last Tuesday, and not last Wednesday.

of language and non-verbal cues in a way that will facilitate the accuracy of our communications.

Explicit/conscious and implicit/tacit/subconscious aspects of communication

As anaesthetists we are familiar with the terms 'implicit', 'tacit' and 'explicit'. These terms are usually used in discussions concerning memory or awareness. In the context of this and several other chapters, explicit communications are interpreted consciously, while implicit or tacit aspects of communication are interpreted subconsciously. No matter how conscious the message appears to be, there are always subconscious components which have the potential to influence meaning. Usually the content or intent of the communication is obvious—for example, '*Pass me the bougie*'. Although this statement seems a simple request, the implicit message may be that the anaesthetist is experiencing a degree of difficulty which may be well recognized by an experienced skilled assistant, or go completely unrecognized by other members of the theatre team. All statements will contain additional, complex meanings regarding the person communicating and, when listened to carefully, can provide valuable insights that facilitate useful responses.

The tone, pitch, volume, pacing and body language all combine to give information regarding the person's cognitive and emotional state, indicating their confidence, comfort, sense of well-being, pain, fear, guilt, depression or anxiety.

In short, paraphrasing the song, 'It's not (only) what you say it's the way that you say it!' it's also not only the words but their implicit intent, that largely determines how they are perceived by the listener. This is what the Calgary–Cambridge model terms 'Process' communication as opposed to 'Content'[1,2]. The way we communicate will inevitably, and to a variable degree, change perceptions, feelings and behaviour of our patients, our colleagues and ourselves.

Human interaction: the patient and anaesthetist

It is very attractive for the anaesthetist to develop a paternalistic model of care as much of the anaesthetist's interaction with patients is when they are unconscious. The anaesthetist is then de facto *in loco parentis* with the patient. The anaesthetist's responsibility for the safety of the patient, whether conscious or unconscious, is always present. However, the authoritative model of the paternalistic role, while necessary at times, has the potential to erode the patient's perception of control, and limits the choices available to both parties.

Anaesthetists are human and, as such, subconscious responses can kick in to dissociate oneself at times from the patient as a fellow human being. Anaesthetists do not choose consciously to dehumanize patients. This serves as a protective mechanism to maintain an emotional distance that allows the clinician to function optimally in technically difficult and emergency situations. Examples of dehumanizing language are when we think in terms of the patient as a procedure—for example, '*a difficult intubation*', an extension of our anaesthetic equipment such as '*connect him to the drip*' or the body as a container, '*fill him up with fluids*' as a metaphor to assist with maintaining hydration during or prior to surgery[3]. This dehumanizing behaviour is of course not restricted to anaesthetists. However, understanding why some dehumanizing behaviours occur allows us to recognize how it might inadvertently creep in to everyday practice. Recognition allows the insight to prevent objectification of the patient, and minimizes misunderstandings and offence which may lead to patient complaint. This recognition of dehumanizing behaviour facilitates re-engaging with the patient as a person as soon as possible after such protective mechanisms are no longer required. Similarly, highly technical language can be off-putting with some patients and is likely to promote miscommunication and, in some contexts, can adversely affect patient safety[4].

Patient rapport

Rapport is one of the most important features or characteristics of subconscious human interaction[5]. It is commonality of perspective: being 'in sync' with, or being 'on the same wavelength' as the person with whom one is talking. Rapport in the context of anaesthesia is the harmonious relationship engendered between anaesthetist and patient. The development of patient rapport will inevitably facilitate all other anaesthetic interactions. We all have our own different mechanisms of establishing rapport, such as the use of humour, authority, confidence and empathy. Rapport allows the patient to develop confidence in the anaesthetist's abilities and conversely facilitates developing confidence in the anaesthetist of patients' abilities to cooperate and assist with their care.

Many patients have the skills and abilities to cope with potentially painful or distressing surgical procedures. They may feel out of control but fail to realize they have psychological resources that have been useful and readily available to them in other aspects of their lives. These could be utilized successfully in the anaesthetic context, for example, the patient who is frightened of pain after surgery yet has previously fractured a femur during a rugby match without any pharmacological pain relief and later ran a marathon.

Communications that enhance patient autonomy and the perception of control

The first step in enhancing autonomy is to give patients a perception of control. Whether this is real or imagined is immaterial. An example is the superior satisfaction scores reported with patient-controlled analgesia (PCA) use despite there being little or no improvement in analgesia as measured by pain scores. There is a fine balance between recognizing and respecting a patient's autonomy and fulfilling our ethical duty to care for them in the most effective and safest manner possible. Our perception of the risks and benefits may involve making a decision that is radically different from that of the patient. It is our acceptance of the patient's 'alternative reality' that enables us to communicate in a way that maximizes the patient's understanding of the issues and enables a solution to be found.

Understanding and accepting different realities

We experience the world in our own individual way through different perceptual filters depending on context. We frequently make the assumption that everybody sees what we see, values what we value, and believes as true what we believe is so. Nevertheless, there are an infinite number of realities and truths. Contrary to the saying; '*Seeing is believing*', the concept of realities being discussed in many of the chapters is one of '*Believing is seeing*'. This concept becomes very obvious when one shows the needle-phobic patient a 24G neonatal intravenous (IV) cannula. If the first premise were true, the patient would not subsequently describe the cannula as a '*molten hot poker piercing their body*', '*a knitting needle*' or a '*horse needle*'.

For the purposes of improving and teaching anaesthetic communication skills, just three realities need to be considered. The first reality is that of the anaesthetist. The second reality is that of the other person, be it patient or colleague, with whom the anaesthetist is communicating. This reality may or may not overlap (see the above needle-phobic example) to a variable degree with the first, dependent on topic and context. Finally there is a third reality that encompasses an infinite number of alternative ways of communicating. This reality is useful to appreciate as being always available even when there seems no alternative or other choice to consider during an interaction between two individuals or groups. This concept implies that there is a wavelength at which communication could successfully take place, it just hasn't been found in this particular context yet.

For example, during IV cannulation:

1st Reality—Anaesthetist: '*Just a little sting with a needle*'.
2nd Reality—Patient (hiding): '*Oh my god it's a harpoon!*'
3rd Reality—Anaesthetist: '*We all feel what we feel!*' Or '*We'll all have a whale of a time then!*'

(Patient laughs as cannula is inserted.)

Patient advocacy

Patient advocacy is a core role of all doctors and other healthcare workers. The most effective form of advocacy is when patients are empowered to be their own advocate. However, when patients are rendered unconscious, there is an implicit onus transferred to the anaesthetist to advocate for them temporarily. One not infrequently hears the words; '*I am the patient advocate*'. Unfortunately the implication here is that everybody else in the vicinity—usually theatre—is not the patient's advocate. This may impair team communication and achieve the opposite of what is intended.

Being a patient advocate requires the anaesthetist to establish rapport with the patient, have some understanding of their wishes and concerns, and to act and behave 'below the radar'. Paradoxically, an essential component of being a patient advocate is not drawing attention to the fact that this is what the anaesthetist is doing. This behaviour demonstrates almost above all else what professionalism is about. The '**LAURS**' concept will facilitate understanding and working with both patients and the surgical team.

The 'LAURS' of communication and a 'GREAT' way to structure interactions

There are two major concepts used in many of the chapters that follow. The first of these can be used in part or whole, as a means of developing and maintaining rapport during an interaction—the '**LAURS**' concept.

Listening reflectively

Acceptance

Utilization

Reframing

Suggestion

The second of these concepts provides a learnable template that can be used to structure any interaction—the '**GREAT**' template.

Greeting, **G**oals

Rapport

Evaluation/**E**xplanation

Acknowledging/**A**ddressing concerns

Tacit agreement and **T**hanks

These acronyms provide a common structure and framework, both implicitly and explicitly, throughout the book in a whole range of interactions.

The 'LAURS' concept

The '**LAURS**' of communication are an easy way to remember the key concepts of effective therapeutic communication when our usual strategies or words are either not working or not coming to mind easily. The application of the '**LAURS**' concept may occur as individual components or as a whole.

The first part of the 'LAURS' concept is to ***Listen. The three steps to improving communication skills are:***

Step 1 Listen

Step 2 Listen

Step 3 Listen

Listening reflectively

Learning how to teach and utilize communication more effectively in clinical practice requires one skill above all others, namely to listen [6–8].

What are the steps for effective listening?

1 Observe yourself and recognize your role as a listener.
2 Note whether you are thinking about your response to the patient or colleague rather than listening to what is being said.
3 Resist the temptation to interrupt or second-guess what the patient is thinking.

4 Recognize that silence or pauses can be useful to both anaesthetist and patient.
5 'Check in' to seek clarification regarding your understanding of what the patient means, and their understanding of what you mean (see below).

As doctors, we are used to telling patients what we need them to do, rather than listening to them and responding to their needs. Listening to what patients or colleagues are saying involves more than hearing what one thinks has been said. Listening whilst observing is one of the most important aspects of communication. It consists of a series of observations—looking at the patient's demeanour and posture while noting tone, pace, volume and pitch of the voice, as well as the words used. It is not just about being silent while the patient is talking.

There are four questions to ask when listening reflectively. First, did you hear what was said? Second, did you understand what was meant? Third, does the patient know that he/she has been heard? Finally, does the patient know he/she has been understood? To determine the answer to these questions requires a 'checking in' process. Please note: this takes seconds rather than minutes.

How not to listen:

Patient: *'I don't want to feel anything during the caesarean'.*
Anaesthetist: *'Look, we can't guarantee that! It is a bit like the surgeon doing some washing up in your belly'.*
Patient: *'I really don't want to feel anything!'*
Anaesthetist: *'Look you'll be alright ... there is nothing to worry about—you'll be fine'*

Alternatively ...

Listening reflectively:

Patient: 'I *don't want to feel anything during the caesarean'*
Anaesthetist: *'What do you mean by that?'*
Patient: *'Will I feel any pain?'*
Anaesthetist: *'Your block is working beautifully so you should be nice and comfortable but if not, let me know!'*

Listening for content

This concept involves hearing the words. For example, a woman came for elective caesarean section—for grade IV placenta praevia—with a list of demands, as she had desperately wanted 'natural childbirth'. Her demands included: *'I want three support people in the room during my operation'*, having been told that it was hospital policy only to have one person in the OR during a caesarean; *'I want the drapes down for the entire procedure'*, having been told that this was not sterile and wouldn't be allowed for safety reasons. She wanted her partner *'to video the procedure and birth'* despite video cameras being prohibited in the theatre.

The content of these statements was interpreted by the anaesthetic registrar as having to meet these demands literally or else ...!

Listening for process

How could these words be reconciled with hospital policy and safe clinical practice? The answer began by listening not only to the actual words but how they were being vocalized. The woman was in fact not necessarily asking for the actual words of the demands being met, but was asking for some sense of control and choice over what was happening to her and her baby.

Listening and 'checking in' for meaning

For this woman, the meaning of the various statements began to be understood by gaining patient rapport. The first step was accepting the importance to her of having any concerns and wishes addressed as fully as possible in the context of her and the baby's safety.

> '*I want three support people in the room during my operation*'.

When the woman was asked what the role of each person was, she said that she wanted her partner to, '*see the baby being born*', and her two best friends to be with her to '*provide support*' through the operation.

These requests were addressed by asking: '*Would it be OK if one friend was with you for part of the operation and the other could take over at a time you decided was best for you?*' It transpired that the partner did not want to be in the operating room and the woman was informed that '*he could still be there to see the baby being born*' as there was a glass partition where he could observe the baby's birth.

When asked why she wished the drapes to be down she replied that she wanted this so as '*to see the baby being born*'. This was easily addressed as this is standard practice and she was informed that as soon as the baby was about to be delivered, '*we will lower the drapes for you so that you can see the baby being born*'. Finally she was informed that as many still pictures as she liked could be taken by her partner or support person. There was no further mention of video.

The second part of the '*LA URS*' concept is to ***Accept***.

Acceptance

Acceptance of another person's alternative reality is sometimes a difficult concept for anaesthetists to grasp. It is the concept of being open-minded and having a non-judgemental attitude to other people. This can be a hard philosophical issue, especially if the patient's beliefs run counter to those of the anaesthetist and seem illogical or even stupid. There is little point arguing with patients logically if they are stressed or distressed, as their responses are primarily subconscious. They are frequently unable to accept reason or logic at this time.

Patients may present to the anaesthetist with behaviours and perceptions which run counter to the anaesthetist's own beliefs and experiences. Take, for example, patients with easily visible veins on the dorsum of the hands who have an 'irrational' fear that they will experience excruciating pain when a 22G cannula is inserted. Acceptance of alternative realities is a fundamental prerequisite for communicating effectively and is a core communication skill when attempting to gain patient rapport. In this example, the anaesthetist might be tempted to dismiss the patient's concern by saying something like, '*Don't worry, you'll be fine*', or, '*There is nothing to worry about—it's only a little needle*'. Such statements invariably are unhelpful as there is disparity between the anaesthetist's and the patient's perception of the experience. For further details on how to manage such disparities see Chapters 4, 9, 10, 14 and 20. In a patient with 'no veins' who has to have frequent injections or cannulas, the realities of the anaesthetist and patient are usually congruent and it is therefore much easier to accept the patient's concern of pain on cannula insertion.

Acknowledging the same concern and engendering empathy is harder when there is discordance between the differing realities of the patient and anaesthetist or the surgeon and anaesthetist, as this frequently leads to miscommunication and conflict. This is particularly so when there is a strong emotional attachment to a belief.

Anger is usually a demand for recognition of emotions or views, and the patient or a colleague may be indirectly expressing that they do not feel that they have been listened to or their viewpoint appreciated. When appropriate, venting of the patient's emotions can be encouraged. This involves accepting the emotion, be it crying or anger, in a non-judgemental way.

Anaesthetists may also need to recognize that there is a danger that their own anger or frustration may emerge as a subconscious response. Once recognized, these 'knee-jerk' responses can be interrupted and behaviours or emotions altered. This break in the normal pattern of one's own subconscious behaviour allows logical consideration as to whether some other more useful communication strategy could optimize patient care. Awareness, mindfulness, emotional intelligence, self-reflection and taking responsibility for communications that are not going well are all fundamental techniques that can be used to gain mastery of the challenging situations that anaesthetists increasingly find themselves confronted with.

A temporary acceptance of the patient's beliefs or emotions, no matter how strange they appear, allows the anaesthetist to gain rapport and then move on to a situation that is more therapeutic for the patient. For example, a patient in established labour was shouting at the anaesthetist as he entered the room. She stated that there was no way she could sit up to allow epidural catheter placement for analgesia. The dialogue continued:

> **Woman:** '*I can't sit up. It's too painful!*'
> **Anaesthetist:** '*That's OK, you don't have to sit up during this contraction but in a moment when you are ready for the epidural to be placed as comfortably and as quickly as possible, you will find* ***you can do this***'.
> **Woman:** '*I can't, I can't, I can't!*'
> **Anaesthetist:** '*I know you can't just now, but during the next rest or the one after, you will find you can sit up as comfortably and still as you can be for just now, without even thinking about it*'.

The anaesthetist acknowledges the present reality of the patient's inability to sit still and, has utilized an alternative reality that the patient can do more than she thinks she can in the very near future, within one or two contractions, without her necessarily appreciating consciously this future reality herself until she finds herself doing it! (see also Chapter 9). In this way, the anaesthetist is in a position to engage with the patient in a more cooperative and constructive manner.

Another example is the pain patient who is severely distressed and expressing pain, despite having no obvious organic basis or diagnosis for being in this position. Unless the patient's reality of being in pain is accepted and believed as true, we are not allowing ourselves the opportunity to engage with patients in a way that facilitates the treatment of their problem.

The third part of the '*LAURS*' concept is to ***Utilize***.

Utilization

The neuro-linguistic programming (NLP) principles which have emerged over the last 20 years have contributed to an understanding as to how language is structured and how this can be used to tailor communications with others.

Our perceptions are frequently communicated in the form of sensory perceptual language, usually of the three main senses: visual; kinaesthetic; and auditory. Visual language incorporates phrases such as '*I'm not **looking** forward to my surgery*' or '*I **see** what you mean*'. Kinaesthetic phrases include '*It doesn't **feel** right*' or '*It's like a **weight off** my shoulders*'. Examples of auditory language are '*I **hear** what you say*' or '*That **sounds** clear to me*'. Much less commonly, gustatory or olfactory language is utilized, such as '*It leaves a bad **taste** in my mouth*' or '*It doesn't **smell** right*'.

Utilizing the patient's perceptual world is likely to increase rapport and allow the anaesthetist to reframe negative perceptions and experiences. For example a patient might say,

> '*I am not **looking** forward to the anaesthetic. I'm a bit worried I won't wake up*'.

Rather than respond with a platitude such as, '*Of course you will wake up*' or '*It's very unlikely that will happen*', the anaesthetist can use the patient's perceptual language and reframe it into something useful such as, '*You may not be **looking** forward to the anaesthetic but you can **look** forward to **waking** up in recovery surprised that it was a little easier than you had thought*'.

Developing an ear for patients' or colleagues' preferred communication modality and style can lead to engagement with other people in a way that increases the chances of being heard and understood. Almost anything a patient or colleague says or does can be utilized therapeutically. The only limiting factor here is the anaesthetist's imagination—for example, when the anxious patient asks whether the anaesthetist will be in theatre there all the time or asks,

> '*How will you know if I'm asleep?*'

These concerns can be utilized by explaining all the different types of monitors in some detail and then utilizing the experience. For example,

> **Patient:** '*How will you **know** I'm OK?*'
> **Anaesthetist:** '*When you are lying in the operating room we will position a number of monitors to ensure you are as safe and comfortable as possible throughout the procedure, and for when you wake up in the recovery room. For instance, we will place some ECG stickers on your chest and a blood pressure cuff on your arm to monitor your heart, a pulse monitor on the finger to check the oxygen level in the blood. **Knowing** how closely we are looking after you will help you relax*'.

Utilizing patient strengths

All patients will have strengths and abilities, qualities and experiences that have been used effectively in other contexts such as at work, at school or playing sports. These can be utilized and emphasized in the context of the challenge anaesthesia and surgery represents. If patients have had good or successful experiences while in hospital previously, these can be focused upon—for example, the patient who has managed to mobilize effectively on the day of previous similar surgery. This success can be encouraged by saying that now the patient knows what to do for this success to be repeated.

The fourth part of the 'LAURS' concept is to ***Reframe***.

Reframing

The reframe is a concept whereby a patient's concern that is generating a thought, perception or behaviour that is unhelpful—for example, anxiety—is reframed in a way that generates a thought, perception or behaviour that is helpful or therapeutic—for example, relaxation. If an anxious patient is stating that he is very stressed and that there will be '*too many people*' in the operating room, the anaesthetist can reframe this concern by utilizing this perception. A reframe can be communicated that '*Every person in the operating room will have a job to do that will help you feel as safe and comfortable as possible*'. Then, no matter how many people there are in the room, the patient can be reassured that there will be only enough people to do their job and no more.

The fifth part of the '*LAURS*' concept is to ***Suggest***.

Suggestion

See also Chapters 3, 4, 15 and 20.

Suggestions are verbal or non-verbal communications that can lead to subconscious, non-volitional responses in mood, perception or behaviour. Patients and people generally are in large part subconscious beings. This is the basis of how the consumer society is targeted by the advertising industry. It is also the '*raison d'être*' for poetry, art and prose.

At times, the ability of people to respond to communications in a subconscious way is termed suggestibility. Suggestibility increases when patients are highly anxious, distressed or when in pain. It also increases in pregnancy[9,10] and is higher in the paediatric population[11]. We tend to focus on, and associate with, what is being suggested. This is highly relevant in the recovery room after surgery, when the patient is repeatedly asked for their pain scores. This encourages an association of the surgery with injury, rather than the healing process of recovery[12].

The importance of ***expectancy*** and how ***positive expectancy*** can enhance the anaesthetic experience is a highly relevant communication tool in the practice of anaesthesia.

Positive suggestion A positive suggestion is a communication that has the potential to elicit a positive therapeutic response. For example, '*Most people find it is more comfortable than they thought*' is an indirect positive suggestion to elicit the perception of comfort.

Negative suggestions (see Chapter 3) Lang et al. have shown that the ubiquitous use of language with negative emotional content is likely to increase patients' anxiety, pain and distress[13].

A 'GREAT' structure for an interaction

Many anaesthetists will already have working, implicit templates for many aspects of their anaesthesia practice.

Greeting, Goals

The 'greeting' confirms the identity of persons in the interaction. 'Goals' confirms or negotiates the purpose of the interaction and ensures mutual understanding as the interaction progresses.

Rapport

The 'How to' of developing rapport, whether it be with colleagues or patients, is using the '**LAURS**' concept. This concept can be used throughout the interaction as a means of maintaining and improving rapport. Although to communicate effectively does not necessarily require the people involved to like or respect each other, it does require listening and an acceptance of the other's reality, and recognizes that cooperation is required to achieve a common goal. Any therapeutic process or complex interaction can reasonably be seen as a journey in which there are 'potholes in the road'. A good relationship involving trust copes better with such obstacles, minimizes unnecessary delays and can prevent complete derailment.

Evaluation, Expectations, Examination, Explanation

An example of evaluation is the traditional taking of a history. If not already clarified during the greeting phase, expectations should be explicitly addressed at this stage. Following examination, explanation of management choices, for example, therapy or procedure recommended, can occur.

Asking and Answering questions, Acknowledging and Addressing concerns

The issue here is to address matters both explicitly and implicitly while being aware of control and vulnerability. It is during this stage that something highly relevant usually surfaces.

Tacit agreement, Thanks, Termination

The end of most interactions frequently involves a tacit agreement that a relationship has been formed and an agreement reached as to where to go from here. Termination of the interview can be followed by thanking the other party.

Key points

1. The more we learn about what is 'useful communication', the more we realize that there are common specific processes involved that have structure, can be readily understood and therefore can be taught.
2. The '**LAURS**' concept can facilitate the anaesthetist's communications, in ways that are likely to optimize patient care.
3. The anaesthetist is in a unique and powerful position and needs to recognize at all times the patient's vulnerability.
4. Listening involves managing concerns and helps prevent misinformation and misperceptions.
5. Increasing or allowing patients some control over what is happening to them can decrease anxiety, increase patient autonomy and allow the patient to cooperate more fully with their anaesthetic care.

References

1 Silverman J, Kurtz S, Draper J (2005). *Skills for communicating with patients.* 2nd edn. Abingdon, UK: Radcliffe Publishing Ltd.

2 Kurtz S, Silverman J, Benson J, Draper J (2003). Marrying content and process in clinical method teaching: enhancing the Calgary–Cambridge guides. *Acad Med,* **78**(8), 802–9.

3 Shafer A (1995). Metaphor and anesthesia. *Anesthesiology,* **83**(6), 1331–42.

4 Babitu UQ, Cyna AM (2010). Patients' understanding of technical terms used during the pre-anaesthetic consultation. *Anaesth Intensive Care,* **38**(2), 349–535.

5 Anon (2010). *Rapport.* Wikipedia, http://en.wikipedia.org/wiki/Rapport. (Accessed 14 March 2010).

6 Cericola SA (1999). Communication skills: the art of listening. *Plast Surg Nurs,* **19**(1), 41–2.

7 DiBartola LM (2001). Listening to patients and responding with care: a model for teaching communication skills. *Jt Comm J Qual Improv,* **27**(6), 315–23.

8 Willen J (1986). The skills of listening. A review of helpful communication techniques. *Am J Hosp Care,* **3**(4), 39–41.

9 Tiba J (1990). Clinical, research and organisational aspects of preparation for childbirth and the psychological diminution of pain during labour and delivery. *Br J Exp Clin Hypn,* **7**(1), 61–4.

10 Alexander B, Turnbull D, Cyna A (2009). The effect of pregnancy on hypnotizability. *Am J Clin Hypn,* **52**(1), 13–22.

11 Olness K, Gardner GG (1978). Some guidelines for uses of hypnotherapy in pediatrics. *Pediatrics,* **62**(2), 228–33.

12 Chooi CSL, Nerlekar R, Raju A, Cyna AM (2011). The Effects of Positive or Negative Words when Assessing Postoperative Pain. *Anaesth Intensive Care,* **38** (in press).

13 Lang EV, Hatsiopoulou O, Koch T, Berbaum K, Lutgendorf S, Kettenmann E, et al. (2005). Can words hurt? Patient–provider interactions during invasive procedures. *Pain,* **114**(1–2), 303–9.

Chapter 3

How words hurt

Allan M Cyna and Elvira V Lang

'If you assume there is no hope, you guarantee there will be no hope'.
Noam Chomsky

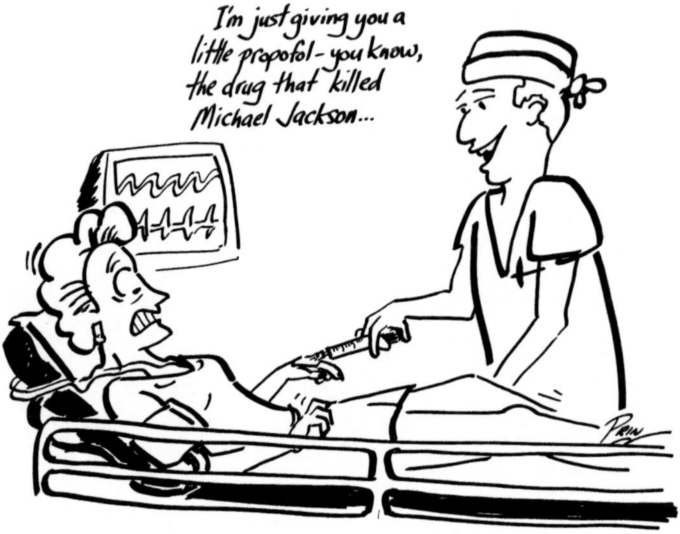
I'm just giving you a little propofol - you know, the drug that killed Michael Jackson...

What this chapter is about

Negative suggestions and how to look out for them

Suggestions are statements that evoke an image in the listener's mind. They may be positive, evoking an image of peace and hope or a desirable mood and behaviour, or they may be negative, eliciting thoughts of pain and doom.

Once mentioned, the suggestion is front and centre: '*You probably even didn't think of an endotracheal tube before we mentioned it right now—even if we had instructed you not to do so or just reminded you that there is absolutely no need to think of it right now*'.

When anaesthetists tell patients that a procedure such as intravenous or arterial line placement '*will hurt*', the communication itself increases the likelihood of this possibility, and the perception referred to becomes more likely to be experienced as pain[1–3].

Fortunately, suggestibility can also be used in a positive way[4]—for example, telling patients that there are ways to improve their comfort such as coughing during IV cannulation[5] or that breathing exercises after abdominal surgery[6] can make things more comfortable. Also just not mentioning words with negative connotations significantly reduces pain and anxiety associated with potentially painful stimuli such as injection of local anaesthetic[1,7]. Remaining factual '*I will give you the local anaesthetic now*' or '*the numbing medicine*' as some prefer, will suffice.

In times of stress, patients assume a focus of attention that leads to a hypnotic frame of mind that is highly suggestible to communications from the anaesthetist, whether the communications are negative or positive[8]. Hence an important step is to avoid wording with negative connotations.

Often, however, even well-meaning comments are misunderstood. Many words have double meanings, and in this setting patients will cling to the more pessimistic interpretation[9]. '*I will put you to sleep*' may conjure images of the veterinarian euthanizing a pet. Also interpretations are highly individual. We (EL) had one patient who objected to being made '*numb*' since '*numb*' meant '*dumb*' for him.

Placebo and nocebo effects

The effects of suggestion become all too evident when considering the widely recognized phenomenon of placebo. Placebo analgesia represents a situation where the administration of a substance known to be non-analgesic produces an analgesic response when the subject is told that it will make him or her comfortable. Interestingly, the type of suggestion-concordant response can be analgesic or antalgesic. When the suggestion elicits a negative response the phenomenon is usually called the nocebo effect[10]. Such effects follow negative suggestions where verbal or non-verbal cues lead to negative patient responses in terms of their perceptions, mood (affect) or behaviour. For example, offering the patient a sick bowl (emesis basin) in case of nausea can result in the patient feeling nauseous or even vomiting. More than two-thirds of an unselected sample of 34 college students reported mild headaches when told that a non-existent electric current was passing through their heads. Reports such as these are consistent with a view that clinical focusing on pain may of itself be a cause of pain[11]. Suggestion, intentional or not, must be taken into consideration when considering both placebo and nocebo effects[12].

In patients undergoing interventional procedures for lumbar facet joint pain, placebo effects were found in 13–15% of patients[13]. This is highly relevant in the practice of anaesthesia where successful doctor–patient relationships can mitigate nocebo responses. Negative beliefs are probably the single most important factor generating the nocebo effect, which is increasingly being recognized as both important and a major challenge to modern medicine[14]. Negative reactions to placebo medications (drugs without an active ingredient) are well documented, and similar responses can be induced in patients presenting for anaesthesia care where the use of negative language tends to increase patients' stress, negative expectations and perceptions. Several common language traps have been examined with a view to formulating alternative ways to communicate with patients[15].

Anaesthetists are in a position to enhance or sabotage the pharmacological effects of their drug administrations. For example, the side effects of propofol can be exaggerated if patients are advised during the injection that the propofol '*will sting*' or '*hurt*' as it is injected. Alternative communications could be that propofol gives, '*a warm or a cool feeling*' during its administration. We have heard of anaesthetists suggesting that the propofol '*sparkles*' as it is experienced—a sensation frequently appreciated by patients in a pleasant way as they are being induced. If one is concerned about whether anaesthetists could honestly describe the perception of propofol in a positive way, a more neutral alternative could be that it is: '*a powerful anaesthetic that may or may not be experienced or noticed as it begins to have an effect*'. Even more neutral could be '*I am starting the propofol now*', and leaving the patient the right to his or her own experience and description. Some anaesthetists may feel that they need to warn everyone regarding injection pain and propofol, despite the fact that the incidence of pain is under 40%[16]. If the types of communications given prior to injection are not controlled for, it is likely that the very act of suggesting pain may have an effect on the results of research in this topic[7].

Minimizing words and negating words

Minimizing words such as, '*a bit*', '*a little*', '*tiny*', '*just*' or '*only*' have no effect on mitigating the patient's response to negative suggestion. The image is already created in the mind, and modifiers do not displace its adverse effects. For example '*Just a tiny* ***sting*** *that will only* ***hurt*** *for a bit*' already sets the stage for stinging and hurting[7,17,18].

Negating words—when '*Don't worry*' means there is '*Something to worry about!*'

Negating words also fail to mitigate the effects of negatively valued words. Saying '*this won't hurt*' is double jeopardy. The suggestion in itself brings attention to hurting and if it then indeed hurts, the anaesthetist has lost credibility. Similarly when asking a patient '*not to move*', rather than '*stay still like a statue*', will probably lead to a subconscious response '*to move*'.

Try—the failure word

'Try' is a word that suggests anticipated failure of what is being asked. For example, '*Try to ignore the sound of the drill*' is likely to focus the patient's attention on the drill—just as being asked as the reader to '*Try not to think of an ampoule of propofol!*' (see also Chapters 4 and 20).

Therapeutic communication

Communications by the anaesthetist can provide information to the patient regarding the reason behind what otherwise might be perceived as an uncomfortable experience. Such therapeutic alternative communications could be, '*This local anaesthetic will* ***numb*** *the skin*', rather than '***sting***', or '*The anaesthetist is there to ensure your comfort and safety during the surgery and until you wake up in recovery*' rather than '*... put you to sleep*'. It is implied that comfort is one possible way to interpret a sensation. Similarly patients are reassured that they will be anaesthetized throughout the procedure, and that they will wake up at the end! Alternatively the anaesthetist could say, '*We will keep you under general anaesthesia for as long as necessary, so that you can awake refreshed*', or '*modern anaesthetics really allow us to tailor the effects to your needs whatever they might turn out to be*'. Such suggestions allow patients to experience procedures in ways that facilitate neutral or positive behavioural responses[19].

Case study 1 Negative suggestions have no effect?

An 8-year-old boy was asked in the pre-anaesthetic consultation two hours prior to surgery whether he wanted an intravenous (IV) or inhalational induction. His father stated that he should have the gas as this would help him vomit less. The boy insisted that he didn't want a mask and that he wanted '*the needle*' to go to sleep. The anaesthetist asked the parent whether it would be OK to go along with the boy's wishes as there was no evidence that an IV induction would adversely affect the risk of post-operative nausea and vomiting (PONV). The father reluctantly agreed but stated to the boy, '*As long as you know that you will vomit in recovery, when you wake up, if you have the needle*'. The boy had a smooth induction and an uneventful procedure but woke up in recovery crying and vomiting. His first words were, '*I should have listened to my dad!*'

Children are more suggestible than adults, particularly when stressed[20]. Parents are powerful authority figures and this parent had made a powerful suggestion for the child to vomit in recovery.

Case study 2 Negative suggestions have no effect?

A surgeon walked over to a 21-year-old patient during face mask pre-oxygenation and IV propofol induction. He then began talking to the patient who was scheduled for a circumcision and said that it would; '*hurt like hell in recovery*'. When the anaesthetist asked the surgeon why he had said that to the patient, the response was that, '*It always does hurt*'. Despite a penile nerve block and IV fentanyl, the patient woke up distressed, in pain and needing a prolonged stay in recovery while an analgesia protocol regime was administered.

Surgeons are powerful authority figures and there is a high response rate among patients to their expectations and suggestions. Over the last ten years the same surgeon now regularly tells patients that they '*can wake up comfortably as the wound heals and everything gets better*', and they frequently do.

Case study 3 Negative suggestions have no effect?

Antacid was administered prior to a caesarean section; '*You need to take this. It tastes disgusting and will probably make you feel sick*'. Interestingly the woman hesitated for a moment and then drank the antacid only to grimace and exclaim '*My god! That tastes disgusting!*' A few minutes later she proceeded to vomit on the way to theatre.

The patient actually used the same words as the anaesthetist administering the antacid where the negative suggestion was then perceived as a negative experience which subsequently led to the behavioural response of vomiting as she was transferred to the operating room. An alternative communication could have been used such as, '*Please take this. It is an antacid which pleasantly coats the stomach and helps you stay safe if you need a sleeping anaesthetic*'.

Interestingly, our anecdotal experience suggests that when patients are provided with an explanation of why they are being asked to drink the antacid rather than suggesting how bad it tastes, they frequently make no comment on the taste. This is the subject of future research. If there are still any doubters out there of the effects of negative suggestion, excerpts from the following verbatim transcript of a taped recording of one of the author's (EL) colleagues injecting local anaesthetic prior to a procedure[18] illustrates the point most effectively. (Case study 4 is reprinted with permission[18].)

Case study 4 Negative suggestions have no effect?

The patient is draped and the doctor is about to inject local anaesthetic prior to large core breast biopsy.

Dr A: '*OK, you are going to feel a* ***pinch*** *and a lot of* ***burning*** *and* ***stinging****. This is a* ***pinch****… a* ***pinch****…OK?* ***Burning*** *and* ***stinging****. How are you doing? Doing OK?* ***Pinch*** *and* ***sting****, Do you feel that? More* ***stinging***'.

Patient: '*I can still feel a needle in there*'.

Dr A: '*You feel a* ***needle*** *but do you feel any sharp* ***pain****?*'

Patient: '*I am OK, I just feel a needle*'.

Dr A: '*You feel a something moving but nothing* ***painful****, nothing* ***sharp*** *right?*'

Patient: '*Oh. … I feel prickly… Yeah*'.

Dr A: '*What was that?* ***Sharp****? …****Sorry***'.

Patient: *'That hurts!'*
Dr A: *'**Sorry**'*
[The doctor removes the needle].
Patient: *'That kills, it hurts, ...it hurts, it hurts'*.
Dr A: *'There is nothing there'*.
[The doctor places a gauze on the puncture site]
Dr A: *'Does it **sting**?'*
Patient: *'It didn't sting before...weren't you doing it before?'*
Patient: *'Wait, wait, wait. What did you just do? The last three times you injected me it didn't hurt. It stung a little but this time it feels like you are cutting the flesh out of my chest'*.
Dr A: *'Sorry about that, is it **burning** now?'*

The ethics of communication

It is just as inadvisable to say something '*will hurt*' as it is to say it '*will be comfortable*' when there is a possibility that it will do neither. One is then left wondering what to say when the patient asks, '*Will this hurt?*' Since the patient's response to stimulation cannot be known upfront there really is no honest truthful answer. If the anaesthetist responds by saying, '*It is quite variable. Some people experience discomfort, others tell me how surprised they are to feel more comfortable than they thought they would be*', this is entirely consistent with honesty with the added benefit of giving an indirect positive suggestion[19].

Similarly, if a patient asks, '*Will I have much pain after my operation?*' the anaesthetist can and should always respond honestly, and yet avoid the use of negative suggestions wherever possible. Adding a measure of control is also helpful, thus a response might take the form of, '*The healing response is highly individual. Some patients may experience **discomfort*** (instead of 'pain'), *while some people are surprised that the sensation of the wound healing is more comforting than they had thought. And if there should be some discomfort, there is no need to fight it, just to admit it, and most importantly to let us know right away. You can have as much medication as you wish within the limits of safety, to recover as quickly and comfortably as possible*'.

Choosing the word '*discomfort*' rather than '*pain*' and reframing '*pain*' as '*a healing sensation*' changes the meaning of the sensation from one of disability, to one of recovery. Addressing the patient's concerns is always paramount and these need to be dealt with. Note the use of the indirect suggestion '*some people...*' This implies indirectly that the patient too may feel more comfortable than expected. There sometimes is concern regarding the ethics of not telling patients something will hurt when the anaesthetist thinks that it might do. However, the best available evidence suggests that, the patient's and the anaesthetist's expectations, in some part, determine the experience[2].

The patient may hear you even if you don't think so!

Some patients under general anaesthesia may hear, although not necessarily recall, what was being said about them in the surgical theatre, particularly when rude remarks have been made. This has the potential for adverse effects during the post-operative course[21] (see Chapter 15).

Clinical researchers have traditionally tended to talk of positive and negative suggestion in terms of placebo and nocebo effects. There is an increasing recognition that patients who believe they will get better tend to realize this self-fulfilling prophecy, while the nocebo effect serves to make patients feel worse[22]. Anaesthetists are in the privileged position of influencing their patients' perceptions, mood and behaviours in powerful and subtle ways. Awareness is increasing of words and phrases that can lead to adverse patient responses such as increased anxiety and pain. Negatively framed language can nearly always be reframed in a way that can lead to a therapeutic rather than an adverse patient response. Research in the radiology setting of invasive procedures[23] and various anaesthetic settings has found that an understanding of how communications function as suggestions can minimize sabotage and harm caused by inadvertent negative language. Communications can then function as a valuable additional tool for the anaesthetist's armamentarium in selected patients.

Key points

1. Negative suggestions are ubiquitous in hospital practice in general, and in anaesthesia in particular.
2. There is now clear evidence from both observational and randomized controlled studies that negative suggestions increase pain perception and anxiety.
3. 'Try' is a failure word and should be used with caution.
4. Using positive language and suggestion can help generate positive outcomes.
5. Anaesthetists need to be aware of nocebo effects on outcomes such as pain, anxiety and PONV.

References

1 Varelmann D, Pancaro C, Cappiello E, Camann W (2010). Nocebo-induced hyperalgesia during local anesthetic injection. *Anesth Analg*, **110**(3), 868–70.

2 Dutt-Gupta J, Bown T, Cyna AM (2007). Effect of communication on pain during intravenous cannulation: a randomized controlled trial. *Br J Anaesth*, **99**(6), 871–5.

3 Lang EV (2005). Letters to the Editor, Response to Cyna and Andrew. *Pain*, **117**, 236–43.

4 Bjenke CJ (1996). Painful medical procedures. In: Barber J (ed.) *Hypnosis and suggestion in the treatment of pain: a clinical guide*. pp. 209–61. London: WW Norton.

5 Usichenko TI, Pavlovic D, Foellner S, Wendt M (2004). Reducing venipuncture pain by a cough trick: a randomized crossover volunteer study. *Anesth Analg*, **98**, 343–5.

6 Egbert LD (1986). Preoperative anxiety: the adult patient. *Int Anesthesiol Clin*, **24**(4), 17–37.

7 Lang EV, Hatsiopoulou O, Koch T, Berbaum K, Lutgendorf S, Kettenmann E, et al. (2005). Can words hurt? Patient–provider interactions during invasive procedures. *Pain*, **114**(1–2), 303–9.

8 Spiegel H, Greenleaf M (1963). Current perspectives on hypnosis in obstetrics. *N Y State J Med*, **63**, 2933–41.

9 Ewin D, Eimer B (2006). *Ideomotor signals for rapid hypnoanalysis.* Springfield, IL: Charles C. Thomas Publishers.

10 Benedetti F, Lanotte M, Lopiano L, Colloca L (2007). When words are painful: unraveling the mechanisms of the nocebo effect. *Neuroscience*, **147**(2), 260–71.

11 Schweiger A, Parducci A (1981). Nocebo: the psychologic induction of pain. *Pavlov J Biol Sci*, **16**(3), 140–3.

12 Bangert J, Tolksdorf W (1984). [Pain diagnosis and pain measurement. II. Clinical aspects]. *Anasth Intensivther Notfallmed*, **19**(5), 226–30.

13 Manchikanti L, Pampati V, Damron K (2005). The role of placebo and nocebo effects of perioperative administration of sedatives and opioids in interventional pain management. *Pain Physician*, **8**(4), 349–55.

14 Eccles R (2007). The power of the placebo. *Curr Allergy Asthma Rep*, **7**(2), 100–4.

15 Schenk PW (2008). 'Just breathe normally': word choices that trigger nocebo responses in patients. *Am J Nurs*, **108**(3), 52–7.

16 Kam E, Abdul-Latif MS, McCluskey A (2004). Comparison of Propofol-Lipuro with propofol mixed with lidocaine 10 mg on propofol injection pain. *Anaesthesia*, **59**(12), 1167–9.

17 Corydon Hammond D (1998). Formulating hypnotic and post-hypnotic suggestions. In: Corydon-Hammond D (ed.) *Handook of hypnotic suggestions and metaphors.* pp. 11–44. Chicago, Illinois: American Society of Clinical Hypnosis.

18 Lang EV (2009). Avoiding negative suggestions. In: Lang EV, Laser E (eds) *Patient sedation without medication.* pp. 56–63. Oxford: Trafford.

19 Cyna AM, Andrew MI, Tan SG (2009). Communication skills for the anaesthetist. *Anaesthesia*, **64**(6), 658–65.

20 Olness K, Gardner GG (1978). Some guidelines for uses of hypnotherapy in pediatrics. *Pediatrics*, **62**(2), 228–33.

21 Goldmann L (1988). Information-processing under general anaesthesia: a review. *J R Soc Med*, **81**(4), 224–7.

22 Kasdan ML, Lewis K, Bruner A, Johnson AL (1999). The nocebo effect: do no harm. *J South Orthop Assoc*, **8**(2), 108–13.

23 Lang EV, Benotsch EG, Fick LJ, Lutgendorf S, Berbaum ML, Berbaum KS, et al. (2000). Adjunctive non-pharmacological analgesia for invasive medical procedures: a randomised trial. *Lancet*, **355**(9214), 1486–90.

Chapter 4

Language and the subconscious

Allan M Cyna, Marion I Andrew, and Suyin GM Tan

'This chapter is so subconscious that you don't even know that you know it!'
AMC

What this chapter is about

Many of the communications commonly encountered in anaesthetic practice elicit subconscious responses, and, because this is so, they frequently go unrecognized. This form of communication involves verbal and non-verbal cues also known as suggestions that can elicit automatic changes in perception or behaviour. Much of this chapter is based on language structures that are thought to make subconscious changes in perception, mood or behaviour more likely[1], both with patients and anaesthetists themselves. Recognizing subconscious responses will facilitate communication. As is discussed later, anaesthetists can communicate with patients and colleagues in ways that utilize subconscious functioning. To all intents and purposes this looks like intuitive communication, when in reality it has structure and therefore can be learned and taught.

The conscious and the subconscious

The conscious and unconscious states are familiar to all anaesthetists. However, it is frequently unappreciated that all patients, whether in an unconscious or conscious state, will also be functioning subconsciously (see Chapters 2, 3, 15 and 20). In the unconscious patient it is well recognized that subconscious activities still occur—for example, in implicit awareness (see Chapter 15).

Most people would appreciate that there are times during consciousness when they switch off the 'logical brain' and enter 'daydream'-type thinking or they 'tune out'. People including anaesthetists tend to function subconsciously most of the time—for example, during routine activities such as driving home on 'autopilot' and arriving home without realizing it consciously. The ability we all have to function automatically—that is, subconsciously—frees up the conscious part of the mind to focus on other things such as planning tomorrow's 'neuro' case.

The teleological basis for this ability lies in being able to filter the massive amount of information continuously presented to the individual. This allows the conscious mind to focus on what it perceives to be important—facilitating learning, logical thinking and problem solving.

During activities where logical thinking is not a requirement, the subconscious comes to the fore. This is characterized by dissociation from the external environment—being 'in your own world'. Paradoxically, at times of extreme stress, the subconscious tends to take over when the conscious part of the mind becomes so overwhelmed by external inputs it ceases to function logically. An example of this is going into an exam and not being able to recall or vocalize the dose of morphine.

The conscious mind responds to logic and direct command, and is under volitional control. Subconscious processes are not usually considered to be under volitional control but can be accessed by using subconscious communication. The language of the subconscious is contained in metaphor, imagery, symbolism (see Chapter 5) and suggestion.

Subconscious communication is 'below the radar' and awareness of it requires a shift in thinking—once recognized, subconscious communication can be utilized therapeutically.

When patients are extremely anxious they are sometimes unable to obey a conscious command such as '*Lie still*'. In this situation, the use of suggestion is frequently more effective. For example,

> '*In a moment, you will find that you will be able to lie still*'.

Subconscious non-verbal cues would include the anaesthetist's own calmness, posture, vocal tone and confidence being conveyed to patients while managing their distress or pain effectively. An example of an inadvertent negative subconscious cue would be handing a patient a sick bowl '*in case you feel nauseated*'.

Subconscious responses

The first step in perceiving subconscious responses is to be aware that all human behaviours and communications have subconscious aspects. When the anaesthetist greets the patient, a subconscious response is elicited that frequently doesn't reach conscious awareness. However, this response can be very potent, and the ability to utilize this aspect of brain functioning represents a powerful tool in the anaesthetists' armamentarium. This effect may exacerbate any anxiety or pain already present (see Chapter 3), or be as anxiolytic as a midazolam premedication[2].

Most of the time, recognizing our own subconscious responses is not particularly important as these responses just allow us to get the job done! Much day to day functioning as anaesthetists, and as people, is subconscious. This is the concept of 'being on autopilot'—that is, the performance of a task without making conscious effort. Examples in anaesthesia include central venous catheter (CVC) placement or intravenous (IV) access. These motor skills are initially performed with varying degrees of conscious effort depending on the experience and skill of the anaesthetist. When we first learn a procedure the initial learning and performance of the skill is conscious, 'clunky', and takes time as the procedure tends to be learned in chunks, as a sequence of steps. With experience the steps become more fluent until they become one smooth action skillfully performed with increasing accuracy and proficiency. This subconscious learning can be used by the anaesthetist clinically—for instance, visualizing a vein prior to its cannulation.

There are times when it is useful for anaesthetists to recognize their own subconscious responses as these can both enhance and detract from performing optimally. Once recognized, the subconscious behaviour can be temporarily curtailed if necessary. There can then be consideration given to whether to use a strategy that may be more helpful or even therapeutic. Examples of subconscious responses that are frequently helpful include intuition, anxiety in moderation and the ability to compartmentalize or dissociate from external stimuli, and focus on a single task—for example, difficult intubation. Subconscious responses that can be unhelpful include excessive anxiety, and dissociation from external stimuli resulting in focusing on a single task, such as repeated attempts to intubate during a difficult intubation when, in fact, the patient is hypoxic and needs mask ventilation with 100% O_2—a 'fixation error'[3]. These responses occur spontaneously and frequently.

Imagery and imagination

Imagery and imagination is one way of communicating with the subconscious and can be used to elicit subconscious responses that allow people to do things that might be thought out of one's control. For example, if one consciously asks the salivary glands to secrete, nothing happens as the autonomic nervous system is not under conscious voluntary control. However communicating subconsciously by imagining, a favourite meal or sucking on a lemon soon causes the salivary glands to secrete. This example can be used as a metaphor that encourages patients to appreciate that they frequently can do more than they think they can.

Some people, especially children, find it very easy to enter an imaginary world where to all intents and purposes this becomes their reality or real world. This is the basis for distraction techniques that allow the patient to dissociate from their immediate environment.

For example, an anxious patient waiting to go into the operating room said,

Patient: '*I wish I could run away but I can't*'
Anaesthetist: '*Well, if you could run away. Where would you run to?*'
Patient: '*I'd run up the stairs*'.
Anaesthetist: '*What would be at the top?*'

Patient: '*A beautiful view*'.
Anaesthetist: '*Tell me about the view ... is it night time or day time?*'
Patient: '*It is night time I can see the lights... it's beautiful!*'

The anaesthetist has listened reflectively, accepted the patient's reality and utilized the patient's desire to run away, in order to facilitate an imaginary 'escape'. By entering the patient's world the anaesthetist has helped the patient distance herself from the stress of the immediate environment and allowed her to relax and cooperate with her care.

The question then arises—are there other ways that anaesthetists can use the subconscious with patients in a therapeutic way?

Suggestions

Suggestions are the single most useful form of subconscious communication. When the conscious mind is focused on something else, suggestions are not processed in a logical way. This provides the anaesthetist with an opportunity to communicate with the subconscious and elicit therapeutic responses.

Anaesthetists may recognize that they routinely use suggestions all the time so they might as well make them useful and therapeutic.

Direct suggestions

These tend to take the form '***You*** *will find that...*', '***You*** *will be able to...*' or '***You*** *may be surprised that...*' For example, at induction of anaesthesia, the anaesthetist could suggest to the patient,

'*You will feel better when you wake up*'.

Indirect suggestions

These take the form,

'*Most/some people find that...*' or '*A patient I saw last week found that...*' The implication here is that the patient too will experience the same thing. For example, at induction of anaesthesia, the anaesthetist could suggest to the patient,

'*Patients having this surgery, frequently tell us how much better they feel when they wake up*'.

Linked suggestions

Suggestions may involve linking two perceptions or behaviours with one another. This means that when you do one thing that is conscious, something else will happen that is subconscious. For example,

'*When **you** focus on your breathing* [conscious], *each time **you** breathe out you will find yourself relaxing automatically* [subconscious]'.

A direct suggestion tends to capture the attention of the conscious mind, gets logically processed and can then be rejected. However, patients are more likely to respond to a direct suggestion under extreme stress when the conscious mind is focused elsewhere.

Indirect suggestions are more permissive. For example,

'*When **people** focus on breathing, each time they breathe out they find themselves relaxing automatically*'.

This indirectly implies that if the patient focuses on breathing, then relaxation will also occur.

Repetition

Repetition in a variety of forms is one of the most useful ways that people retain important information, both consciously and subconsciously. This learning response can be facilitated by using a variety of phrases that mean the same thing. For example, during pre-oxygenation, if the anaesthetist's suggestion for relaxation with breathing appears to be effective, this can then be reinforced by saying; '*That's good!*', '*Well done!*' or '*That's right!*' coinciding with the patient's exhalation.

Seeding an idea

As the phrase suggests, seeding an idea prepares the patient in a way that enhances the probability of a response occurring with a suggestion. Examples of seeding are expressions of confidence in the anaesthetist made by nursing staff and others, prior to the pre-anaesthetic visit.

Nurse: '*Dr S is really good at putting drips in—you won't feel a thing...*'

This generates an expectation that the cannulation will be comfortable and straightforward.

Reversed effect

The harder one tries to do something, the less chance there is of succeeding. This is especially the case with anxious patients who try not to feel anxious. When patients find themselves unable to cooperate with anaesthetic care, asking them to do the opposite of what is required frequently allows them to respond in a useful way. For example, a patient who says, '*I can't relax*' can be asked '*not to relax*', as a way of facilitating a subconscious 'relax' response. Similarly during an inhalational induction of anaesthesia, children can be asked ***not*** *to blow up the balloon too hard.* This will usually result in the child taking deeper breaths and therefore speed up the induction (see also Chapter 10).

The word '***not***' isn't processed by the subconscious. This means that when the anaesthetist asks the child, '***not*** *to blow up the balloon too hard*', this is a subconscious suggestion for the child to blow harder!

Failure words

'***Try***' is a failure word and should be used with caution. It implies an attempt, with the probability of failure. However, the two words 'try' and 'not' can be used therapeutically. For example, when the anxious patient is asked to, '*Try not to relax*' the patient consciously will fail '*not to relax*' but subconsciously the patient will relax, as the 'not' isn't processed by the subconscious. The confusion this statement generates tends to facilitate the non-logical processing of the subconscious. Another example is if an anxious patient states that he cannot keep his arm still during arterial line placement, the anaesthetist can ask him, '*Try not to stay too relaxed and still and it will just seem to* *happen all on its own!*' This type of statement frequently leads paradoxically to the arm relaxing and staying still.

Double binds

Double binds are statements of comparable alternatives that can facilitate a sense of control by allowing stressed patients the perception of choice when there isn't any. This is a technique most successfully used with children. For example, when leading a child in to theatre the anaesthetist can ask the child,

> '*Would you like to climb up onto the bed all on your own or would you like Daddy to help you?*'

Either choice results in the child on the bed. Another example would be,

> '*When you are lying still on the bed, would you like to hold Mummy's left hand or her right hand?*'

If a hand is chosen, the child is subconsciously communicating that they will (probably) lie still on the bed!

Use of metaphor

'Metaphor' comes from the Greek word 'metapherein', meaning 'to transfer'[4]. The term 'metaphor' has two distinct meanings. In one sense it is a story or narrative used to convey meaning other than the literal words used. As a linguistic term it is a figure of speech in which a word or phrase is applied to something to which it is not literally applicable—for example, food for thought. An example of metaphor is '*I'll just put him under*', representing anaesthesia as submersion. Metaphor in all its meanings can help anaesthetists facilitate useful subconscious changes in perceptions and behaviour in the patient (see also Chapters 5 and 20).

Concentrated attention

Concentrated attention refers to the phenomenon that when a person concentrates on an image or experience over and over again, it spontaneously tends to realize itself. For example, the suggestion that patients will find that they can lie perfectly still during an anaesthetic procedure can be far more effective than reasoning with them.

An example where communications with patients are likely to concentrate attention in a negative way is when patients are repeatedly asked whether they are '*in pain*' or '*feel sick*' or for their '*pain scores*' when they appear to be, or state that they are, perfectly comfortable (see Chapter 3).

Truisms and the development of a 'Yes set'

A truism is a statement that is difficult to refute—for example, '*Oxygen is good for you!*' Truisms can be utilized to elicit subconscious '*Yes*' responses as each truism is heard and taken on board.

A 'Yes set' is elicited by making a series of truisms which generate subconscious '*Yes*' responses. These can be utilized to elicit therapeutic perceptions and behaviours that would otherwise be difficult to achieve. For example, prior to IV cannula insertion, rather than suggest that the patient's arm can go numb, the anaesthetist can suggest a series of small changes in perception that culminate in numbness. For example, the anaesthetist can say,

> '*As the tourniquet is placed on the arm, a change in sensation may occur* (subconscious 'yes').
> *Then, as the tourniquet tightens the arm starts to tingle* (subconscious 'yes').
> *Then, it feels a little more different* (subconscious 'yes'),
> *a little sleepy* (subconscious response leading to a perceptual change),
> *perhaps heavy ... and then it goes numb* (perceptual response to the suggestion).
> *This tends to allow the drip to be inserted more comfortably*' (see Chapters 9, 10 and 14).

Time—distortion and progression

'*The experience of an individual appeared to us arranged in a series of events; in this series the single events which we remember appear to be ordered according to criterion of "early" or "later"*'. This quote from Einstein refers to our innate sense of the passage of time to which we also attribute a magnitude—for example, a '*short*' or a '*long*' time. Time, as we experience it, is different from 'clock time', and this phenomenon can be explored by comparing 'experiential time' with 'clock time'. When this occurs we experience time as much shorter or longer than 'clock time'. This is referred to as 'time distortion'. During periods of boredom, time appears to pass much more slowly. Likewise in dreams it is common to experience a large number of events in a very short time span. Hence the expressions,

> '*Time flies by when you're having fun*'

or, alternatively,

> '*A watched kettle never boils*'.

Our perception of time, like other perceptions, is open to alteration by suggestion. In circumstances where the anaesthetist may wish to emphasize benefit and de-emphasize negative aspects of an experience for a patient, suggestions can be made to associate and affect time in a positive and helpful way. For example, as stated in Chapter 9, the woman in labour can be asked to focus on the 'rest' that follows each contraction and it can be suggested that,

> '*in this way the rests can start seeming to last longer than they really are and the contraction to last for shorter periods...*'.

Our sense of passage of time combined with memory and imagination can allow us to think into the future, and this expectance can generate useful perceptual and behavioural experiences in itself. For example, suggesting to patients that they can,

> '*look forward to a rapid recovery*'

where they,

> '*can look back on the experience and feel it all went a little easier than they had thought.*'

Key points

1. A shift in thinking is required to become aware of subconscious communications and then to utilize them therapeutically.
2. Suggestions make up many of the communications commonly encountered in anaesthetic practice and acute care.
3. Language structures that act therapeutically can be readily learned.
4. Language structures of particular value to the anaesthetist include, double binds, developing 'Yes sets', and the use of time distortion or progression.

References

1 Corydon-Hammond D (1998). Formulating suggestions. In: Corydon-Hammond D (ed.) *Handook of hypnotic suggestions and metaphors.* Chicago, Illinois: American Society of Clinical Hypnosis.

2 Lang EV (2009). *Patient sedation without medication.* Oxford: Trafford.

3 Fioratou E, Flin R, Glavin R (2010). No simple fix for fixation errors: cognitive processes and their clinical applications. *Anaesthesia,* **65**(1), 61–9.

4 Compact Oxford English Dictionary (2006). 3rd edn. Oxford: Oxford University Press.

5 Kroger WS (2007). *Clinical & experimental hypnosis in medicine, dentistry, and psychology.* Philadelphia: JB Lippincott.

Chapter 5

Narrative and metaphor

Audrey Shafer

'If I can ease one Life the Aching
Or cool one Pain...
I shall not live in Vain'.
Emily Dickinson, Complete Poems[1]

What this chapter is about

Narrative and metaphor can be viewed as literary terms without much use in the world of medicine other than to prettify language and decorate ivory tower treatises on medical esoterica. However, since narrative and metaphor are integral to how we think, how we analyse and process information, how, in fact, we perceive and thus act, it would be naive and arbitrary to exclude such concepts from an understanding of the practice of medicine[2,3]. Furthermore, with its compression and crystallization of communication with the patient, the complex interplay between human and machine, the draconian consequences of poor communication and the emotional toll of a high stress environment, the practice of anaesthesia lends itself well to a closer look at how narrative and metaphor imbue and inform what anaesthetists do.

Narrative and story

The relationship between narrative and story is largely determined by context. Interchangeable in some respects, the terms both mean an account of events, and each can be contained in the other. For instance, a narrative can be woven from various stories and a story can contain narratives of various characters. The term narrative is mostly used here primarily because it encompasses text, however fragmentary, dialogue, and the study of narrative in medical education and practice, termed 'narrative medicine'[4]. Nonetheless, 'story' is also understood here, and is a useful term, particularly in relation to a point of view or a retelling of an experience, in Rashomon fashion, from differing perspectives. As noted in Chapter 2, inflection and emphasis change the meaning of even a single sentence.

The idea of differing perspectives deserves special attention in the anaesthetist–patient relationship. The 'narrative incommensurability'[5] between doctor and patient is one of the prime driving forces behind the need for good communication pre- and post-operatively. That is, the unknowableness of another person, indeed a stranger, for whom we anaesthetists assume vital and personhood responsibilities during the operation, makes clear and comprehensive communication that much more important.

People develop not only as individuals, but also as social beings. Just as we try to understand another's actions through, among other ways, the mirror neuron system, we try to understand another's perspective, all the while recognizing that we are, by definition, distinct[6].

During the course of the anaesthetist's relationship with patients, the patient's perspective is essentially and dramatically changed by what we do. We cloud the patient's sensorium to a degree not achieved (legally or routinely) by other physicians. The dynamics of the change in the patient's perspective, and his or her ability to convey desire and choice, are what make us, in part, guardians of what we knew of the patient prior to induction.

The idea of story, of a beginning, ending and middle, is also particularly germane to the practice of anaesthesia, and may well be part of the attraction of the profession to its practitioners. There is something tidy and satisfying about induction and emergence as beginning and ending, with maintenance of general anaesthesia as the middle, and perhaps the pre- and post-operative periods as preface and epilogue.

The patient also experiences these time points, but may place them in the larger history of his or her medical journey. One of the telling differences in narratives written by surgical patients, and by anaesthesia residents asked to imagine they were the patient just cared for, is the framing, in the patient narratives, of the operative and perioperative experience in the context of previous surgeries and recovery processes[7]. Furthermore, patients are far more likely to rank highly concerns about their family as a cause for pre-operative anxiety compared with what surgery or anaesthesia residents imagine are their patients' top concerns[8]. A patient is apt to place the surgical experience not only in the continuum of his life, but also in the middle of his experience of life—family, work, and other aspects of life which hold meaning and significance. A surgeon, however, begins the progress note as, for example, POD #4 (the fourth day after the operation) no matter how long the patient had been hospitalized prior to the day of surgery, when the diagnosis was made or any number of other time points which may begin the patient's story of illness.

It is human nature to seek meaning in life. A recitation of a series of events is enlivened by the connections, perceived or imagined, behind the series. This is plot.

This is meaning-making. From the moment we start thinking about a case, to the closure we feel at the end of the day when all has gone well, we try to tie all the pieces of anaesthesia care together into a coherent whole. We notice something odd—for instance, the patient lying in the holding room has the blanket pulled over his mouth, and we think, perhaps he is embarrassed because his false teeth are out. Our approach to that patient is altered. And this is just the beginning of the complex dynamic that characterizes the series of interconnected events as we interact with the patient, the operating room team, other staff and the 'props'—various devices and machines.

Life is messy and demarcations blurred, which is why telling the story of a trip is easier than recounting what you did during a week some months prior to the trip. The boundaries of typical anaesthesia care make it journey-like. If all goes well, drama and conflict are prevented. A smooth, seemingly easy anaesthetic makes even the remarkable nature of what we do appear routine. We do not seek to make bestseller adventure tales of our anaesthetics; nonetheless, the natural boundaries of daily anaesthesia care make even an 'uneventful' anaesthetic story-like, punched out of the rest of our lives and of our patients' lives.

Narrative as a way of knowing

When compared with 'logicoscientific knowledge', knowledge gained from an appreciation of narrative has been touted to honour the individual—that is, 'to illuminate the universally true by revealing the particular' rather than by 'transcending the particular'[9]. Narrative knowledge, then, is similar to case-based ethics, or casuistry, in that the particular, archetypal situations on which the reasoning is based are given prominence.

However, medical knowledge, even the *au courant* evidence-based medicine, is more narrative based than may be suspected[2]. The power of anecdotal experience cannot be overestimated, whether it is one's own, or 'told' to one via informal story, or via formal presentation at a morbidity and mortality conference or by reading a case report. These narrative-based experiences underlie anaesthesia skill building, such as interpretive reasoning, clinical judgement, as well as storing and retrieving information and knowledge. Furthermore, medicine is a practice. We 'know' to decrease sedative doses in the elderly because of observing the effect of titration. We also 'know' to decrease such doses from reading the anaesthesia literature, which is filled with studies of individuals coalesced into groups. For instance, pharmacokinetic and dynamic studies are performed using individual patients and volunteers. Any translation of those results needs to be applied back to the particulars of the patient before us—his age, habitus, debility, organ function, and so on.

Knowledge is iterative, reinforceable, malleable and imperfect. If knowledge were not, then the delivery of anaesthesia care would be formulaic and robotic. We would gain nothing from the phenomenon of 'eyeballing' a patient—that is, comparing the 'paper' version of the patient described in the chart with the person before us—and we could do push-button anaesthesia. By acknowledging that much of science is based on probabilities (the proverbial '*P*-value'), one acknowledges that determining where the particular patient is on the continua of anaesthesia–stimulation–consciousness–paralysis–pain perception, and so on, is an acceptance of the importance of the particulars of that patient at that moment. This is narrative knowledge.

The anaesthesia record is a valuable form of communication which is largely non-narrative in form. It can be extremely reassuring to view a checkmark notation by the previous anaesthetist for a particular patient with a potentially difficult airway, indicating no difficulties with laryngoscopy and intubation. However, a brief narrative as adjunct to the formulaic record is an effective form of communication across time for those circumstances where unexpected difficulties arose and the patient now requires another anaesthetic. Similarly, the narrative given to the recovery room nurse or intensive care team is formulaic in nature, but the specifics of the pre-operative status of the patient and intraoperative events make the narrative unique to the patient[10].

Narrative in education, well-being and reflection

Just as one cannot fully understand mathematics by reading a chapter in a textbook, one cannot understand the impact of narrative without doing the problems, in this case telling stories, playing with language and possibly even facing the terror of the blank page. Writing has been touted as a way of improving reflective practice, sharpening critical thinking skills and preventing professional burn-out[11]. Anaesthesia trainees asked to write narratives of challenging informed consent situations they had encountered can use those narratives as the basis for improving pre-operative communication with patients[12]. Acknowledging the challenges we face via narrative tools can enhance our ability to recognize and respond to similar situations as they arise in future anaesthetics[13].

A growing literature on possible health benefits of writing about emotionally troubling experiences has led to initial investigations of the effects on patients of writing about their cancer pain[14]. Conceivably, therapeutic writing can provide an adjuvant means of communication for patients under the care of pain specialists. Even professional writers lament the difficulty of verbalizing the experience of pain[15]. A fascinating study of the use of a personal diary for patients in the intensive care unit invited entries by staff and relatives of the patient. In this study, designed to address problems of long-term psychological trauma of survivors of critical care and their family members, intensivists found that both writing and the document itself were therapeutic[16].

Other uses of narrative include the inculcation of professional values, such as a commitment to optimal patient care, via reading or relating historical tales of remarkable anaesthetists[17]. These tend to be complete narrative texts. At the other end of the spectrum are the so-called unruly or post-modern texts, those which use electronic media in the form of blogs, postings, mixed media, and multiple authors whose only connection is via cyberspace[18]. These websites or other electronic media all rely to some extent on narrative, which is used for intradepartmental communication, patient information, community building, social and professional networking and a host of other purposes.

Narrative comments are also used for performance evaluation, largely in training programmes. Of particular note is the correlation between the presence or absence of negative comments on professionalism—including communication skills—and overall performance. No anaesthesia resident whose overall performance was evaluated as excellent (top 30%) had received negative comments during training regarding professionalism (as had 21% of residents)[19]. Analysis of narrative comments, particularly negative ones, may be especially important as faculty can be reluctant to communicate concern about negative traits. Indeed, throughout medicine, competency and communication skills are inseparable[20].

Metaphor: ubiquity and import

Neuroscience is, more and more, informing many branches of knowledge, from business structure to computer science to courtroom evidence regarding criminal motivation. Hence, it is not surprising that neuroscientific tools are being used to investigate language, and more specifically, metaphor processing[21]. In a fractal-like spiral, metaphor, which is essentially connection-making between two or multiple concepts, is being studied by imaging which neural centres and interconnections activate on functional scans as people 'process' metaphors[22,23]. Depending on how figurative or literal the metaphor, how novel or hackneyed, how open-ended or closed the context, and how reinforced or negated by gestural or non-verbal cues, different brain loci are recruited[24,25].

Therefore, the range of metaphor presented in now classic texts, such as Lakoff and Johnson's *Metaphors we live by*, constitutes a probable range of neuroexcitory responses. There are a number of classification systems for metaphor depending on the historical, philosophical or linguistic bent of the academic. Neurolinguists study brain activation patterns for different types of metaphor; for instance, whether a metaphor is nominal—noun based, such as '*the recertification exam was a breeze*'—or predicate—verb or motion based, such as '*the patient sailed (or flew) through the anaesthetic*'[26]. A metaphor embedded in our language, such as '*under anaesthesia*', makes anaesthesia into a 'something' one can be within and below—that is, an ontological and orientational metaphor[27]. This form of metaphor would most probably be processed quite differently from a metaphor which is novel, innovative or surprising, and which more directly conjures up a host of associations. For instance, if the anaesthetist describes the anaesthetic plan in an uncommon way, saying, for example, '*I'll be your bartender for the next hour, here's your first drink*', the anaesthetist should be aware that multiple brain loci are stimulated to process the metaphor due to the less common metaphor employed, let alone possible negative connotations associated with alcohol by a particular patient.

This is not to say that humour has no place in anaesthetist–patient communication. On the contrary—humour can be extremely useful, not only as a distraction or to lessen the stress of the moment, but also as a way to connect, person-to-person. Humour can instill confidence, if used appropriately, and imply that the anaesthetist is so comfortable with her own abilities that she can handle multiple tasks such as starting the intravenous line and joking about something else. Much of humour relies on metaphor and forming new, off-beat connections between ideas, words and situations. Just as one would not tell off-colour jokes to a patient in the holding area and risk alienating and angering that patient, the anaesthetist should think about what one says to and how one speaks with the patient in terms of metaphoric implications, including possible negative effects.

Metaphor: dehumanizing, patronizing, yet persistent

Common classifications of medical metaphors include war, parental, and machine or engineering metaphors[28]. Because of the physical nature of anaesthesia practice and the alterations in patient sensorium we cause, anaesthetists can readily view the patient as an object; something to be controlled. This overlaps with aggression/war metaphors, something that resembles a container and/or something mechanical[27].

The direct connections between our patient and the anaesthesia and other machines, including infusion pumps and computerized record-keeping machines, make the anaesthetized patient particularly prone to mechanical descriptors and human–computer metaphoric transformations which have increasingly been reviewed in cultural studies of embodiment[29]. The projection of people-related terms onto their environments, including machines—for example, '*a virus infection*'—is a natural outgrowth of human conceptions of their world. But the obverse, machine onto person—for example, a productive academic '*churns out papers*', and an efficient surgeon can be called '*a machine*' with a short procedures room likened to '*a factory*' with patients '*on an assembly line*'—contributes to the linguistic blending of humans and machines. The translation of the patient into physiological data represented on the anaesthesia monitors can mean a temporary metaphoric transformation of patient into machine. When the surgeon asks how the patient is doing, we glance at the vital signs and say '*Fine!*'. Further, when we present a case at conference, the patient 'becomes' the projected anaesthesia record.

Some examples of metaphor used in anaesthesia are listed below.

War

'*Arterial stick or stab*'

'*Patient is resistant to the drugs*'

'*Knock out the patient*'

Machine

'*Tube the patient*'

'*Hook the patient up to the monitors*'

'*Patient is on cruise control*'

Patients also use metaphors to organize their thoughts and desires regarding healthcare. If they have a medical problem, they expect the doctor to '*fix it*'. They might have something wrong with their '*ticker*' or '*plumbing system*'. They may ask for the '*knock-out*' drugs, or feel '*like a pincushion*' after multiple intravenous line attempts. Terrain metaphors are common as well, after all, sick patients enter not only the hospital but also the land of the ill, leaving '*a country as far away as health*'[30] where '*the memory of your health is like an island, going out of sight behind you*'[31]. Patients may ask to go to '*la la land*'.

No matter the classification system, metaphors which turn the patient into an object can be particularly dehumanizing. Jargon shortcuts used to communicate with other professionals frequently employ metonymy—for example, part for the whole—'*He's a Mallampati 3*'. It is not always wise to assume the patient is oblivious to the shop talk around him. For instance, as you enter the room with the patient, a nurse asks for later charting purposes, '*What's his ASA?*', and the anaesthetist responds '*He's a 2*'. This exchange may not be interpreted by the awake patient in a positive way. Even if the patient is fully anaesthetized or not present, it is wise to think about the language used to describe patients and cases as we communicate with colleagues. '*He's a full stomach!*' '*Tank him up!*', '*It was a peek and shriek*' or '*Open and shut case*'—a metaphor for an exploratory laparotomy/oscopy aborted due to tumour load.

A prime reason to consider the objectifying language that we use is to sort out emotions when something goes awry. If one is used to always describing patients as if they were body parts, then when one encounters airway difficulty, for example, it is easier to slide into blaming the patient for the oxygen desaturation or other problems—'***He is** a difficult airway*' rather than '***He has** a difficult airway*' or '***His airway** is difficult*'.

It is unrealistic to believe or even desire the end to jargon, shortcut language or metonymic references. But it is realistic to examine one's own practices. What language choices are made? In what context? To whom? Who else is in earshot? We make and try to interpret language choices constantly. Not only figurative but literal language also requires interpretation—what does it mean that the radiologist wrote 'not enlarged' for the aorta, rather than 'normal'[20]?

The point is not to avoid metaphor—metaphor is too integral to how we think and talk and it enables communication. When we begin relating a case to a colleague by stating '*What a train wreck!*' we have set the stage for the narrative of the difficult case that ensued. Our colleague instantly knows what we mean, sympathy is generated and the specifics of the arduous anaesthetic are better appreciated. Yet we should also realize that by comparing the patient with a disaster zone and the image of massive railway carriages jackknifed off track, we have instinctively protected ourselves from some of the blame, stress, second-guessing and other negative effects of being a provider of anaesthesia care, even when we feel we've provided the best possible service.

Using metaphor to understand difficult communication situations

Rather than shy away from communication in difficult situations, such as a demanding patient, a patient with 'Do Not Resuscitate' (DNR) orders who is scheduled for an operation or a patient nearing end of life, it behoves us to take the time and emotional energy to deal with them[32]. Understanding the anaesthetist–patient relationship in a metaphoric way can help explain why difficult situations are so complex. Discussions about patients who are near the end of life are fraught with emotion, such as patient fears of abandonment (a charged and associative word), a lack of clarity about 'informed' consent where the gambling metaphors of 'odds' and 'risks' can be understood differently by different individuals, and various spiritual and moral beliefs[33]. Because metaphor can help clarify an unfamiliar situation by inviting comparison with one more familiar, judicious use of metaphor can open discussion in a non-threatening way[34]. For example, the anaesthetized state can be contrasted to the sleep state to explain why resuscitating drugs and intubation may be necessary for a patient with DNR orders where the need for a general anaesthetic is contemplated as a back-up plan: '*Unlike sleep, sedation and anaesthesia can make your blood pressure go down and your breathing slow down—we will need to be able to treat that*'.

The statement, '*No one dies on my watch*', spoken in response to whether or not DNR orders will be suspended in the operative/perioperative period, is both a military and paternalistic metaphor. Such a statement closes discussion because it assumes:

- the anaesthetist knows best;
- the anaesthetist is at all times in command and control;
- the anaesthetist, just like a general, is not to be questioned.

Death is seen as the enemy, to be defeated at all costs. However, difficult decisions need to open the discussion not close it, to promote interaction, not absolutism.

'*All medical and surgical practices today are "team sports"*'.[35] Team metaphors acknowledge the complexities of interpersonal dynamics, goals, procedures, and practice. There are loyalty and leadership issues. Metaphors need scrutiny, but not necessarily flat-out rejection, at points of murkiness or failure[36]. In fact, rigidly adhering to metaphor connections as if they were one-for-one analogies limits the imaginative force and meaning-making inherent in metaphor. For instance, if one continues with the sports team metaphor, one wonders where the patient fits in; as another team member? As playing field?

Metaphor: embedded in practice, perception and research

Examples of deeply embedded metaphor in anaesthetic practice occur in the presentation of data by, for example, anaesthesia machines, and our interpretation of that data. In essence, this is communication between machine and anaesthetist. The metaphor, proximal is similar (and the opposite—dissimilar is far apart), is found in language such as '*even though she's a first-year resident, her skills are close to a third year's*'. Our natural and manmade environments generate and reflect this concept—think of a flock of birds or the organization of syringes in one drawer of the cart. This metaphor, along with 'up is more', guides much of the visual displays of the monitors, for instance, the grouping of ventilatory data in one part of the screen. We find controls or displays which do not follow such basic metaphors to be counter-intuitive or illogical.

Because, however, we bring objects close to each other in order to search out differences, purely visual comparisons can accentuate our perception of difference when objects are physically close[37]. The benefits of arranging similar-looking vials into proximate bins in an anaesthesia cart drawer because we will be more likely to scrutinize the label and avoid a drug swap may, however, be outweighed by the lack of muscle memory of reaching for lookalikes in disparate parts of the drawer.

The 'up is better' metaphor underlies the synaesthetic translation of the colour of oxygenated blood to pitch[27]. Other auditory stimuli in the operating room, such as loud music, can reduce the effectiveness of this beat-by-beat communication of patient well-being. 'Red means stop' is used for colouring visual alarm status and as an aid to how much to pump up the pressure bag. The lack of colour coding standardization of gas cylinders internationally, or even across manufacturers in a single country, is a failure to use a consistent colour metaphor (e.g. in the USA, oxygen is life is green), and has led to faulty communication and catastrophic error.

Tidiness in the anaesthesia workspace is used as a metaphor for competence of anaesthetic care. In legal proceedings, the anaesthesia record can be regarded 'as a metaphor for the care provided; an illegible, scantily completed chart infers care that was likely substandard and inattentive'[38].

Lastly, embedded metaphors influence how well research results are communicated and how accurately we interpret those results. Theories of visualization emphasize the importance of underlying metaphors on data presentation—for example, treemap (nested rectangles) versus node-link charts—for user comprehension[39]. Algorithms, such as those for the difficult airway or pre-operative cardiac testing for non-cardiac surgery, rely on branching metaphors, or decision-tree visualization. Anaesthesia researchers can affect practice by understanding what visual metaphors are assumed when communicating research results via graphs and charts.

From the moment we are consulted or look at the operating room schedule and start thinking about a case, we begin placing the care of that patient in the context of our experience and knowledge. We build the story by reading the patient chart, reviewing prior anaesthesia records, and talking with and examining the patient. We set the scene in the operating room, preparing our equipment and pharmacopoeia for whatever twists we envision the plot of the anaesthetic care may take. We relay the story, using a wide variety of narrative constructs, to a relief anaesthetist, a recovery room nurse, the patient and family, or, potentially, to colleagues at a morbidity and mortality conference. Metaphor is embedded in the language we use, how we think about mechanisms underlying anaesthesia, and how we translate data into patient care. Examining the narrative and metaphoric structures which underpin our thought processes can clarify such processes and improve communication.

Key points

1. Language is integral not only to how we express our thoughts, but also to how we think.
2. Narrative structure and the elements of story, such as character, tone, plot and context, are fundamental to medical knowledge, recall and clinical reasoning.
3. The essentials of anaesthesia care—make such care both story and journey like.

Key points *(continued)*

4. Metaphors are ubiquitous in language and gesture; how we process various types of metaphors is under intensive investigation.
5. Attention to the metaphoric basis of what we say and how we interpret sensory input can make us aware of the potential effects of such metaphors, including both positive and negative effects on subconscious perceptions, mood and behaviours.

References

1 Dickinson, E (1890, 1960). 'If I can stop one Heart from breaking' poem 919. In: *The complete poems of Emily Dickinson.* Boston, MA: Little, Brown & Co.

2 Montgomery K (2006). *How doctors think: clinical judgment and the practice of medicine.* New York, NY: Oxford University Press.

3 Lakoff G, Johnson M (1980) *Metaphors we live by.* Chicago, IL: University of Chicago Press.

4 Charon R (2006). *Narrative medicine: honoring the stories of illness.* New York, NY: Oxford University Press.

5 Hunter KM (1991). *Doctors' stories: the narrative structure of medical knowledge.* p. 123. Princeton, NJ: Princeton University Press.

6 Iacoboni M, Mazziotta JC (2007). Mirror neuron system: basic findings and clinical applications. *Ann Neurol,* **62**(3), 213–8.

7 Shafer A, Fish MP (1994). A call for narrative: the patient's story and anesthesia training. *Lit Med,* **13**(1), 124–42.

8 Shafer A, Fish MP, Gregg KM, Seavello J, Kosek P (1996). Preoperative anxiety and fear: a comparison of assessments by patients and anesthesia and surgery residents. *Anesth Analg,* **83**, 1285–91.

9 Charon R (2001). Narrative medicine: a model for empathy, reflection, profession, and trust. *JAMA,* **286**(15), 1897–902.

10 Kopp VJ, Shafer A (2000). Anesthesiologists and perioperative communication. *Anesthesiology,* **93**, 548–55.

11 Bolton G (2007). Narrative and poetry writing for professional development. *Aust Fam Phys,* **36**(12), 1055–6.

12 Waisel DB, Lamiani G, Sandrock NJ, Pascucci R, Truog RD, Meyer EC (2009). Anesthesiology trainees face ethical, practical, and relational challenges in obtaining informed consent. *Anesthesiology,* **110,** 480–6.

13 Shafer A (2009). "It blew my mind: exploring the difficulties of anesthesia informed consent through narrative. *Anesthesiology,* **110,** 445–6.

14 Cepeda MS, Chapman CR, Miranda N et al. (2008). Emotional disclosure through patient narrative may improve pain and well-being: results of a randomized controlled trial in patients with cancer pain. *J Pain Symptom Manage,* **35**(6), 623–31.

15 Woolf V (2002). *On being ill* (original pub. 1926). Ashfield, MA: Paris Press.

16 Bäckman CG, Walther SM (2001). Use of a personal diary written on the ICU during critical illness. *Intensive Care Med,* **27,** 426–9.

17 Bacon DR (2008). The historical narrative: tales of professionalism? *Anesthesiol Clin,* **26,** 67–74.

18 McLellan F (1997). 'A whole other story': the electronic narrative of illness. *Lit Med*, **16**(1), 88–107.

19 Rhoton MF (1994). Professionalism and clinical excellence among anesthesiology residents. *Acad Med*, **69**(4), 313–5.

20 Groopman J (2007). *How doctors think*. New York, NY: Houghton Mifflin Company.

21 Giora R (2007) Is metaphor special? *Brain Lang*, **100,** 111–4.

22 Shibata M, Abe J, Terao A, Myamoto T (2007). Neural mechanisms involved in the comprehension of metaphoric and literal sentences: an fMRI study. *Brain Res*, **1166**, 92–102.

23 Mashal N, Faust M, Hendler T, Jung-Beeman M (2009). An fMRI study of processing novel metaphoric sentences. *Laterality*, **14**(1), 30–54.

24 Cornejo C, Simonetti F, Ibáñez A, Aldunate N, Ceric F, López V, et al. (2009). Gesture and metaphor comprehension: electrophysiological evidence of cross-modal coordination by audiovisual stimulation. *Brain Cogn*, **70**, 42–52.

25 Schmidt GL, Seger CA (2009). Neural correlates of metaphor processing: the roles of figurativeness, familiarity and difficulty. *Brain Cogn*, **71**(3), 375–86.

26 Chen E, Widick P, Chatterjee A (2008). Functional–anatomical organization of predicate metaphor processing. *Brain Lang*, **107**, 194–202.

27 Shafer A (1995). Metaphor and anesthesia. *Anesthesiology*, **83**, 1331–42.

28 Coulehan J (2003). Metaphor and medicine: narrative in clinical practice. *Yale J Biol Med*, **76**, 87–95.

29 Skara D (2004). Body metaphors—reading the body in contemporary culture. *Coll Antropol*, **28**(Suppl 1), 183–9.

30 Plath S (1960). 'Tulips'. In: *Collected poems*. pp 160–2. New York, NY: Harper & Row.

31 Hoagland T (1992). 'Emigration'. In: *Sweet ruin*. pp. 69–70. Madison, WI: University of Wisconsin Press.

32 Kirklin D (2007). Truth telling, autonomy and the role of metaphor. *J Med Ethics*, **33**, 11–14.

33 Hug CC Jr (2001). End-of-life issues and the anesthesiologist. *Int Anesthesiol Clin*, **39**(3), 39–52.

34 Periyakoil VS (2008). Using metaphors in medicine. *J Palliat Med*, **11**(6), 842–4.

35 Hug CC Jr, Palmer SK (2007). Practical ethics for caring for patients with DNR requests. *ASA Newsletter*, 71(5) Available at: http://www.asahq.org/Newsletters/2007/05-07/hug05_07.html (Accessed 14 March 2010).

36 Evans HM (2007). Medicine and music: three relations considered. *J Med Humanit*, **28**(3), 138–48.

37 Casanto D (2008). Similarity and proximity: when does close in space mean close in mind? *Mem Cognit*, **36**(6), 1047–56.

38 Crosby E (2007). Medical malpractice and anesthesiology: literature review and the role of the expert witness. *Can J Anesth*, **54**(3), 227–41 (quote p. 231).

39 Ziemkiewicz C, Kosara R (2008). The shaping of information by visual metaphors. *IEEE Trans Vis Comput Graph*, **14**(6), 1269–76.

Section 2

Routine clinical applications

Chapter 6

The pre-anaesthetic visit

Vincent J Kopp

'Chance favours the prepared mind'.
Louis Pasteur

What this chapter is about

This chapter addresses deficiencies in pre-anaesthesia communication. Here, the use of medical narrative illustrates communication-enhancing techniques and attitudes that may help anaesthetists anticipate and respond to the biopsychosocial content, extant in the pre-anaesthesia assessment setting[1].

By any measure, the pre-anaesthesia evaluation sets anaesthesia care in motion. Until now, little has been written about the development of a learnable framework for effective communication, in this or any other anaesthesia care setting[2]. With respect to pre-anaesthesia communication, the need for heuristics or 'rules of thumb' is ever acute to improve rapport, elicit and respond to questions, manage ambiguity, as well as to obtain valid consent. Furthermore, anaesthetists have to communicate effectively with patients about conflicting advice, prior negative anaesthetic experiences and fears about awareness and intraoperative death[3] (see also Chapters 12 and 15).

Anatomy of a suboptimal pre-anaesthetic communication

A 56-year-old man scheduled for an elective left inguinal herniorrhaphy meets his anaesthetist minutes before surgery is to begin. Three days before, the patient presented to hospital with his hernia incarcerated. It was easily reduced. A follow-up office visit with his surgeon preceded the surgery. The patient's sole co-morbidity is benign prostatic hypertrophy. On the morning of surgery this otherwise healthy-appearing man, accompanied by his wife, meets the anaesthetist for the first time. After record review the patient is told three anaesthetic options exist—local anaesthesia with intravenous sedation, general anaesthesia and spinal anaesthesia—and that '*spinal is the way to go*'. Unquestioningly, the patient agrees to spinal anaesthesia. The spinal block is easy to place. The surgery is uneventful.

Post-operatively, the patient cannot urinate. His discharge from the day-surgery unit is delayed by hours. He is told it is because of '*the spinal*'. Bladder catheterization ensues. The rest of his recuperation is uneventful, except for lingering feelings of betrayal, distrust and disappointment. He wonders why he was not told spinal anaesthesia might cause urinary retention. He becomes angry. He resolves never to use that anaesthetist's or hospital's services again. His wife even urges him to sue them both for pain and suffering.

What could have been done to effect a more positive outcome for the patient, the anaesthetist and the hospital? The answer lies, at least in part, in improved communication. This requires a commitment to self-education, and a willingness to consider systemic change, and practice by the anaesthetist[4].

Using templates to improve pre-anaesthesia communication

Each anaesthetist should consider developing a workable, reproducible communication template for pre-anaesthesia evaluation. The template should guide and direct one's interactions without limiting the ability to improvise. In essence the template is analogous to a difficult airway algorithm or a cardiopulmonary bypass weaning routine. In use, adjustments are made as required by dynamic circumstances.

The template could include interview phase features such as: salutations; preamble; medical interview; physical examination; anaesthetic choice review; questions; acknowledgment of concerns; appropriate reassurances; assents and consents; summary questions; covenant establishment; expressions of thanks.

As will be evident from the narrative example, separation of phase features is artificial and never neat. Each phase can allow time for maximum response from the patient. It also calls for maximum flexibility. The anaesthetist may be required to bring back straying conversation to its objectives, which are, pre-anaesthesia evaluation, eliciting patient trust and rapport, and preparing patients in a way that facilitates anaesthetic care.

The '**LAURS**' (Listen, Accept, Utilize, Reframe, Suggest) concept and values as elaborated in Chapter 2 can be incorporated during template construction and script enactment. Many anaesthetists may already have working (implicit) templates for their anaesthesia practices, including pre-anaesthesia evaluation. One such template using the mnemonic '**GREAT**' as detailed in Chapter 2 is presented.

Greeting the patient includes confirming identity. ***Goals*** refers to the assessment of the patient for anaesthesia.

Rapport development can include utilizing one or more aspects of the '**LAURS**' concept to gain patient rapport (see Chapter 2).

Evaluation, Expectations, Examination, Explanation includes the medical interview, physical examination and anaesthetic choice review.

Asking and Answering questions; Acknowledging and Addressing concerns at any stage again uses '**LAURS**' where appropriate.

Tacit agreement/Thanks/Termination results in 'covenant establishment' as the assessment ends with overt consents and tacit agreements, verbalized in a way that indicates the anaesthetist will competently and compassionately care for the patient.

Beyond training, anaesthetists' opportunities to witness how colleagues do things diminish. Because few anaesthetists witness how colleagues conduct pre-anaesthesia evaluations or pre-induction consent discussions, this chapter provides an extensive narrative example to help fill this gap. It illustrates an approach to the pre-anaesthetic evaluation that may serve as a model for others.

Using 'GREAT' to structure the pre-anaesthesia evaluation

The following narrative illustrates how template elements can be scripted to achieve a '**GREAT**' evaluation. Composed of phrase sets commonly used by the author in actual practice, the script can be adapted to any patient care situation.

Greeting, Goals

Greeting the patient includes confirming identity and the nature of any procedure.

Dr A: '*Good morning, I'm Dr A. Are you Mr P?*'
Mr P: '*Yes, sir*'.
Dr A: '*How you doing this morning?*'
Mr P: '*Fine. Thank you*'.
Dr A: '*Good. May I call you Mr P or do you prefer a different name?*'
Mr P: '*You can call me anything you want, you're the doctor, but my friends call me B*'.

The patient has given the anaesthetist permission to call him by the name used by his friends. ***Listening*** to the patient can allow the anaesthetist the opportunity to ***accept*** what the patient is saying and ***utilize*** the use of the name B. The use of B at this stage by the anaesthetist may facilitate building rapport at an early stage in the consultation. However, it is perfectly acceptable for the anaesthetist to maintain a more formal relationship if that is more comfortable.

Dr A: *If it's all the same to you I'll just call you Mr P. Maybe once we get to know each other better I'll call you B.*
Mr P: '*Suit yourself. I'll answer to anything that's got food at the other end*'.
Dr A: '*I know what you mean. Before we begin I need to make sure we are all on the same page. Can you tell me in your own words what you are having done today?*'
Mr P: '*Yes sir, a hernia repair*'.
Dr A: '*Would that be on the right or the left side?*'
Mr P: '*Left*'.
Dr A: '*Fine. That is what I read on your surgical consent form: left inguinal herniorrhaphy—is that your understanding?*'
Mr P: '*Yes, if that's what herniorrhaphy means. I can't never say it quite right*'.
Dr A: '*Well you've done a nice job. I sometimes have trouble with it myself*'.

The anaesthetist has confirmed the proposed surgery and side with the patient and has made a first step towards establishing rapport by acknowledging the patient's difficulty with the technical term 'herniorrhaphy'.

Dr A: *'Mr P, I will be your anaesthesia doctor today. These are the other members of your anaesthesia care team today: Ms M, my assistant, and Mr J, my technician. At various times other care team members may also be involved as well'.*
Mr P: *'That's fine. I don't care who takes care of me as long as y'all do your job and don't kill me'.*
Dr A: *'Understood. We'll all work to take good care of you today'.*
Wife (laughs): *'You better, or he'll come get you!'*

This piece of dialogue suggests that the patient and wife recognize death as a possible complication and express anxiety and concern in the form of humour. The anaesthetist acknowledges the concern and reassures the patient and wife that the whole team will '*take good care*' of him.

Rapport

Rapport development includes utilizing the '**LAURS**' concept to gain patient rapport and assess the patient's mood. Reflective listening and the '**LAURS**' concept is balanced with the need to complete, within an appropriate time frame, the communication tasks required prior to anaesthesia. Sometimes one can be easily sidetracked. It is important to get back on track as soon as the opportunity arises, as the anaesthetist does in this case.

Dr A: *'Did you have any trouble getting in here this morning?'*
Mr P: *'No. Thank you for asking. Everything went fine. Everyone's been so nice, so far'.*
Dr A: *'Good. Did you have far to come?'*
Mr P: *'Oh, about thirty miles. My wife and I got up about 5 this morning. It took us about forty minutes to get here. It wasn't so bad'.*
Dr A: *'Good. Kind of hard to get up early if you're not used to it. And then to miss your coffee, too ....'*
Mr P: *'You got that right, doc'.*
Dr A: *'So, what did you have for breakfast this morning?'*
Mr P: *'Are you kidding? Nothing! They told me not to eat anything'.*
Dr A: *'Well, that's the right answer. You must be hungry'.*
Mr P: *'You bet I am. I haven't had a thing to eat since last night'.*

This is an example of rapport building as the anaesthetist confirms the patient's fasting status and acknowledges the implicit response from the patient that he must be hungry.

Dr A: *'How about to drink?'*

The anaesthetist then goes on to 'check in' with the patient to confirm that he has really understood that the patient is fasted and has not just had a milky coffee!

Mr P: *'That neither. My throat is burning'.*
Dr A: *'Well, we can fix that by giving you some fluids in the drip. Most people find that they can have a cool drink as soon as they feel like it after coming out of surgery'.*

The patient's 'burning throat' is ***acknowledged***, ***utilized*** and ***reframed*** as only temporary. The anaesthetist's response has the advantage of utilizing the '*burning*' sensation with a '*cool*' indirect positive suggestion utilizing the patient's own kinaesthetic language for anti-emesis afterwards (see Chapter 4).

Evaluation, Examination, Explanation, Expectation

This involves the medical interview, physical examination and anaesthetic choice review.

> **Dr A:** '*Are you in any pain or discomfort right now?*'
> **Mr P:** '*Yeah, my left nut hurts—sorry, dear—but not as much as it did the other night when that ER doc mashed on it. I guess it's OK today. I just want it fixed*'.
> **Dr A:** '*I understand. Is there anything I can do to make you more comfortable now?*'
> **Mr P:** '*No. Let's just get started*'.
> **Dr A:** '*OK. Before we talk about your anaesthesia options, I want to ask you questions about your overall health. Then I need do a limited physical exam. After that we'll discuss what might work best for you*'.

No part of a '**GREAT**' evaluation should be sacrificed to another. The anaesthetist strives to move seamlessly from greeting and rapport establishment to substantive discussion surrounding evaluation, examination, explanation and seeding expectations. Success in creating seamless transitions facilitates completion of the evaluation. By continually setting conditions where questions can be asked and answered openly, tacit agreements are forged, thanks communicated and termination of discussions can be achieved with each party feeling they were treated with dignity and respect.

> **Mr P:** '*I've already talked to the surgeon. Can't you get my stuff from the medical record? He's already poked and prodded me. I'm ready to get started. I want to get out of here, get me some sausage, grits and eggs and a big cup of coffee*'.
> **Dr A:** '*I'd like to do that myself. Can I go with you?*'
> **Mr P:** '*Suit yourself*'.

This example of acceptance and utilization shows empathy with the patient but also curtails small talk in order to move forward with the work at hand.

> **Dr A:** '*My questions and exam will be a bit different. What I will do is focus on things that might affect the anaesthesia side of your procedure. I want to make sure I know about your health so we can develop a plan you can accept, one that will keep you safe during surgery and get you home comfortably and quickly*'.

Dr A's statement does much at once. It highlights differences between anaesthesia and surgery, and the separate roles of anaesthetist and surgeon. It also accomplishes a tonal shift in the dialogue toward some serious subjects such as safety, comfort and expeditiousness in the patient's care.

> **Mr P:** '*I appreciate it, doc. I've never had surgery before. No one has ever told me about it before. You're the first one. I've never even been to the doctor much except for my prostate. I don't know about these things*'.
> **Dr A:** '*I understand. So, what kind of prostate problem do you have?*'

As this dialogue shows, the right words at the right time can re-direct conversation without shutting it down entirely. Here the transition is made to an open-ended question that puts the patient back in the lead while directing the conversation along lines required by the anaesthetist.

Mr P: *'I have to get up at night a lot to pee. The doctor says I have an enlarged prostate but no cancer. I'd have trouble peeing then my nuts would hurt—sorry, dear—so I strained and that's when I caused the rupture, when I was trying to pee'.*
Dr A: *'That must have been uncomfortable. I've reviewed your chart and don't see mention of any other problems'.*
Mr P: *'No, I'm otherwise healthy'.*

The anaesthetist can then proceed to the rest of the evaluation and examination.

Asking and Answering questions, Acknowledging and Addressing concerns

Dr A: *'Do you have any questions so far?'*
Mr P: *'Yes, sir. What kind of anaesthesia are you going to use on me today. The surgeon said you would tell me about that'.*
Dr A: *'Did you and your surgeon have any discussion about anaesthesia options?'*

Implicit and expressed expectations are examined and addressed. Here, for example, the anaesthetist's open-ended question discerns whether any information provided by the surgeon regarding anaesthesia requires supplementing before the pre-anaesthesia evaluation can be completed successfully.

Mr P: *'Not really. He said he'd leave that up to me and you. My brother-in-law, though, he said he thought I should get knocked out. He said he had a friend who got a needle in his back for a hernia and now he has back pain'.*
Dr A: *'That's interesting. We can talk some more about that. What are you thinking you'd like?'*

How quickly the evaluation conversation can shift! Here the anaesthetist negotiates an articulated bias fed to the patient by a relative without refuting or acknowledging the role a spinal needle might play in possible back pain. This skilful manoeuvre keeps the evaluation on track.

Mr P: *'Well, I don't want to see or hear nothing. As long as I don't have to know nothing I'll be fine. And I don't want to die, neither. Or be paralysed and awake'.*
Dr A: *'I hear you. Fortunately these are very rare problems'.*
Mr P: *'So there's a chance?'*
Dr A: *'Yes, but very small. Nothing in life is 100 per cent'.*
Mr P: *'I hear you. Good'.*
Dr A: *'Understood. Let me examine you now then we'll discuss your anaesthesia more. May I see where the surgeon said the operation will be?'*
Mr P: *'Right down here'.*
Dr A: *'Let's review what we've already discussed. Sounds like you want to be asleep throughout the procedure and safely wake up at the end so that you can recover as quickly as possible from the operation so that you can soon be walking out of hospital. But otherwise you don't have any strong feelings—is that correct?'*

As the interaction proceeds, the anaesthetist has used the patient's concerns and reframed what he '***does not***' want to outcomes that he '***does***' want: the negative risk discussion of '*paralysis*' to '*walking*' and '*awake*' to '*sleep*'. The conversation then moves towards tacit agreement about options and the final phases of the pre-anaesthesia evaluation.

Mr P: *'Well sort of. What do you think I should do?'*
Dr A: *'Based on your medical history and physical exam I think you are a reasonable candidate for just about any kind of anaesthesia. Let me go over the pros and cons about each. The first option is to numb the place where the surgeon is operating with local anaesthetic. We also give you medications through the drip to make you feel comfortable and sleepy. This is called IV sedation. If for any reason we need to give you more anaesthetic to keep you comfortable, this is usually very easy and straightforward to do'.*
Mr P: *'What are my other options, doc?'*
Dr A: *'The second option is to do a spinal block combined with IV sedation'.*

The anaesthetist describes the spinal anaesthesia technique plus associated risks and benefits in detail commensurate with patient's preferences.

Mr P: *'That don't sound too good to me. I've got a big prostate. Isn't that a problem? You said I might not be able to pee afterwards and then I'd have to get a tube put up into my bladder. That doesn't sound like very much fun, especially if I'm awake. I don't think I want that'.*
Dr A: *'Let's talk about your third option before you decide. Your third option is general anaesthesia. That's what most people think of as being "knocked out"...'*

The anaesthetist describes a general anaesthesia technique as with prior options.

Dr A: *'Whatever anaesthetic you choose, we aim to do everything possible to keep you safe and comfortable. Fortunately the vast majority of people have an anaesthetic that is more comfortable and straightforward than they anticipated. Unusual things can and do happen, so I can't tell you there's not a risk'.*
Mr P: *'How do you know if I'm really asleep?'*
Dr A: *'General anaesthesia—it's not the same sleep you experience at night in your bed. It works so you won't feel anything, remember anything or move suddenly during surgery. It makes you feel like little or no time goes by between the time you go to sleep and the time you wake up in the recovery room. We follow your vital signs and look for signs that you are not getting too much or too little anaesthesia. We sometimes use a brain-wave monitor though it, like all monitors, is not 100 per cent effective. Nothing in medicine is. But we* ***will do*** *everything we can to keep you safe and comfortable'.*
Mr P: *'I believe you* ***will****'.*
Dr A: *'Do you have any questions about what we have discussed so far?'*
Mr P: *'No. You've told me everything and more than I wanted to know'.*
Dr A: *'Do you have a better idea of what kind of anaesthesia you want today?'*
Mr P: *'Yes. I don't* ***think*** *I want the spinal. I couldn't handle* ***watching*** *someone put something in my penis if I couldn't pee after surgery'.*
Dr A: *'Well, that's also a possibility with general anaesthesia though I don't* ***think*** *it's quite as common. We'll* ***watch*** *how much IV fluid we give you'.*

It's interesting to note how the anaesthetist matches the patient's language as a method of increasing and maintaining rapport—see also below.

Mr P: *'Well, I'll take my chances. I appreciate that. I also don't like the idea of waiting for the spinal to wear off or not being able to move around after the surgery. I don't want to have to wait to go home. I'll want to eat. I think I want to try that local block with sedation. If that* *doesn't work then you can just knock me out. I'm OK with that. I'm not scared of dying. I know you'll* ***take good care of*** *me. At least I'll know you tried. I think I'd like that better than a spinal or general anaesthesia as my first choice. I understand any of it can kill me if it goes wrong so let's try the first one. Hell, if I don't do something this hernia could kill me, according to the surgeon. He said I better get it fixed now. Next time it could get stuck and then I'd have to have emergency surgery. What would my choices be then? I'd just have to be put to sleep. Then what? I could die even more that way'.*

Dr A: *'Well, we will* ***take good care of*** *you and work with you to make the first option work the best we can. You're healthy and sensible so I think we can work it out. Do you have any other questions?*

Mr P: *'No. You've been very thorough'.*

Dr A: *'Great. Let me reassure you: your goal and our goal are exactly the same, which is for you to be safe, comfortable throughout, and for you to get out of here as quickly as possible with only one thing changed and that is what you came in here for. Everything we do is designed to enhance your safety and comfort and minimize any risks'.*

The '**GREAT**' template allows a structured approach to eliciting from the patient the required facts for safe anaesthesia and interweaving the skills necessary to improve trust and rapport while acknowledging that power and control differences exist between physician and patient. Thus, when the anaesthetist repeatedly uses words in different ways to reassure the patient that his safety and comfort are primary outcomes of anaesthetic care, the building blocks are put in place of a workable medical care covenant.

Tacit agreement, Thanks, Termination

Dr A: *'Do we have your permission to do what we need to do to make sure you are safe and healthy during your anaesthesia?*

Mr P: *'Of course'.*

Dr A: *'Mind if I call you B?*

Mr P: *'Doc, I'd be honoured if you would'.*

Dr A: *'Thanks for letting me take care of you, B. We will do everything we can to keep you safe and comfortable'.*

Mr P: *'I believe you will'.*

Anaesthetists need excellent communication skills. As Shafer notes '*Anesthesiology, in so many ways, is crystallized medicine. We rarely, if ever, have the luxury of multiple office visits to connect with the patient and family*'[5].

Anaesthetists can enhance or teach communication for the pre-anaesthesia interview using the '**GREAT**' structure for the interaction and the '**LAURS**' principles to improve rapport as described here and in Chapter 2. As the above narrative illustrates, these tools can be used to facilitate communicating in ways that respect each patient's unique circumstances. Without sacrificing the traditional focus on safety and comfort, patients will tend to hear best what is said to them when they feel anaesthetists really care about them as people. The goal is to treat everyone as special but no one as different. This can be enhanced through the use of communication that takes into account the patient's vulnerability that exists where the ability to make choices and maintain a modicum of control rises to the level of utmost importance.

Key points

1. Pre-anaesthesia communication demands respect for each patient's unique circumstances.
2. Patients interact best with the anaesthetist when they feel cared about as people.
3. The goal is to treat everyone as special but no one as different.
4. Anaesthesia communications need to take into account patient vulnerability.
5. The ability to make choices and maintain some control is, to many patients, of the utmost importance.

References

1 Engle GL (1980). The clinical application of the biopsychosocial model. *Am J Psychiatry*, **137**(5), 535–44.

2 Cyna AM, Andrew MI, Tan SGM (2009). Communication skills for the anaesthetist. *Anaesthesia*, **64**(6), 658–65.

3 Waisel DB, Lamiani G, Sandrock NJ, Pascucci R, Truog RD, Meyer EC (2009). Anesthesiology trainees face ethical, practical and relational challenges in obtaining informed consent. *Anesthesiology*, **110**(3), 480–6.

4 Kopp VJ, Shafer A (2000). Anesthesiologists and perioperative communication. *Anesthesiology*, **93**(2), 548–55.

5 Shafer A (2009). "It blew my mind": exploring the difficulties of anesthesia informed consent through narrative. *Anesthesiology*, **110**(3), 445–6.

Chapter 7

Consent

Alan F Merry and Sally N Merry

'If it is not right do not do it; if it is not true do not say it'.
Marcus Aurelius

What this chapter is about

The language with which many doctors describe their interactions with patients can be very revealing. A sense of needing to comply with onerous procedural requirements is often more apparent than any enthusiasm over opportunities for positive communication. This was well illustrated by a friend and colleague who picked us up from the airport in a distant city, and said, '*Do you mind if we drop by the hospital on the way home? The thing is—I have a list tomorrow and I still need to gloom up the patients*'.

This sort of negativity probably reflects a widespread tendency to place undue emphasis on the legal implications of consent. Lawyers have advocated ticking a checklist to ensure legally robust documentation of the information provided. This idea has merit, especially given recent data showing that documentation of informed consent is often poor[1]. Nevertheless, the fact that such documentation might be seen as the central element of the process says much about how far the concept of informed consent has moved from its proper place. Ideally, informed consent should not be seen in a legal context at all, but rather as an important part of patient–doctor relationships founded on a commitment to patient-centred care.

Patients' contact with anaesthetists is often short term and brief, and they are often anxious and would like to know what to expect. It follows that the provision of information in a way that can be understood and assimilated, and in a setting where questions can be answered, is the central part of gaining consent. This is an important role for anaesthetists. Skilled communication at this stage will also facilitate the subsequent management of all the other aspects of anaesthesia and perioperative care, thereby repaying the required time and effort involved.

Outside medical settings, much of what anaesthetists do to patients falls within the law of trespass, which includes battery and assault. In the context of medical and surgical treatment, consent is a defence against actions in trespass. In fact, actions based on failures of informed consent are infrequent, and successful actions are even less common. In general, the risk of a complaint or lawsuit is very much a function of how patients feel about their doctor. Adverse events associated with negligence in healthcare lead to lawsuits only infrequently, while at the same time lawsuits are often brought over adverse events which have occurred in the absence of negligence[2]. The one factor that seems to reduce substantially the risk of a lawsuit or complaint on any grounds is a patient's sense that the doctor cares; 'glooming up' one's patient is not an attractive opening gambit for establishing a good relationship. Neither is conveying the sense to patients that the anaesthetist has just attempted to forestall any possibility of a complaint by a legalistic approach based on the fear that this might actually occur.

Trust is essential in any relationship, and honesty is a sound basis for building trust. One problem is that individuals have different beliefs, realities and expectations which may make it difficult for anaesthetists to reconcile their views with those of some patients, and vice versa.

Given the legal and regulatory environment of healthcare today, it is of course understandable that some anaesthetists are preoccupied with ensuring that they have complied with requirements for informed consent by documenting the process, and getting a signed consent form in countries where this is a requirement. Patients, on the other hand, will have a very different reality, with concerns frequently not appreciated by the anaesthetist. It is interesting to consider what a typical patient might think important.

- *'Who is this person to whom I am going to entrust my life? Is he/she trustworthy?'*
- *'I feel vulnerable and will be unconscious, in a small gown that flaps at the back with no "undies"—will this person treat me with respect and not make fun of me?'*
- *'What will actually happen?'*
- *'Will it hurt, how much and how often?'*
- *'What should I expect when I wake up?'*
- *'How bad will I feel?'*
- *'When should I worry? Will the staff be clued up enough to pick up any problems?'*
- *'How dangerous is all this anyway?'*
- *'How quickly can I expect to recover?'*

Risk of anaesthesia in context

The risks of any procedure can only be evaluated in relation to the realistically available choices. It is important to recognize what these choices are. In reality, the choice over whether or not to have an anaesthetic in the first place cannot be considered in isolation. This point could be made by asking, '*Would you like the operation with or without an anaesthetic?*' Patients really need to be able to weigh up the risks of the whole procedure—the risks of the surgery and the anaesthesia as a package deal. Thus the question may be, '*What are the risks if one has the proposed operation under general anaesthesia?*' '*What are they under regional?*' But also, and significantly, '*What would they be if the operation were declined altogether?*'

It is clear, for example, that declining a laparotomy for an acute abdomen has very different implications from declining an arthroscopy for a painful knee. The potential benefits of a minor and entirely elective procedure may not be worth the risk of an anaesthetic, whereas considerable anaesthetic risk may be acceptable for a potentially life-saving operation.

Thus context has a bearing on the way in which disclosure should be approached. To make good choices, patients need to feel comfortable with the decisions they make and that these decisions are congruent with their own reality and belief systems. This requires being given appropriate information, in such a manner, at such a time and in such a setting, that they can reasonably assimilate it. Ideally they should have the opportunity to reflect on their options, and to discuss them with their close family or friends if they wish. For some, it may mean making a decision which, from the viewpoint of the anaesthetist, is illogical.

Patient autonomy should be respected in all aspects of anaesthesia care including the provision of information related to risk. There is enormous variation in what patients wish to know and in how much detail. Many anaesthetists have no doubt that an explanation of the relevant risks of anaesthesia should be given to patients, and that this would usually include mentioning the possibility of death. Others argue that the risk with this approach is that patient's autonomy could be undermined since it does not take into account the patient's needs and desire for this information. However, important and potentially worrying information can be conveyed in ways that are compatible with maintaining a positive relationship and avoiding undue anxiety.

Patients need to be helped to understand the relevant issues and to put the key facts into context; and they need to be given guidance and support. It is true that they must be allowed, and even encouraged, to make their decisions autonomously. Nevertheless, autonomy is only one virtue, and there are others that also need to be considered. Autonomy has little value if the outcome is a poor decision for the person concerned, judged from his or her own perspective and in hindsight. A good decision is one for which the patient remains happy with the process of decision making, whatever the actual outcome.

Few decisions in life are predicated on hard logic firmly grounded in facts. People function through a complex mix of rationality and instinct. They typically form emotional relationships, make major purchases, and pursue lifelong careers not because of careful decisions formulated on the basis of weighing up probabilities and percentages, but because of the way they *feel*. It is reasonable to assume that decisions about anaesthesia or surgery are unlikely to be different.

Obtaining informed consent is only one part of preparing patients for anaesthesia, and should be integrated with the other objectives an anaesthetist may have when seeing a patient preoperatively.

Risk disclosure

The legal requirements for disclosure of risk in the UK, Australia and in many similar jurisdictions today arise from the landmark Australian case, Rogers v Whittaker[3]. They have been expressed as follows:

> 'Doctors should give information about the risks of any intervention, especially those that are likely to influence the patient's decisions. Known risks should be disclosed when an adverse outcome is common even though the detriment is slight, or when an adverse outcome is severe even though its occurrence is rare[4]'.

In practice, many anaesthetists place their own interpretation on the risks to be disclosed, taking their own view of the risks 'the reasonable patient' in the circumstances would want to know, so there is considerable variation in the risks disclosed by individual anaesthetists in particular clinical scenarios[5]. Obviously an assessment is needed of the specific risks related to each individual patient in the context of the proposed procedure and anaesthetic. Nevertheless, we think it is difficult to escape the conclusion that the possibility of death should be disclosed when general or major regional anaesthesia is to be administered, and that the possibility of paralysis should be disclosed when a neuraxial block is to be undertaken.

Is there a way of satisfying the legal requirements of risk disclosure without undue risk of causing or increasing the patient's anxiety? The data suggest that for most people the answer is yes[6,7]. However, achieving this may involve more than one interaction; patients may need time to consider their options, and perhaps consult with others.

Documentation

It is a matter of good clinical practice to document the key medical issues, key specific relevant risks discussed and patient treatment choices. It is relevant to note that in many jurisdictions there is no legal requirement to document informed consent, but policies, precedence and good practice usually establish an onus on practitioners to do this. Some colleges and medical regulatory bodies explicitly require such documentation.

Important elements of informed consent are listed in Box 7.1.

Optimizing the consent process

Time and place can have a significant impact on how effective and easy it is to do this.

It is essential to provide enough time for the preoperative consultation. Timeliness also matters—it is poor practice, and unfair, to present a patient with choices that require consideration of major risks and difficult concepts minutes before an operation is due to start—although there may be no alternative in an emergency. By the time a patient has been changed into theatre garb and wheeled into a holding area, his or her decisions have been substantially made. Supplementary information and confirmation that the patient is still happy to proceed may be appropriate, but it would take considerable moral courage for a patient to stop the 'production line' and ask to get off at the last minute.

Box 7.1 Elements of informed consent

These *elements of informed consent* expressed as patients' rights have been modified from selected clauses of the New Zealand Code of Health and Disability Services Consumers' Rights[8], but would apply in most countries.

- The right to be treated with respect.
- The right to have privacy respected.
- The right to be free from discrimination, coercion, harassment or exploitation.
- The right to effective communication in a form, language and manner that enable understanding of the information provided. Where necessary and reasonably practicable, this includes the right to a competent interpreter.
- The right to an environment that enables open, honest and effective communication.
- The right to the information that a reasonable person, in that person's circumstances, would need to make an informed choice or give informed consent, including:
  - an explanation of his or her condition;
  - an explanation of the options available, including an assessment of the expected risks, side effects, benefits and costs of each option;
  - notification of any proposed participation in teaching or research, including whether the research requires and has received ethics committee approval.
- Where a patient has diminished competence, the right to make informed choices and give informed consent, to the extent appropriate to his or her level of competence.
- The right to have one or more support persons of his or her choice present, except where safety may be compromised or another person's rights may be unreasonably infringed.

With the increasing emphasis on efficiency, and the consequent increase in day-of-admission surgery, this issue has become quite problematic for anaesthetists. Obviously the ideal is for everyone to be seen in a pre-anaesthetic clinic well ahead of time. In practice some institutions find it difficult to justify this for all fit and well patients having minor day-surgery procedures, and there are various ways in which patients can be screened, and given information about anaesthesia.

The environment in which consent is obtained is also very important, and every effort should be made to ensure that this provides adequate privacy, and makes it possible for family members or other support people to be present. Again, restrictions on time and hospital real estate frequently create considerable pressure for anaesthetists to interact with patients in settings that are less than ideal—for instance, in the holding area in the theatre suite. Every effort should be made to avoid such compromises, but, in the end, the setting is less important than how the patient is approached and how the anaesthetic interaction takes place. The key requirements for effective communication to take place are: privacy to be respected; and patients to feel reasonably able to talk about personal and potentially frightening matters, supported by family and friends if they wish.

Using 'GREAT' to structure the consent process

Greeting, Goals

In any interaction, first impressions matter. Every anaesthetist is different, with his or her own style. There is no point in adopting other people's techniques unless one is comfortable with them. Nevertheless the following points are largely a matter of common sense, but often forgotten. Looking at people and smiling at them is a good start. It really does make a difference to stand up when patients come into the consulting room. Shaking hands is good and so is remembering to wash one's hands. This non-verbal communication implies that if you care enough to wash your hands, you probably care enough to do the other important things well too.

In introducing oneself, it is important to be clear about how you wish to interact with patients. In some countries a degree of formality is the norm. In others, informality is more common. One approach is to say something like,

> '*I am Doctor Jones, one of the consultant anaesthetists. Can I confirm your name is....*'

It is then possible to add your first name if you would like it to be used. A good strategy following initial introductions is to get the patient to say why he or she is there. For example, one might ask,

> '*Now, do you have a good idea about the operation you are going to have? Why don't you tell me about it*'.

This has two merits. First, it is the most reliable way of checking that one has the right patient for the right procedure. If one simply says something like, '*You are having a hip operation aren't you?*' patients may acquiesce incorrectly, either because they haven't heard properly, or because they haven't understood, or for other reasons that relate to context and culture. Secondly, it continues to signal that one wishes to listen as well as speak. This helps patients to feel able to speak up if something seems to be wrong. It is surprising how hard this can be, and patients quite often fail to tell nurses and doctors that they are worried about obviously incorrect activities.

The goals related to delivering risk information and the choices available can be made at the outset by saying something like,

> '*I am here to keep you as safe and comfortable as possible, and together we can discuss the various options for your anaesthetic*'.

This statement allows the issue of safety to be 'seeded' at the beginning of the anaesthetic consultation and suggests a therapeutic alliance.

Rapport

It is important to put everyone at ease and to establish rapport. This will provide a platform for giving information and for patients and their families to ask questions and raise issues that are important to them. A good way to do this is to start with some general discussion which has little or nothing to do with the anaesthetic. One example might be to ask,

> '*What would you be doing today if you weren't here?*'

This is a fairly open-ended question that can lead to further questions about school, work and hobbies, all of which can help to build a picture of a patient, and his or her life, while at the same time conveying the sense that he or she matters as an individual. In addition the language used by the patient can be utilized later in the provision of information and the consent process, to promote understanding, and build further trust and rapport. For example, for an accountant, language use could include a 'risk and benefit ledger' with the provision of 'detailed numbers'. In this way patients can feel heard and understood.

There is a lot to be said for making sure everyone is comfortable and at the same height. For a doctor to stand while a patient sits is to set up an undesirable power gradient. This is not a big problem on a quick ward round where the objective is just to establish that all is well, for example, and perhaps, post-operatively, a power gradient of this type is something a sick patient might even welcome. The point is to be aware of the issue, and to realize that if a relaxed and somewhat more equal conversation is to be had, it is best for everyone to be seated perhaps around a patient's bed. Standing for a pre-operative consultation, even at the bedside, will tend to create a sense of limited time.

At every stage it is appropriate to let patients know what is going to happen next and to check that they are happy with this and with the way things are proceeding. This can be very informal. For example, in some cultures people might be offended if someone sat on their bed. In the first instance it is probably better to avoid this as a matter of principle, but sometimes on the ward the patient is already in a chair, the bed is fully made and there is no easy alternative. One could get another chair, but it might be acceptable to say, '*Do you mind if I sit on the bed?*' Similarly, if one is about to take a pulse or listen to a heart, it does help to say, '*Do you mind if I….*'

The point, apart from common courtesy, is that this consolidates trust. It signals that there will be no surprises, and that the patient's autonomy is respected. So that, for example, if an IV is to be inserted later the patient will have some confidence that this will be signalled, and permission obtained. Getting this dynamic right from the start will help the patient relax at every stage in the process. The converse is that failure to gain this trust will tend to increase apprehension, suspicion and anxiety.

Explanation, anaesthetic choices and disclosing risk

At this stage, many patients find it really helpful to receive an explanation of what is going to happen. People don't like surprises, and don't like being kept in the dark. One might say something like,

> '*I have already read your notes. What we are going to do is this: I am going to ask you some questions, listen to your chest and have a look at one or two things. This will all be quite easy. Then we are going to have a chat about your anaesthetic and sign a form, if you are happy. After that I will leave you for a few minutes and then someone will come and get you and take you into the operating room. I will tell you more about what will happen there in a minute. Is all of that OK with you?*'

It is very reassuring for people to have this sort of clarification, and it signals to the patient that he or she is recognized by the anaesthetist as a person—and, furthermore, as a person in an unfamiliar and potentially frightening environment. It is an essential part of building trust.

Probably the part of the pre-operative assessment most anaesthetists find difficult is the explicit disclosure of serious risk. This is made more difficult by the fact that many patients will not have thought about the risks of anaesthesia, and some may not even realize that there are any. Risk disclosure is probably best done in the context of explaining what the anaesthetic options are.

It is reasonable to provide advice, rather than just options. So, for example, there is nothing wrong with saying something like,

> *'OK, so you need to have this hip done. What the surgeon and I usually find best is a spinal anaesthetic. What this involves is.... Of course it is possible to go to sleep for these operations, but we find most people are pretty comfortable with our approach, and a little sedation seems to work pretty well. Do you have a preference?'*

A pause at this stage to allow questions or comments would be appropriate. Then one might continue,

> *'Of course everything in medicine does have risk'.*

It can be quite effective to contextualize the risk information before stating it, rather than after. To do this, after another pause, one might say,

> *'Just like driving to the hospital, really. That has risk. Actually you could die or become paralysed in a car crash? But you usually don't. Anaesthesia is a bit like that. Bad things like that can happen, but they are extremely rare. Do you understand what I mean by saying that?'*

It is argued that anaesthetists should always use explicit words such as 'die', 'death' or 'paralysis' in the interests of honesty and open disclosure. The repeated use of such negatively loaded words can be counter-productive. In the above example, the requirement for explicit disclosure is fulfilled in a matter of fact manner, without the necessity to reinforce the point.

Checking for understanding is very important. Most patients understand the point that risk is involved, and are comfortable with this sort of disclosure. Surprisingly, occasional patients appear to be astonished to hear that there might be risk, and will say so if given the opportunity. If they do respond by indicating surprise, it may be wise to increase the allocated time to discuss the matter in as much detail as is required. A good way forward is to acknowledge that this might be surprising,

> *'Yes—I guess you might not have thought about this'.*

If a patient clearly wants more information, it becomes more important to be explicit.

> *'Yes, anaesthesia does carry risk. Paralysis from spinal anaesthetics, and death, are possible but extremely rare. I think the risks of something really bad happening are extremely low in your case. Other things are more common—for example, nausea post-operatively. But, given what I know about you and given our setup in this hospital, I am expecting that everything will go smoothly for you'.*

This is an example of a deliberate technique, aimed at moving the conversation on from the very unlikely to the more probable scenario that most patients have few problems following anaesthesia. This provides further context to the information about serious risks and helps to get across the difference between things that are likely to happen, and things that really aren't.

There are three points to consider at this stage. First, the message should be personalized. This is not a general discussion of the risks of anaesthesia—it is about a particular patient, in a particular place, for a particular operation, in the hands of a particular anaesthetist. Second, it is essential to be honest. Third, it is important to appreciate that honest disclosure may lead a patient to ask for more time, and the anaesthetist should make it clear that this is available. In fact, it may even lead to a patient declining the procedure, thereby exercising his or her autonomy, which, after all, is the whole point of encouraging informed decision making.

However, the last possibility will be unlikely if the surgery is indeed indicated and the consultation is well managed. It may be useful to come back to the context. For example, one might say,

> '*You know, there are also risks of not having your operation. That is why we are here after all. We think you really need this aortic valve replacement, because you are short of breath. And of course, the real trouble is that the valve is likely to get worse ....*'

Asking and Answering questions, Addressing concerns, giving Advice

These days, with the considerable emphasis on patient autonomy, some doctors have retreated from providing any direction whatsoever. Obviously coercion is unacceptable, but advice is not, in itself, coercion, provided patients realize that one is simply discussing the alternatives and their risks, and that the final decision lies with them.

It cannot be stated clearly enough that advice is important, as well as information. People appreciate being given the facts and advice from an experienced and honest expert. In the end a patient may turn down the advised option, but at least this will be done in the knowledge that it is the advised option, and with the opportunity to explore the reasons for this advice in more depth if desired.

Thanks, Termination

Having disclosed the key risks, established that the patient is comfortable with the proposed anaesthetic, and understands, in principle at least, what his or her choices are, agreement is made. Many countries do not require a signed consent form for anaesthesia. For those that do, getting a signature is a simple matter. One way of doing this is to sum up while adding notes to the form.

For example, the anaesthetist might say,

> '*So I need you to sign a form—this is a hospital requirement. Now the things we have discussed are that you are going to have a spinal anaesthetic...*' (writing it down on the form) '*... and I have just mentioned the risks; they are very rare, but I will just note them, and also that in your particular case we will take particularly good care of your crowns*'.

The signature on the paper is a symbolic representation of the agreement that the patient has accepted the anaesthetist's care and the anaesthetist has accepted responsibility for the patient's care.

Children and adolescents

Children have a right to be consulted and to give consent, and recognizing this helps to establish a relationship with them which will facilitate communication during other aspects of anaesthesia. However, with patients under the age of 16, risks should usually be discussed primarily with the parents, and consent obtained from them. The information provided to the child, and the degree the child should be included in the consent process, depends on his or her developmental level and verbal and cognitive ability (Box 7.2). There are certain circumstances in which parental involvement may not be appropriate even for children under the age of 16, and some judgement may be needed in deciding about this. These situations should be rare, and are beyond the scope of this chapter, but, if in doubt, consultation with a colleague is advisable. As with adults, legislation differs between jurisdictions.

Box 7.2 shows some rules of thumb for obtaining informed consent for anaesthesia for children and adolescents.

Box 7.2 Informed consent for anaesthesia with children and adolescents

- Babies obviously can't be told anything, and are not competent to give consent, but the way in which one interacts with them is important.
- Toddlers and pre-schoolers should be told what is going to happen, with the aim of minimizng stress. Discussion of risk is not appropriate.
- Five- to seven-year-olds should be given a simple explanation of the procedure and what to expect, including likely side effects. Again, explicit discussion of serious risk is seldom appropriate.
- Children between the ages of 8 and 12 may well wish to participate in decisions which affect them, and they should be given increasing amounts of information as they get older and as the risks become more material. It is not appropriate to tell every 8-year-old that death is a complication of anaesthesia, but truthful answers to the questions of a 12-year-old facing life-threatening surgery may well be.
- By adolescence, young people should be actively engaged in all aspects of the consent process and should take a central role. Some argue that early adolescents (aged 13–15) should not need parental consent in addition to their own, but the norm should be for parents to give consent as well. This is primarily because abstract thought is not well developed at this age and the interests of the adolescents will, for the most part, be best served by having the counsel of their parents. It is also important to realize that the decision being made is likely to have considerable importance for the parents as well as for the child. In many societies the role of the family in the decisions of individual members is given great emphasis.

Box 7.2 Informed consent for anaesthesia with children and adolescents *(continued)*

- The age at which young people can give consent themselves varies between jurisdictions. Many people argue that children of 16 and older should not have to have the consent of their parents, and this is the legal position in some countries. However, the late teenage period is an age when young people are impulsive, take risks and feel 'bullet proof', and they are likely to benefit from having the support of parents or other supportive adults in making decisions. Again, parents will also often appreciate this. After the age of 18 people should be treated as adults and this is their legal entitlement in most countries.

Emergencies

The principles discussed above apply in general, but in an emergency the opportunity for discussion may be much more limited. As with any anaesthetic interaction, in serious medical emergencies a patient's best interests are typically served by trusting the doctors. However, there are caveats. First, communication matters more than ever—explaining every step of the way, what is happening and why, is critical for building trust and reducing anxiety. Second, if at all possible someone needs to take the family, or other relevant people, aside and spend time with them explaining the risks in detail, either immediately or as soon as the opportunity arises.

Probably the key points to establish with a patient in an emergency are that the condition is life-threatening, the risks are high whatever one does, and the situation is urgent. One should then determine whether the patient is willing to place trust in the doctors and leave it largely to them to do what they think best. Most people are. Some aren't, and a few may even elect not to go ahead. This last response would need to be respected, but is rare.

Key points

1. The legal requirements for informed consent in many jurisdictions are relatively clear and generally non-negotiable.
2. Meeting them in a manner that builds rapport and reassures patients is usually possible if the process is approached from the principles of good patient care.
3. Key requirements are adequate time, appropriate timeliness, and a setting that provides reasonable privacy and permits support people to be present.
4. Children and adolescents have the right to be informed, and to give consent, in a way appropriate for their developmental stage.
5. Informed consent is part of the ongoing relationship between patients and their anaesthetists, and should be obtained through honesty and sensitivity, recognising both the autonomy and the vulnerability of each individual patient.

References

1 Siddins M, Klinken E, Vocale L (2009). Adequacy of consent documentation in a specialty surgical unit: time for community debate? *Med J Aust*, **191**, 259–62.

2 Localio AR, Lawthers AG, Brennan TA, Laird NM, Hebert LE, Peterson LM, et al. (1991). Relation between malpractice claims and adverse events due to negligence: results of the Harvard Medical Practice Study III. *N Eng J Med*, **325**, 245–51.

3 Rogers v Whitaker (1992)/ 175 CLR 479.

4 National Health and Medical Research Council (2004). *General guidelines for medical practitioners on providing information to patients.* Canberra: Australian Government.

5 Braun A, Leslie K, Merry A, Story D (2010). What are we telling our patients? A survey of risk disclosure for anaesthesia in Australia and New Zealand. *Anaesth Intensive Care*, **38**, 935–8.

6 Inglis S, Farnill D (1993). The effects of providing preoperative statistical anaesthetic-risk information. *Anaesth Intensive Care*, **21**, 799–805.

7 Garden AL, Merry AF, Holland RL, Petrie KJ (1996). Anaesthesia information—what patients want to know. *Anaesth Intensive Care*, **24**, 594–8.

8 Health and Disability Commissioner (2004). *Code of health and disability services consumers' rights.* Auckland: New Zealand Government.

Chapter 8

Perioperative care

Andrew F Smith, Allan M Cyna, and
Suyin GM Tan

'Every breath you take, every move you make, I'll be watching you'.
Sting

What this chapter is about

The perioperative period can be a life-changing event for many patients, the effects of which can be lifelong for better or worse. The anaesthetist's communication at this time can have a profound impact on the care of their patients in the matter of both short-term cooperation and long-term perceptions of their hospital experience.

Induction

Induction of anaesthesia is a stressful time for many patients, young and old. There is an inevitable loss of control when the patient hands this over temporarily to the anaesthetist. In order to enhance cooperation, anaesthetists will reap unexpected benefits by avoiding the use of negative language (see Chapter 3)[1]. Well-meaning staff may, however, sabotage an otherwise smooth induction by telling patients, '*There is nothing to worry about*' with the implicit suggestion that there is '*something to worry about*'. Unfortunately such well-meaning statements, even when directed at children, tend to yield the opposite effect of what is intended.

Patient stress at this time increases suggestibility such that comments frequently function as inadvertent suggestions—be they positive or negative (see Chapters 3, 4 and 20). This can be utilized to enhance the anaesthetist's ability to provide a smooth, safe and stress-free induction. A typical series of pre-induction communications may go something like,

> '*Don't worry we won't drop you*'. As the patient is transferred from a trolley to the operating table.
> '*The blood pressure cuff gets really tight and may hurt and try not to move while it's pumping up*'.
> '*That noise over there is just the nurse checking the drill!*'

Explaining what is happening in simple straightforward non-technical language, and at the same time communicating in a positive way, is invariably the more useful approach. For example,

> '*Welcome to the operating room Mr P*'.
> '*You can relax as we move you to this other bed—you are quite safe*'.
> '*We will place some monitoring leads on so we can keep you safe and comfortable. A pulse monitor gently placed on your finger, an ECG on your chest and a blood pressure cuff on your arm. As the blood pressure cuff tightens and we take its reading this often allows patients to relax knowing how closely we are looking after them*'.

This is an indirect suggestion that the patient too can relax as the blood pressure cuff tightens.

> '*Although operating rooms aren't the quietest places, all this activity is just everybody getting ready to ensure that things go smoothly, safely and, as comfortably as possible for you*'.

Cannulation

Although having an IV cannula inserted is usually straightforward for many patients, negative suggestions are frequently encountered in this context, and theatre staff may require education in how to avoid them. It is useful to ask the anxious patient to focus on a spot with the eyes directed away from the arm that is to be cannulated. Suggestions for subconscious 'arm anaesthesia' (see Chapters 4 and 14) can be elicited in many patients to facilitate comfortable insertion.

Pre-oxygenation or inhalational induction

There are several strategies to consider when using a mask. Many patients feel more comfortable if they are allowed to hold the mask themselves. In any event, the anaesthetist should be wary of placing the mask on the patient's face without permission. It is helpful to avoid touching the face initially while the patient becomes familiar with the mask. This is an excellent time not only to inform patients of the benefits of oxygenation but also to link deep breathing with relaxation, and an element of control.

Pre-oxygenation presents the anaesthetist with an opportunity for some therapeutic suggestions. For example, the anaesthetist could say,

> '*The oxygen is full of goodness. Each time you take a deep breath in you can feel stronger, more in control. Each time you breathe out, feel yourself relax and become a little more comfortable as the mind drifts into a bit of a daydream*'.

As the patient breathes in the anaesthetist can reinforce the effect by saying '*That's right!*' '*Well done!*' '*Good, it's healthy to fill your lungs with oxygen*'.

Inhalational induction is commonly used with young children (see Chapter 10), and with some adults where venous access is limited. Patients can be asked to take slow gentle breaths or, if they prefer, they can blow the gas away. A counting technique can be used for adults as described for children in Chapter 10.

Propofol induction

Intravenous injection of propofol is not infrequently accompanied by a negative suggestion. '*This is going to sting!*' (see Chapter 3). An indirect positive suggestion might include something like, '*People sometimes feel a cool feeling, sometimes a warm feeling*'. A more neutral suggestion might be simply, '*You may feel something in a moment as you drift off to sleep*', or '*You will feel what you feel*'.

Communications at induction that may enhance recovery

Asking patients about hobbies, work, sport, and other activities that they enjoy can be utilized. It can be suggested to patients that when they imagine doing their favourite activity as they drift off to sleep, they can wake up in recovery surprised that things went a little easier than they might have thought[2].

> '*It's OK for you to go off to the beach or somewhere else you would rather be. When people take themselves to a favourite place or do a favourite activity they usually relax more easily and find themselves recovering more quickly*'.

Similarly, imagining eating a favourite food or drink during the induction can be suggested as facilitating eating and drinking as soon as the patient feels like it post-operatively—an anti-emesis suggestion (see also Chapter 20).

The anaesthetist can suggest prior to an anaesthesia induction for a surgical procedure, '*As people wake up from the surgery, knowing that the problem has been dealt with allows them to appreciate that any sensations are telling them they are on the road to recovery as the wound heals*'.

If a urinary catheter or vaginal examination is required prior to induction in an anxious patient, it could be suggested that, '*As you breathe out you will find the legs flop apart without even thinking about it. There is nothing you need try and do and nothing you need think about—as it will just seem to happen all on its own!*'

This suggestion frequently facilitates relaxation of the lower part of the body which the anaesthetist can re-enforce as soon as any positive responses become evident by saying something like '*Good!*', '*Well done!*' or '*That's right*'.

Eyes open or closed

Some anaesthetists insist on asking patients during induction to keep their eyes open for as long as they can. Presumably this is to determine when patients are anaesthetized. This can be uncomfortable for some patients and fails to give them an opportunity to develop an internal focus away from the external environment of the operating theatre—with its bright lights, multiple personnel and visible instruments of 'torture'. A helpful communication might be, '*You can close your eyes if you wish and just take yourself somewhere you would rather be—perhaps a favourite holiday place or just somewhere comfortably at home if you prefer*'. Unconsciousness can be confirmed by asking the patient to take a deep breath, and waiting for a response or not.

Communicating with patients during potentially painful procedures and during procedures under regional block are discussed in Chapters 9 and 20.

Using 'GREAT' in an emergency

One of the biggest problems in an emergency is that communication tends to break down and not infrequently is omitted altogether (see also Chapters 7, 9 and 16). It is at this time that clear communication and the use of a structured approach is at its most useful. The emergency version of '**GREAT**' (see Chapter 2) can be used to communicate effectively within the short time available—usually in less than 3 minutes. For example:

Greeting, Goal

Dr G: '*Hi, I am the anaesthetist, Dr S. Gonzales. I just wish to confirm, you are Mr Ian Extremis?*'

(Pause for response).

Dr G: '*Do you know what operation you are having?*'
Mr E: '*Yes, they are going to cut my belly to repair that big blood vessel*'.

Rapport

Dr G: '*We are doing everything we can to get you through this as safely and comfortably as possible*'.

Evaluation, Expectations, Examination, Explanation

Dr G: '*I need to ask you some questions while I examine you so that the anaesthetic is as safe for you as it can be...* (Dr Gonzales performs a focused history and examination) *I understand that you have been told that this is a life-threatening illness and that we need to act quickly. We are very shortly going in to the operating room and will be placing some monitoring, giving oxygen, blood etc.... As with any anaesthetic there are risks but the biggest risk is that without treatment it is likely you will die*'.

Asking and Answering questions, Acknowledging concerns

Dr G: '*Do you want me to go in to more detail about the anaesthetic risks?...*'
Mr E: '*No, I know I've got to get this done*'.
Dr G: '*Are there any questions you wish to ask?*'
Mr E: '*Does my family know I am here?*'
Dr G: '*Yes, I've been told your wife is outside waiting to see you*'.

Tacit agreement, Thanks, Termination

Mr E: '*I know you will do your best for me*'.
Dr G: '*We will. Thanks*'.

Inevitably in a crisis, there are a lot of communications between team members, which are occurring literally and metaphorically, over the patient's head. The important thing here is to remain aware that everything and anything said may be misinterpreted or inadvertently suggested to the patient (see also Chapters 3, 11 and 15).

Anaesthetist (referring to suction tubing): '*This one's buggered we may have to chuck it!*'
Patient hears: '*I'm buggered and am going to die!*'

The same principles of communication apply in an emergency situation as they do during elective surgery. Explaining what is happening and reassuring patients that everything is being done to ensure their comfort and safety will increase rapport and cooperation.

There is some evidence that communicating with patients using therapeutic suggestions intraoperatively may be of value in improving recovery[2], and further research on this interesting topic is required.

Recovery

As the number and complexity of surgical procedures has increased, immediate post-operative care has developed from a brief period of observation in a convenient area near the theatre suite, to more prolonged and active monitoring and intervention in a specifically designed clinical environment.

The recovery room, where patients can recover from anaesthesia and surgery and be cared for by specialist staff, has been developed as a dedicated area within the operating theatre complex. This section draws on one of the author's (AFS) own research and experience and other published guidance, and aims to encourage anaesthetists and others to think about how they might communicate within the recovery room, and to consider how this can be done more effectively.

The recovery room is known in many countries as the post-anaesthesia care unit (PACU).

The recovery room environment

Despite their presence in all modern hospitals, little has been written about recovery rooms. One exception[3] contains advice suggesting that the design and ambience of the recovery room deserve some thought. The decor should be pleasant and, if possible, there should be windows as natural light both aids accurate observation of patients and allows reorientation to time of day on emergence from anaesthesia. General lighting should not be harsh, and may be supplemented with local lighting to assist clinical examination if necessary. Noise levels should be as low as possible and the ceiling should be sound absorbent.

The ideal state described here is seldom achieved. Noise pollution is inherent to the nature of the recovery room environment. Mechanical devices, excessive personnel and patient traffic, and the acute nature of the medical and nursing care delivered, all contribute to the increased noise level.

As part of a large project investigating knowledge and expertise in anaesthesia, we carried out a number of observations in the recovery room[4]. The utopian vision above is only occasionally realized. The recovery room we observed served up to four operating theatres, where the working pattern is unpredictable, and the transfer of patients from theatres can coincide. Many different members of staff were transiently involved in the care of patients in the recovery area—including porters, operating department practitioners, nurses and surgeons, and as such there was considerable movement in and out of this space. Furthermore, many activities, both clinical and non-clinical, took place simultaneously.

Within the recovery room there are two main communication tasks, communicating with the patient emerging from anaesthesia and communication between staff. For both these tasks, it is necessary to consider both the content and the style of the communication.

Communication with patients

Effective communication must start with setting the right tone. Ideally, patients should return to consciousness in a quiet, softly lit environment, spoken to quietly, and with privacy and dignity maintained. Anyone going through this experience would surely want to regain consciousness in such a way.

It must be a cause for concern that awakening takes place with bright fluorescent lights directly in the supine patient's line of sight and is often accompanied by a tug-of-war with the patient's airway device sound-tracked by shouts of '*Open your mouth! Open your mouth so I can take this tube out!*' We can be grateful that awareness is still clouded by the residual effects of general anaesthesia.

Although there are standards for staffing, equipment, etc.[5,6], published guidance is lacking on how to talk to the patient emerging from anaesthesia. However, the research mentioned above included an analysis of observations of staff talking to such patients[7]. The researchers recorded, with notebook and pencil, the events, talk and behaviour of the anaesthetists and aimed to capture the complexity of anaesthesia practice.

Immediately after the observation session, these notes were expanded and annotated, and then transcribed for analysis. The interviews were carried out on a purposely selected cross-section of anaesthesia personnel—physicians, nurses and anaesthetists' assistants. The analysis began with individual close readings and annotations of the observational transcripts by all members of the project team, looking for recurring patterns of talk, behaviour and interaction. These were reorganized into broader categories and themes.

Thirty-one patients were observed emerging from anaesthesia. Anaesthesia personnel were noted to be talking loudly to patients, as if communicating to the hard of hearing, and usually addressing them by name. This belied a level of familiarity which would be considered inappropriate or even patronizing in any other context.

The types of communication were classifiable into two types of routine according to the words used and their intention. The 'routines' recorded could be classified into *functional*, where the anaesthetist or nurse used talk to assess the patient's clinical state, or *descriptive*, where an attempt was made to describe to patients what they might expect to feel. Illustrations are shown in Box 8.1.

Box 8.1 Examples of emergence communication routines

Anaesthetist: '*Hello my love*'. He looks at the patient's name band. '*Hello. Open your eyes.... good girl!*' He removes the laryngeal mask airway (LMA). The nurse takes the patient into the post-anaesthesia care unit.
(Observation session 3, consultant anaesthetist)

Anaesthetist (loudly, to the patient)**:** '*I'm just giving you some oxygen to breathe till you're properly awake*'. The bed is brought in, and the sheet and blanket from it are placed over the patient. '*You're just coming round from the operation now....*'
(Observation session 7, consultant anaesthetist)

Communication tended to fall into the *functional* category above, as it focused on establishing that the patient was awake—that is, responding to voice or command—and had regained vital physiological functions such as muscle strength, protective airway reflexes and breathing. Some descriptive communication was also observed, where an attempt was made to reorientate or reassure the patient. In some cases, it was the nurses in the recovery unit who spoke to the patient on emergence.

Given that most communication in this setting is informally learned and lacks any evidence on effectiveness or otherwise of different styles, it is necessary to draw on personal experience and judgement in making recommendations. However, it seems kind to suggest that patients should be allowed to wake up naturally, with constant gentle reorientation from those looking after them.

Communication between anaesthetists and recovery staff

Handing over has a number of functions. Within nursing, four have been identified[8]: ***informational***—catching up on patients' progress, maintaining continuity of care; ***social***—social or emotional support, stress relief; ***organizational***—immediate plans for shift, controlled drugs, prescriptions; and ***educational***—both explicit learning and enculturation. We identified two further functions—transfer of responsibility and checking or audit[4]. These are likely to be more evident in the interprofessional context being observed than in, for instance, handover between nurses.

The handovers witnessed took place in the midst of many other potentially distracting activities, as noted above. The length and content of the anaesthetists' handovers varied with the complexity of the patients' conditions and operations. However, they were typically brief, and concerned with the patients' pre-operative state, operation performed, analgesics given in the operating theatre and any problems encountered. An element of familiarity was also seen—anaesthetists often referring to '*my usual*'—a combination of anaesthetic drugs and techniques they favoured, which they expected the recovery staff to know. While a brief handover might be expected for a straightforward case, instances were observed where quite complex problems encountered during anaesthesia were almost glossed over—for instance, an unexpected prolonged drop in oxygen saturation just before extubation of the trachea.

Further, the receiving nurse often had to ask for other information, not always volunteered—for instance, the patient's name. This not only allowed for verification of the patient's identity, but also helped the nurse to begin the patient's reorientation into the social world as consciousness was regained. Written documents were used too. The anaesthetist left the intraoperative anaesthetic record for the recovery staff, who then added to it with their own recordings of the patient's vital signs during the recovery period. The patient's prescription chart and the surgeon's operation note were also to hand, as indeed were the patient's case notes. There was, however, no formal documentation that a handover had taken place.

Nurses and anaesthetists may have differing expectations and sometimes conflicting agendas for the handover. The anaesthetist may be more concerned with the next patient on the list than with a full handover, and may simply trust the recovery nurse to 'pick up' what needs to be known. The nurse, on the other hand, is coming to the patient fresh and with no prior knowledge and wants to be satisfied that all the information necessary to do a good job has been communicated.

This may explain why the location and timing of 'handovers' observed varied considerably. This transfer of responsibility did not always coincide with the transfer of knowledge described above. Sometimes, the anaesthetist passed on information about the patient while the patient was still in the operating theatre, the recovery nurse having gone into theatre to collect the patient. Sometimes, especially if essential details were missing, the nurse had to return to theatre to query a monitor reading or ask for further drugs or fluids to be prescribed, after the anaesthetist had started to work on the next patient.

So the transfer of responsibility must follow the transfer of knowledge. But transfer of knowledge does not in itself oblige the nurse to accept responsibility for the patient if the knowledge is considered in some way incomplete. How this was determined seemed to depend not on any written protocol or procedure but rather on an informal and unspoken arrangement formed by mutual trust and experience.

There is little published work on handover in the recovery room. The Association of Anaesthetists of Great Britain and Ireland[5], for instance, only states: '*It is essential for the anaesthetist to formally hand over care of the patient to a qualified member of the recovery room staff*'. Anwari surveyed 276 patients admitted to the PACU[9]. The quality of handover to the PACU nurse was assessed by scoring four indicators: the quality of verbal information about the patient; the condition of the patient on admission; the professional behaviour of the anaesthetist; and the nurse's satisfaction with the handover.

Five items of information were sought: the preoperative status of the patient; the premedication given; the operation performed; its course and complications; and analgesics administered. The patient's condition was communicated by providing information regarding arterial oxygen saturation, heart rate, systolic arterial pressure, whether the patient was properly covered to maintain warmth and dignity, and whether there was any pain.

Professional behaviour had four elements: whether the anaesthetist stayed to see the first set of monitor readings; whether the patient was left in a satisfactory and stable condition; whether the anaesthetist returned to review the patient; and whether clear instructions for the recovery room care were given. In the study, anaesthetists performed well on the professional behaviour element, but were less likely to hand over all information sought[9].

The study highlights the fact that handover is about more than simply the transfer of information, since both parties need to attend to the wider context for it to work satisfactorily. Box 8.2 lists some recommendations for good handover practice (see also Chapter 17).

Communicating between recovery staff and ward staff

Patients should be transferred to the ward accompanied by a suitably trained member of staff and porter. The anaesthetic record, together with the recovery and prescription charts, must accompany the patient. The recovery nurse must ensure that full clinical details are relayed to the ward nurse, with particular emphasis on problems and syringe pump settings[5]. Another possibility, not often practised, is for the

Box 8.2 Recommendations for good handover practice

- The handover should take place in the recovery room after the monitoring has been reconnected to the patient, and the nurse's full attention can be given to the anaesthetist. The culture should be such that recovery staff feel able to say if they are not happy with a patient's condition.
- Important and relevant information should be communicated verbally to the PACU nurse such as: surgery (drains, catheters, packs, etc.); anaesthetic technique used; drugs, especially analgesics and anti-emetics; blood loss during the procedure; and intravenous fluids given.
- The anaesthetist should stay in the PACU to see the first recording of vital signs and oxygen saturation, and not leave until the patient is in a stable and satisfactory condition.
- Post-operative instructions should be clear to the PACU nurse including: monitoring required; positioning; drugs and fluids prescribed; expected progress; and when to inform the anaesthetist should the patient's condition depart from normal.
- The anaesthetist should review the patient before transfer to the ward. If the anaesthetist intends to leave the recovery room before the patient, it should be established: whether the staff are comfortable with this; how the anaesthetist can be contacted; and which named member of the medical staff has assumed responsibility for the patient in case the need arises.
- Finally, no account of communication in the recovery room would be complete without the mention of an effective emergency call system[5].

anaesthetist (and the surgeon, for that matter) to hand over directly to the ward staff, when circumstances warrant it.

Using 'GREAT' to structure the acute pain round

The pain round is the clinical context which requires the most of an anaesthetist, in terms of communication skills. This section is written primarily from the point of view of doctor–patient interaction, but it is equally important to remember the communication which occurs between members of the pain team and the patient's 'home team', particularly with regard to written documentation of management plans and drug regimes.

The aim of the interactions with patients on the pain round is to ensure adequate analgesia, recognize and treat side effects, promote patient recovery, reassure and comfort patients, and respond to any queries or concerns they may have.

Greeting, Goal

The first step is to orientate oneself to the patients—know their names, the procedure they have undergone and what their analgesic regimens are. Ask patients what they like being called. Secondly, the environment should be optimized. It is never ideal to conduct a pain round assessment through the shower door! Distractions such as the TV should be eliminated where possible. Having confirmed a patient's identity and introduced oneself, the next step is to explain the purpose of the consultation.

> *'Hello Mrs Brown, I'm Dr James from the Anaesthetic Department. Our team visits people after their operations to make sure that they are* ***comfortable****...'*

Careful choice of words helps to avoid negative suggestions which can increase the patient's awareness and expectation of pain.

> *'Hello Mrs Brown, I'm Dr James from the* ***Pain*** *Service, I've come to see how much* ***pain*** *you are in...'*

This generates a totally different expectation. It is not uncommon to see patients who have been happily watching TV or chatting on the phone suddenly begin to wince and grimace once you introduce yourself as the '*Pain Doctor*' and start asking for pain scores! Subconsciously they are responding to the expectation that they should have pain and this is likely to augment rather than diminish their complaint[10,11].

Rapport

Rather than asking '*How much pain have you got?*' or '*Where does it hurt?*', statements that have the potential to increase rapport can be far more helpful. Utilizing open-ended questions such as '*How are you feeling this morning?*' gives patients the opportunity to talk about issues that concern them rather than the doctor setting the agenda[12]. Often patients will utilize this opportunity to air concerns regarding procedures or other aspects of their illness, rather than pain itself.

Evaluation, Expectations, Examination, Explanation

The efficacy of the analgesia regimen, the presence or absence of side effects and relevant physical examination such as checking the epidural site, comprise this part of the interaction. An assessment of the patients' physical capacity to mobilize and cough or breathe deeply adds a further indication of their degree of comfort. Patients are often uncertain as to what to expect in the post-operative period, and offering a brief, positive description of the post-operative course is useful to many patients,

> *'It's now the third day since your operation Mr Smith and I can see you are doing well—you've been up to the shower and you have had your drain removed. I think that by tomorrow you will be drinking and eating and we will be able to replace the PCA with some tablets...'*

Generating positive, realistic expectations of a patient's progress is a powerful way to assist recovery.

Asking and Answering questions, Acknowledging and Addressing concerns

Enquiring of patients, '*What can we do to make you more comfortable?*' often elicits complaints about urinary catheters and nasogastric tubes rather than a request for more analgesia. Obviously if patients have inadequate analgesia this should be addressed immediately and any changes in analgesic regime explained to them.

The ability to reframe a patient's experience in a positive way is very helpful in eliciting a therapeutic effect.

> **Patient:** '*Doctor, I feel terrible—really nauseated—I don't think I can keep anything down....*'
>
> **Anaesthetist:** '*That's okay Mrs Brown, I note the surgeons have reviewed you this morning and are pleased with your progress. Lots of people feel like this after surgery. Just remember you haven't eaten for more than twenty four hours. A body needs fuel to keep it going and to heal wounds. Perhaps you might feel better if you have a little something to settle your stomach ...*'

It is important of course to ensure that a surgical complication is unlikely. In this therapeutic communication the doctor is reframing the patient's nausea as a need for the body to have food. There is an acknowledgement of the complaint '*That's OK*' followed by a general statement—'*lots of people...*' This is then followed by a more specific and yet generally true statement regarding the patient's need for food. Having engaged the patient's subconscious responses of '*yes*' to the preceding statements, the suggestion that eating may be beneficial is more easily accepted by both the conscious and subconscious mind. This also allows the patient to take a more active role in controlling their nausea rather than being a passive recipient of ondansetron.

Of course, some anaesthetists may throw up their hands in horror and think '*Why not just give some anti-emetic?*—Yes, anti-emetics do work, but may cause side effects and often are no more effective than a placebo. The generation of a positive expectation of the treatment or therapeutic suggestion is the key to eliciting an effect[10]. So, whether the patient has some food or some ondansetron, or even both, the suggestion that '*something will settle the stomach*' is likely to help.

Symptoms such as pain and nausea, the two problems most commonly encountered on the pain round, are inherently subjective, have a strong emotional subconscious component and are therefore usually most amenable to therapeutic suggestion (see Chapters 3, 4 and 20).

Tacit agreement, Thanks, Termination

The interaction ends with a tacit understanding that the patient's needs have been met and that follow-up will ensure that this is maintained.

> **Anaesthetist:** '*OK Mrs Brown—it seems that we are both comfortable with that! Dr Smith will be reviewing you tomorrow and we are happy to call by anytime you feel we can help*'.
> **Patient:** '*Thanks!*'

Some dos and don'ts

- Don't ignore or belittle patients' concerns or complaints.
- Do listen to what they have to say, even if it appears irrelevant or minor, acknowledge the problem and check that you have understood—for example, '*So the way I understand it is—you've been having difficulties getting the nurses on night duty to give you the Oxycodone …*'
- Do be careful when 'normalizing' a patient's experience. Whilst educating a patient as to what to expect post-operatively, and thereby taking the opportunity to generate positive expectations, it is important that pain and nausea are ***not*** presented as inevitable, and therefore 'normal'.

  > '*After your operation, the chest drain is usually left in for a couple of days. Everyone feels differently—some people take a while to get up and about, but most people are getting up to shower on the next day*'.

  rather than,

  > '*Well of course the chest drain is excruciatingly painful for the first couple of days, but once it's out, you will feel much better!*'

  This is seeding the idea that the pain won't go until the drain is removed. The subconscious often latches onto these seemingly innocuous comments, so be aware that words can hurt but words can also heal! (see Chapter 3).
- Do allow the patient autonomy in controlling symptoms. A blood pressure of 230/120 mmHg requires treatment even if the patient is asymptomatic. A pain score of 6/10 or even 8/10 isn't quite the same thing[11]. Often the process of acknowledging symptoms, excluding underlying pathology (e.g. wound haematoma), reassuring the patient and discussing treatment options helps to allay patient anxiety and relieves distress.

While analgesic pharmacotherapy should be given where indicated, the use of therapeutic communication and the generation of positive expectations is likely to help to enhance analgesic efficacy as well as diminish side effects[12].

Key points

1. Communications with patients at induction can have a profound impact on anaesthetic care in the matter of both short-term cooperation and long-term perceptions of their hospital experience.
2. Anaesthetists and patients will reap unexpected benefits by avoiding the use of negative language at induction.
3. Patients emerging from anaesthesia should expect to be able to do so in a calm, quiet environment with reassurance and reorientation.
4. A good handover to recovery staff is not only in the patient's interest but will also mean that the anaesthetist is less likely to be interrupted by queries while inducing the next patient on the list.
5. A structured approach to communicating on the pain round enhances the quality of anaesthetist–patient interactions.
6. The use of communications that generate a positive expectancy is likely to augment analgesia and recovery.

References

1 Lang EV, Hatsiopoulou O, Koch T, Berbaum K, Lutgendorf S, Kettenmann E, et al. (2005). Can words hurt? Patient–provider interactions during invasive procedures. *Pain*, **114**(1–2), 303–9.

2 Evans C, Richardson P (1988). Improved recovery and reduced postoperative stay after therapeutic suggestions during general anaesthesia. *Lancet*, **2**(8609), 491–3.

3 DeFranco M (1985). Planning the physical structure of the recovery room. In: Frost EAM (ed.) *Recovery room practice*. pp. 251–69. Boston: Blackwell Scientific.

4 Smith AF, Pope C, Goodwin D, Mort M (2008). Interprofessional handover and patient safety in anaesthesia: observational study of handovers in the recovery room. *Br J Anaesth*, **101**, 332–7.

5 Association of Anaesthetists of Great Britain and Ireland (2002). *Immediate postanaesthetic recovery*. London: AAGBI.

6 American Society of Anesthesiologists (2004). *Standards for postanesthesia care*. Available at: www.asahq.org/publicationsAndServices/standards/36.pdf (Last accessed 14 March 2010).

7 Smith AF, Pope C, Goodwin D, Mort M (2005). Communication between anesthesiologists, patients and the anesthesia team: a descriptive study of induction and emergence. *Can J Anesth*, **52**, 915–20.

8 Kerr M (2002). A qualitative study of shift handover practice and function from a socio-technical perspective. *J Adv Nurs*, **37**, 125–34.

9 Anwari JS (2002). Quality of handover to the postanaesthesia care unit nurse. *Anaesthesia*, **57**, 484–500.

10 Schweiger A, Parducci A (1981). Nocebo: the psychologic induction of pain. *Pavlov J Biol Sci*, **16**(3), 140–3.

11 Nguyen T, Slater P, Cyna AM (2009). Open vs specific questioning during anaesthetic follow-up after Caesarean section. *Anaesthesia*, **64**(2) 156–60.

12 Pollo A, Benedetti F (2009). The placebo response: neurobiological and clinical issues of neurological relevance. *Prog Brain Res*, **175**, 283–94.

Section 3

Specific clinical contexts

Chapter 9

The obstetric patient

Marion I Andrew and Allan M Cyna

'I have nothing to offer but blood, toil, tears and sweat'.
Winston Churchill 13 May 1940

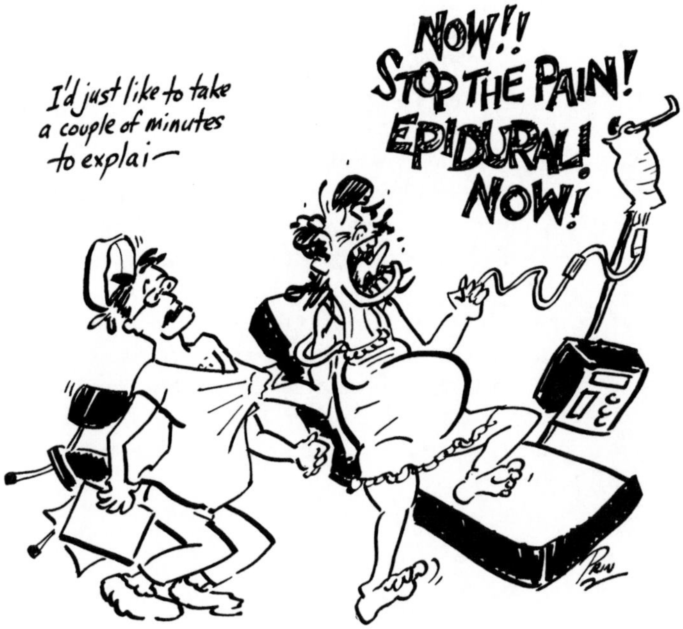
I'd just like to take a couple of minutes to explai—
NOW!!
STOP THE PAIN!
EPIDURAL!
NOW!

What this chapter is about

Addressing unique concerns in obstetric anaesthesia

The obstetric anaesthetist's clinical practice is concerned with the safety of not one, but two intricately interwoven individuals, and much of this takes place in the presence of a third party—partner, friend or relative. Pregnancy and birth are natural and normal processes in the lives of most people. In this context, communication might be expected to be a matter of common sense and somewhat intuitive. How we communicate with women is a pivotal factor in determining their experience and, although recognized as such by many within the midwifery community[1], this is perhaps less so by doctors.

Advances in medicine and changes in society over the last 100 years have resulted in a safer but, socially and technologically, a more complex experience for both women and their babies. Communication in childbirth originally occurred between women caring for each other, but this subsequently became dominated by an authoritarian medical machine, which has left some women feeling vulnerable and 'processed'. Recognition of the importance and value of patient rights and satisfaction has been responsible for a cultural shift in many maternity units. However, the medicalization of childbirth continues to take over even when labour is proceeding normally[2]. Anaesthetists are perfectly positioned as providers of analgesia and anaesthesia, within a multidisciplinary team, to communicate with women in a way that empowers them and supports their autonomy.

Antenatal preparation

Women become highly focused on the pregnancy and labour as the evidence looms ever larger in front of them. Pregnancy and childbirth usually represent a challenging psychological and physiological experience. This focus of attention on the pregnancy makes women highly suggestible to subconscious communications[3]. For this reason, messages received can function as powerful determinants of how women perceive their pregnancy, and respond during childbirth. Central nervous system (CNS) changes occur that reduce anaesthesia requirements during pregnancy and increase hypnotizability[3], dissociation, daydreaming and an ability to use imagery to experience labour in a fulfilling way.

There is a range of emotional responses to pregnancy. For some, there is joy and excitement, while for others there is no excitement—just fear and anxiety. Overlaying this, there may be pre-existing generalized anxiety, social concerns, obstetric problems and other complications. In addition, women may receive negative suggestions (see Chapter 3) from well-meaning relatives and friends who regale them with stories of their own experiences. '*I was in labour for 48 hours, it was awful!*' Whilst we are unable to change the messages that are conveyed to mothers from friends and family, the anaesthetist can communicate in ways that encourage patient autonomy and control.

The first step when preparing women for childbirth is to encourage the woman's own abilities, resources and potential, so that she has more choices and consequently more control to enable her to experience childbirth in as fulfilling a way as possible.

For very good reasons athletes train to optimize physical performance and mental capabilities. This allows them to reframe experiences in a positive way despite the considerable effort, and sometimes pain, involved. After 9 months of pregnancy the mother is, in essence, a finely tuned 'athlete'. She does not quite know the day of the event or whether she is in for a 'sprint' or a 'marathon', what she does know is that by the end of pregnancy her body is optimized physiologically to cope with the demands of labour and childbirth.

Written information is useful on several accounts. First, it gives women plenty of time to think about their analgesia and anaesthesia options. Secondly, risk information can be given in a non-threatening way and women can be encouraged to read it and ask questions or raise concerns which can then be addressed by the anaesthetist. The language of such information should avoid negative suggestions where possible.

The clinical scenario running through this chapter illustrates some of the communication techniques of use throughout pregnancy and childbirth based on the '**LAURS**' concept (see Chapter 2).

Sophie is pregnant with her first child, and is very anxious about the approaching labour. She asks to see the anaesthetist in the antenatal clinic at 36 weeks gestation. She expresses trepidation at the thought of experiencing any contractions at all, and wants to know if she can have an epidural the minute she comes into the hospital. She is '*extremely frightened of pain*' and says she has been called a '*wimp*' all her life.

Sophie: *'I'm due in four weeks and I'll need an epidural as soon as I come in—can I book it now?'*

Possible standard replies might be:

Anaesthetist 1: *'Of course, if you can't cope—you can have an epidural as soon as you come in. We have a 24 hour epidural service. No problem!'*

or

Anaesthetist 2: *'You can have an epidural but you may not necessarily get it right away—and anyway, you would be best to wait till you are 3 cm dilated'.*

Neither of these responses addresses the real issue of fear of not coping. Anaesthetist 1 re-enforces Sophie's negative belief that she can't cope and offers the epidural as a panacea to all her problems. Anaesthetist 2 similarly fails to take the opportunity to offer any other support and 'buys in' to the view that an epidural is the only answer to Sophie's belief that she will not cope.

Is there really an alternative?

Anaesthetist 3: *'You may feel you need an epidural straight away (pause)…'*

Anaesthetist 3 has listened, reflected back—and then pauses to allow a response from Sophie.

Sophie: *'Yes… I was told by one of my friends that labour is the worst pain imaginable. I don't feel I could* ***cope*** *nor does my partner'.*
Anaesthetist 3: *'I understand that this is a whole new experience… and you aren't sure that you can* ***cope****'.*

Anaesthetist 3 accepts Sophie's reality and utilizes her language.

Sophie: *'Yes. My friend was in labour for over 24 hours. I would never manage that. I don't want to be out of* ***control****'.*
Anaesthetist 3: *'It is a little unusual to have a 24 hour labour…'*

The anaesthetist accepts Sophie's reality—rather than suggest that her friend is exaggerating—but says it's unusual.

Anaesthetist 3: *'Spontaneous labour begins gradually with rest periods between the contractions that can seem quite long—you may be surprised how "in* ***control****" you can be, using some very simple techniques'.*

The utilization of the 'need for control' is recognized

Anaesthetist 3: *'As anaesthetists our job is to ensure you and your baby are comfortable and safe. One of the ways we can do this is to put in an epidural but many women find that if their labour is progressing normally, this may not be required'.*

This is an indirect suggestion that Sophie may not need one either.

Anaesthetist 3: *'Everybody's labour is different but one of the things women notice is that they lose track of time when they are in labour and often things happen more quickly than they thought. Your body has been preparing itself for nine months to do this task without you even realizing it. This usually allows women to* ***cope*** *and feel more comfortable with the experience'.*

Anaesthetist 3 has, by listening attentively and reflectively to Sophie, utilized the concern about prolonged labour and suggested an alternative experience. The anaesthetist has also established that the issue here is one of confidence, the ability to cope and control.

Sophie: *'I'm still* ***not sure****'.*
Anaesthetist 3: *'It's OK to be "****not sure****" as in that way you have left all your options open, so that you can do whatever needs to be done when the time is right. By discussing this now you know that you will be able to make an informed choice and have had time to think about it'.*

By utilizing Sophie's uncertainty and reframing it into flexibility, choices, and autonomy, the anaesthetist is able to provide suggestions that she can be more confident in her own abilities and take time in making informed decisions regarding analgesia and potential side effects. This is not to say that women should not have epidural analgesia if they desire or need one at any time, but rather that communicating with patients in a manner that reflects our confidence in them reinforces their own resources and allows them more choice.

Labour

Anaesthetists' contact with women in labour is usually in the context of providing epidural analgesia. Communication with highly distressed women in labour is particularly challenging. Labouring women are frequently in a dissociated state and respond poorly to logical communication. Therefore, different forms of language are often necessary if useful responses are to be elicited.

Epidural analgesia

No opportunity to meet the labouring woman is ever wasted as the anaesthetist can begin to establish rapport. To this end it is often helpful for the anaesthetist to be visible as part of the team attending labour ward rounds and making anticipatory visits in situations where an intervention is likely to be required. Open communication channels occur when the anaesthetist engages with the patient and her partner in a way that shows respect for autonomy.

Women in labour are nearly always relieved and delighted to see the anaesthetist. Establishing rapport on this basis is usually straightforward, with introductions and acknowledgement that pain relief can be given as quickly as possible. The unhurried, cool, professional anaesthetist talking confidently, gently and encouragingly is a source of great relief in itself.

In obstetric anaesthesia practice, verbal—and in some jurisdictions, written—consent needs to be obtained prior to insertion of an epidural catheter during labour. In many maternity units, written patient information is now provided which women can read prior to labour. Written consent might then be obtained in the antenatal clinic, where explanations of the material risks pertaining to that particular woman may be given more fully (see Chapter 7). This solution provides factual information, but does not address the woman's immediate concerns which may be largely unknown to the anaesthetist. The more important aspect of consent is not so much the facts and figures, but the human interaction based upon trust and confidence in a competent professional. Which risks are 'material'? What should be discussed? How should this information be presented? Although there are no easy answers to these questions for every patient there are some things that are worth considering.

Competency

It has been argued that it is impossible to obtain informed consent when women are in labour on the basis that they are not competent to give consent—that is, to undertake informed decision making when in the throes of labour[4]. If the partner or support persons are present, they can hear the information being provided when the anaesthetist talks between contractions. In the absence of a clear definition of 'competent', this remains controversial. But what is apparent is that the patient is vulnerable, is asking for help, her needs are relatively urgent and she wants to feel confident that the doctor is able to perform the procedure as safely and quickly as possible. With very few exceptions, labour is not an emergency, and the insertion of an epidural is not a life-saving procedure. The issue of 'competence' arises because, in distress, the patient, and frequently the anaesthetist and midwife, perceives the situation as an emergency and may behave in a way that suggests that she is irrational and unable to listen to explanations. A labouring woman is often exhausted and may have the 'mental fog' of other medications. Though the woman may appear to be distracted by contractions she is usually capable of listening to a brief focused explanation of the procedure, its benefits and risks in the context of the specific situation. The anaesthetist then needs to confirm her wishes as to whether to proceed or not.

Sophie is now at term and has been admitted to the labour ward with spontaneous rupture of membranes and is in active labour.

> **Anaesthetist:** '*Hello Sophie, my name is Dr B, I'm one of the anaesthetists—I've come to help you.* (Shakes hand of patient and partner). *What can I do to help?*'

This allows the woman to state her wishes and verbally request rather than have the partner, relative or midwife tell you what they believe the woman wants or needs.

> **Sophie:** '*I want a f*** ing epidural!—quick just do it!*'
> **Anaesthestist:** '*We will do this for you as quickly and as safely as possible.* (Waits till the end of the contraction). *Do you have any particular concerns that I need to address before we start? We need to be sure you understand the risks of an epidural as well as the benefits before we proceed. Of the more common risks a bad headache is the main one you need to know about… rarely paralysis, epidurals don't always work perfectly…, but the good news is that epidurals usually allow women to become very comfortable and feel more in control…*'

While it is important to avoid negative language (see Chapter 3), this is nearly impossible when providing risk information (see Chapter 7). Focusing on the benefits of epidural analgesia immediately after the risk discussion can be helpful. For consent to be informed, risks need to be presented in a way that facilitates a decision as to whether or not to proceed with epidural analgesia. The consent process is directed at supporting the patient's autonomy and is not just about 'covering the anaesthetist's back'. Unnecessary repeated emphasis of major risks can reduce patient cooperation by escalating anxiety in an already fraught situation. A 'jumpy' patient is more likely to have complications if she is focused on things going wrong rather than on things going right.

Enhancing patient cooperation during epidural insertion

Women often say that they are unable to cooperate and, while they may be begging for relief, they may insist that they are unable to keep still or move to position themselves. It is particularly in these circumstances that the acceptance of the patient's perception is essential.

Some anaesthetists become irritated and insistent—'*Well, you will have to sit up and keep still otherwise I can't do this. If you move we could damage your spinal cord*'. Although this is one strategy to terrify the woman into sitting still, there are gentler alternative communications that can be used. Also anger and frustration are unlikely to help the woman cooperate with her anaesthetic care. Consider the following example where the anaesthetist accepts the woman's perception and reality and, utilizes this to empower her so that she maximizes her abilities and control.

Sophie has agreed to proceed with an epidural and the midwife is setting up the necessary equipment.

> **Anaesthetist:** '*While we're getting everything ready, I'll tell you how we can make this as safe, quick and as comfortable as possible for you*'.
> **Sophie:** '*Oh no here comes another one! No! Aaaaaargh—just put it in!*'
> **Anaesthetist:** '*OK, let's get on and do this safely, comfortably and as quickly as we can*'.

The anaesthetist communicates with the patient to emphasize '*safety*'—his concern—and '*speed*'—her concern.

> **Sophie:** '*Yeah, yeah I can be paralysed! Please HELP ME—I can't **listen** to anything anymore!*'
> **Anaesthetist:** '*That's OK—you don't have to **listen** because you will **hear** everything you need to allow yourself to relax and sit still, while we place the epidural and get you comfortable*'.

The anaesthetist is accepting that Sophie can't '***listen***', utilizes her language and reframes it so that even though she can't '***listen***' she can still '***hear***' what is being said. The anaesthetist then suggests that Sophie will be able to '***relax and sit still***'.

> **Anaesthetist:** '*Would you like to sit up now or after the next contraction?*'—double bind (see Chapter 4). '*In a moment I will be asking you to tell me when you are having a contraction—I can then insert the epidural during the rest between contractions whilst you are sitting still. I will use local anaesthetic to numb the skin and then you may or may not feel some pressing on the back*'.

The anaesthetist puts research evidence[4] into practice by avoiding the use of negative language '*it will sting*' and encourages the patient at each stage with the expectation that she will be able to achieve what is being asked even if she doesn't believe it herself.

Communicating with women during a contraction

Communicating in a way that helps women to stay still while they are having strong contractions represents a pinnacle of achievement for the obstetric anaesthetist. Some practical dialogue follows to illustrate some possible techniques that can be used when required.

Women can be asked to focus on their breathing by counting their breaths silently during a contraction. This can be communicated in a number of ways depending on circumstances. An indirect approach may be used by saying,

> '*Most women find that as they count their breaths during the contraction it allows them to feel stronger and more in control. Each time they breathe in, they breathe in a little strength and control they didn't even realize they had, and each time they breathe out, they find themselves blowing away a bit of tension or discomfort into the atmosphere and start feeling more in control and more relaxed*'.

If at the end of the contraction the woman has found that she has managed to count her breaths, when the rest is about to eventuate, she can be asked '*to let go of that last contraction and enjoy the much longer rest*'. For the woman who doesn't complete the counting of breaths in her mind before the contraction finishes, it is important for the anaesthetist still to reframe this as a 'success'. For example:

Anaesthetist: *'How many breaths did you count in that last contraction?'*
Sophie: *'Three, the contraction was too painful to concentrate'.*
Anaesthetist: *'Good, well done! Many women can't get past "one" the first time they attempt this. As each contraction passes you will find there comes a point when you will find yourself able to keep counting right through to the end of the contraction. The contractions then start to move into the distance as you feel more comfortable and more in control'.*

This encouragement to focus the woman's attention allows her to dissociate further from the pain of the contraction and become even more responsive to the sensation moving in to the distance.

Time distortion (see Chapters 4 and 20)

In their dissociated mental state, labouring women are often able to accept suggestions in a very concrete and unquestioning way.

'As you know each contraction tells you that you are getting closer to seeing your baby. The other thing you know is that each contraction is followed by a rest. Interestingly, women find that they can cope with each contraction one at a time and enjoy each rest as they build up their strength and confidence. You can notice how the rests start seeming much longer than they really are and the contractions start seeming much shorter than they really are as they move into the distance'.

The suggestion of a much longer rest period is accepted concretely and experienced as a perceptual change which aids relaxation. It should be noted that it is important to use the word '*seeming*' as some highly suggestible patients may reduce the frequency of their contractions with this suggestion.

Reframing contractions

The reframe involves a communication that provides an alternative meaning or interpretation of an experience (see Chapter 2). Table 9.1 shows different interpretations of the same experience.

Metaphor can be particularly useful in this context where the contractions can be described in a way that is positive. A contraction might be described as '*powerful energy that brings the baby closer*' or as '*a powerful wave*'—thus guiding the woman to focus on seeing the baby as the goal rather than enduring the contraction.

Caesarean section

The dynamic and acute nature of childbirth means that sudden changes may result in an emergent situation. A clear understanding of the procedure is achievable when communication is provided calmly, honestly and with sensitivity to the patient's distress, fatigue, and vulnerability to the effects of negative suggestions.

Regional anaesthesia is nearly always the anaesthetic of choice as it is safer for the mother, and allows both parents to participate in the birth. Having an operation while

Table 9.1 Different interpretations of the same experience

Experience	Positive interpretation	Negative interpretation
Labour onset	*'When contractions are regular and the cervix is dilating you are in established labour and well on the way to having your baby'.*	*'We can place an epidural before the contractions become too painful'.*
Labour contractions	*'One step closer to seeing the baby'.* *'The stronger the more effective'.*	*'An increasingly painful experience that is absolutely terrifying and almost unbearable'.* *'The stronger the more painful'.*
Rests between contractions	*'Focusing on the rests can allow them to seem longer than they really are and the contractions seem shorter than they really are'.*	*'The contractions seem continuous and ever more painful and excruciating as labour progresses'.*
Cx 3–4 cm	*'At this stage most women are entering the accelerated phase of their labour where the contractions become much more effective'.*	*'This stage of labour starts getting really painful and most women will need an epidural!'*
Full dilatation	*'This is the exciting part of labour where women are no longer passive observers but become active participants in the birth of the baby'.*	*'Most women find at this stage they are too tired to care as the pain becomes even more unbearable'.*
Pushing and crowning	*'All the rests that you have had during the first stage of labour has given you more than enough energy to push in the most effective way possible for you and your baby'.* *'As skin stretches it usually becomes numb and anaesthetic, allowing the birth to be as comfortable and safe as possible'.*	*'Most women at this stage are too tired to do anything let alone push'.* *'As skin stretches, it burns and the burning sensation is the worst experience of the entire birth'.*

awake is nevertheless an uncommon experience for most people, and naturally enough some women and their partners are anxious. Others may be delighted to have escaped an arduous labour. A few women may feel cheated of the natural birth option. The anaesthetist can establish at the very beginning of a discussion what the woman's perspective is, build rapport by demonstrating a willingness to listen and allow the woman and her partner some degree of control over the consultation and, by implication, the anaesthetic and hospital process.

Despite our own familiarity with regional techniques, it may be a daunting prospect for some women. There is a natural tendency to expect that others will be concerned or frightened about the same things as we would, and to address each woman as if this were the case. Appreciation that vast differences occur between women allows the anaesthetist to focus attention on where the woman's concerns lie, and to tailor communication accordingly. This allows the woman to have an experience that is comfortable, safe and as fulfilling as possible.

Knowing what to expect is an important part of the preparation for women. The mind will naturally rehearse all sorts of scenarios—often negatively—as a survival mechanism (see also Chapter 3).

Sophie has been in labour for 12 hours and has failed to progress. The obstetrician has decided that she requires a Caesarean section. Her epidural has worked well and it has been 'topped up' for the procedure. Sophie is now in the operating room.

> **Anaesthetist:** '*We have talked about what you might* ***feel*** *and I am now going to test the anaesthetic block so that we are both happy that it is working as it should be. We will only begin the Caesarean when we are all confident that it is working well. First of all you can expect to feel touch*'.

Anaesthetist places a hand on the abdomen.

> **Sophie:** '*I can* ***feel*** *touching on my tummy*'.
> **Anaesthetist:** '*Yes that's what you can expect to* ***feel****. You can also expect to* ***feel*** *pressure*'.

Anaesthetist presses firmly on the abdomen.

> **Sophie:** '*Yes*'.
> **Anaesthetist:** '*You can expect to* ***feel*** *pushing and pulling*'.

Anaesthetist maintains firm pressure on the abdomen while moving hand side to side and cephelad and caudad.

> **Anaesthetist:** '*Is that OK?*'
> **Sophie:** '*I can* ***feel*** *that*'.
> **Anaesthetist:** '*Good, I am reassured that you can* ***feel*** *that*'.

The anaesthetist is using repetition '*you can expect*' and listening to Sophie's response, utilizing her own words to reassure her that the block will be adequate. Testing the level of block can then take place as per usual practice.

The drapes are placed, and Sophie is assessed as having a block to T3 with ice.

> **Sophie:** '*I don't think I* ***can do*** *this!*'
> **Anaesthetist:** '*That's OK. I have tested the anaesthetic and am confident that the block will ensure you are comfortable and safe during the procedure. There are things you* ***can do*** *to help yourself. One of the things women* ***can do*** *is to imagine seeing their baby for the first time. How much hair, the little fingers and fingernails, the palm of the baby's hand, the eyes? Even if you don't realize it yet, you know you* ***can do*** *this*'.

'***You know***' is a generalized suggestion that the woman subconsciously knows she can manage getting through the Caesarean and also '***knows***' there are things she ***can do*** to help herself.

> **Anaesthetist** (as the baby is being born)**:** '*You may feel some pressure at the top of the abdomen to help the baby be born more easily. Any pulling and pushing you might feel can remind you that your tummy muscles are still strong even though you thought they didn't exist anymore*'.

Communication with a borderline block when the mother expresses a strong desire to avoid general anaesthetic

Many anaesthetists will not entertain allowing surgery to proceed in a situation where the block appears less than perfect. However, many mothers are highly motivated to be conscious for the birth of their baby and may be very able to cope with some degree of discomfort or pain during the procedure. The importance of 'checking in' with the patient is the key to managing the patient with a less than perfect block successfully.

> **Anaesthetist 1:** '*Although I think the anaesthetic is working reasonably well up to here* (e.g. T6) *it would be better if you were numb up here as well* (e.g. T4). *I appreciate how important it is to you to see your baby being born. What do you think?*'
> **Woman:** '*Does that mean I might feel pain?*'
> **Anaesthetist 1:** '*Yes, you might feel pain but if you are not coping I can put you to sleep*'.

Alternatively—

> **Anaesthetist 2:** '*Not necessarily..., we can help you stay comfortable with extra local anaesthetic if it is required and give other medications into the drip to keep you comfortable once the baby is born. I am ready to give you a sleeping anaesthetic at any time you feel you want it. Is it OK with you to proceed? I am right here*'.

Anaesthetist 1 acknowledges that the woman might feel pain and offers general anaesthesia (GA) as the only solution, with a negative suggestion that she might not be able to cope.

Anaesthetist 2 informs the patient of a range of anaesthetic options available while at the same time supporting the patient's autonomy. Negative suggestions such as '*pain*' are avoided.

Communicating with the partner is usually helpful, and a joint decision is preferred where possible. Similarly the obstetricians need to be informed of the borderline nature of the block (see Chapter 17), especially as they may be requested to infiltrate with local anaesthetic if required. If testing of skin anaesthesia is adequate, the obstetricians can proceed and, once the skin incision is made, the patient can be asked whether she is comfortable. Checking in at regular intervals can occur throughout. If the woman complains of pain there are three options. First, the woman may not desire any other analgesia despite complaining of pain. Second, she may request additional analgesia. Finally, she may request a GA. In all cases the primary consideration is maternal safety and autonomy—not the anaesthetist's fear of litigation! Once the baby is born and is presented to the mother it is unusual for a GA to be required or requested, especially if the baby can stay with her and she can be reassured that the operation will soon be completed. The anaesthetist can inform the obstetrician, where necessary, that this is not the time to be teaching a junior trainee.

Communicating with fathers and partners

On occasion partners do not wish to be present for the birth, and this choice should be respected. However, far more commonly, there is an expectation that the father of the baby will be present at the birth. This raises the emotional stakes and means that anaesthetists now have to be aware of the communication occurring between themselves, parturients and their partners. Some fathers take easily to this situation and can immediately find themselves at home in this role. Others are less comfortable and may be unsure how to help or support their partner. Unfortunately a lack of confidence can manifest itself as agitation or even aggression. Fathers are under a good deal of pressure and stress themselves; they are often tired and hungry—an explosive mixture for some!

It can be helpful for the anaesthetist at the time of introductions to encourage partners to be active participants, providing information, and explaining procedures or obtaining consent. Partners should be advised that they may be asked to leave the operating room if required, '*As more space and personnel are needed for the mother and baby's safety*'.

Tips and tricks

It is not uncommon for women to have various concerns during the surgical procedure. It is important for the anaesthetist to deal with these in a supportive and a positive way with, of course, the avoidance of negative suggestion. Often women are merely seeking reassurance and explanation as opposed to pharmacotherapy.

Example 1 Managing nausea

Woman: '*I'm feeling a bit sick*'.
Anaesthetist: '*Here's the vomit bowl*'.

Alternatively—

Woman: '*I'm feeling a bit sick*'.
Anaesthetist: '*It's because your blood pressure is a bit low. I have just given you something to help the blood pressure and that will help you too*'.

Example 2 Difficulty breathing during Caesarean section

Woman: '*I can't breathe!*' or '*It's hard to breathe*'.
Anaesthetist: '*That's OK. Sometimes when the anaesthetic is working really well we lose the sensation in the chest that we are breathing even when we are. Can you place the palm of your hand on your chest and take a deep breath—and feel the chest move up and down each time you breathe. The breathing soon will start to feel much easier*'.

While it is important to ensure that this isn't an early sign of a total spinal, this is unlikely if the woman is vocalizing.

Example 3 Pruritus with neuraxial opioids

Woman: '*I'm really itchy*'.
Anaesthetist: '*That's excellent. This means the pain relief is working really well, and knowing that allows women to put it into the background. Is that bothering you?*'
Woman: '*No*'.
Anaesthetist: '*Is there anything extra you would like me to do about this?*'

Using 'GREAT' for an emergency GA Caesarean section

Because emergency GA for Caesarean section is a stressful and technical challenge for the anaesthetist, good communication skills tend to be forgotten. Communication with patient, partner, obstetrician and theatre team in these circumstances is a vital component of quality care.

A phone call to the emergency theatre alerts staff that there is a Category I call for prolapsed cord. Thirty seconds later the theatre doors swing open and amidst shouts of '*Don't push!*' the woman on a trolley is wheeled hurriedly towards the operating table. The midwife, with one hand in the vagina, asks for a foetal heart monitor.

Greeting, Goals

Anaesthetist: '*Hi, my name is Dr Gonzales. I'm the anaesthetist. We clearly need to be working quickly here. We are here to keep you and your baby safe and I will be giving your anaesthetic. While I'm putting the drip in and the nurses are placing some monitors, can you tell me what you like to be called?*'
Patient: '*Susie ... Is my baby going to be OK?*'

Rapport

Anaesthetist: '*Susie, all these people here are doing everything possible to make sure you and your baby are OK*'.
Susie: '*I'm scared*'.
Anaesthetist: '*It's OK to be scared*'.

The anaesthetist is acknowledging concerns and letting her know that she has been heard and understood.

Evaluation, Expectations, Examination, Explanation

Anaesthetist: '*I just need to ask you quickly some questions. Have you ever had a problem with anaesthetics?... teeth?... on any medication?... allergies?.... Can you open your mouth for me? ...etc. ...in a few moments we will be giving you some oxygen and some medicine to get you off to sleep...*'.

Asking and Answering questions, Acknowledging and Addressing concerns

Anaesthetist: '*That's good. Have you anything to ask before we start your anaesthetic?*'
Susie: '*Is the anaesthetic going to affect my baby?*'
Anaesthetist (Pre-oxygenating): '*Sometimes anaesthetic does make the baby a little sleepy too, but most of the time the baby is born before the anaesthetic reaches them. The "baby doctor" is here to look after your baby when he is born*'.

Tacit agreement, Thanks, Termination

Anaesthetist (Pre-oxygenating): '*Just let me know when you are ready for us to start...*'

Key points

1. The anaesthetist can communicate in ways that encourage patient autonomy and control.
2. Women who may appear distracted by contractions are usually able to listen to a brief focused explanation of the procedure.
3. The anaesthetist should 'check in' with the patient at regular intervals to confirm her wishes.
4. Women in labour can usually do more than they think they can and frequently respond to 'suggestion'.
5. Verbal and non-verbal communications by the anaesthetist delivered confidently and calmly can rapidly help defuse an otherwise fraught situation.
6. Communicating in a way that helps women to feel in control, and cooperate with anaesthesia care, represents a pinnacle of achievement for the obstetric anaesthetist.

References

1 Burnard P (1998). Effective communication: sharpening your skills. *Pract Midwife*, **1**(3), 12–3.

2 Johanson R, Newburn M, MacFarlane A (2002). Has the medicalisation of childbirth gone too far? *BMJ*, **324**, 892–5.

3 Alexander B, Turnbull D, Cyna A (2009). The effect of pregnancy on hypnotizability. *Am J Clin Hypn*, **52**(1), 13–22.

4 Varelmann D, Pancaro C, Cappiello E, Camann W (2010). Nocebo-induced hyperalgesia during local anesthetic injection. *Anesth Analg*, **110**(3), 868–70.

Chapter 10

The paediatric patient

David Sainsbury and Allan M Cyna

'I had six theories about bringing up children; now I have six children, and no theories'.
John Wilmot

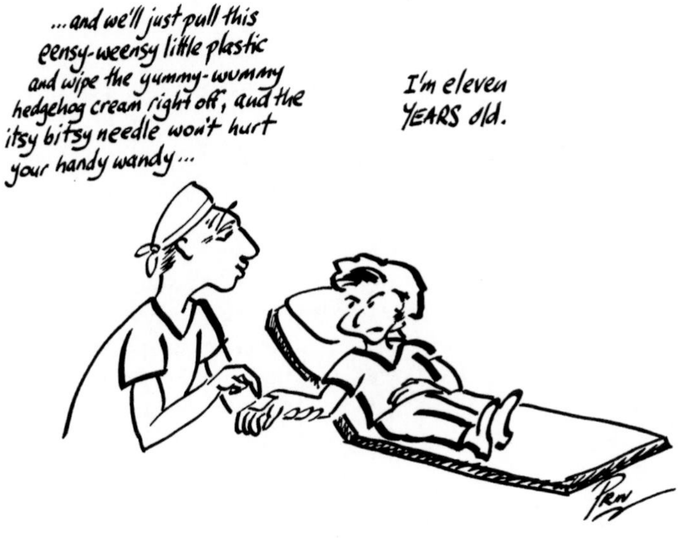
...and we'll just pull this eensy-weensy little plastic and wipe the yummy-wummy hedgehog cream right off, and the itsy bitsy needle won't hurt your handy wandy...
I'm eleven YEARS old.

What this chapter is about

How to make communicating with kids child's play!

Anaesthetists usually develop their communication skills through experience over many years of trial and error. Much angst can be avoided by learning some simple techniques that can facilitate interactions during the delivery of anaesthesia care. Caring for children from newborn to adolescence provides the anaesthetist with unique opportunities to use communication to improve anaesthesia care.

To a parent, the matter of handing over control and protection of their child to the anaesthetist is invariably difficult, emotional and can lead to significant distress. This is irrespective of whether the surgical intervention is major or not. For their child to attend the hospital for a procedure, families have frequently made unspoken and intricate arrangements in their schedule. Making these arrangements adds to the other stresses of coming in for surgery. Being mindful of this can help the anaesthetist communicate in a way that recognizes the possible complexity for some families of even attending the hospital on time.

In recent years the increasing popularity of day-surgery admission has meant that many parents meet their child's anaesthetist for the first time only minutes before the procedure. However, much can be done to enhance patient and parent rapport even when only a short time is available. Flexibility in approach is paramount. The age of the child determines how the '**LAURS**' of communication (outlined in Chapter 2) can be implemented to facilitate patient rapport, trust and engagement during anaesthesia care.

Children or adults: same—same but different!

Communicating with children is similar to, yet differs from, communicating with adults[1]. Children live in a subconscious world of play and make-believe. They are highly responsive to suggestion, and the use of subconscious language and non-verbal cues is frequently more effective than the usual adult logical communication most doctors are familiar with. Because of this, children often do not appear to be paying attention and instead frequently behave spontaneously, subconsciously or contrary to what is being asked of them. Adults when stressed will often do this too. As with adults, the aim of communicating effectively with children is to promote autonomy and a sense of control.

Social development in the communication context

The process of having surgery and anaesthesia inevitably involves interaction with strangers and the separation of the child from their primary caregiver. It is helpful to have a basic understanding of how different age groups are likely to respond to these processes. This allows the anaesthetist to behave in a flexible way that is more likely to optimize anaesthetic care.

The stages of development can be very variable for any particular patient. An 8-year-old may have a higher level of social development than a 12-year-old (see Case study 1 below). Such variability is usually a reflection of many factors including family dynamics, intelligence, cultural, gender and prior or current illness.

Pre-verbal stage

Children in the pre-verbal stage of development—and their parents—do not cope well with separation, although babies less than 6 months old invariably cope with this separation better than their parents. The non-verbal less than 2 age group generally respond to soothing and soft repetitive sounds. Understanding precedes the ability to verbalize. This group are most likely to be responsive to your singing, providing it is a gentle lullaby and not the latest Rap Hip Hop ditty.

2–4 years

The 2–4 years age group are still predominantly attached to their primary caregiver and do not tolerate physical separation from their parents easily in the company of strangers. Whether it be for an intravenous (IV) or inhalational induction, these children are usually more easily induced on the parent's lap.

5–10 years

By the age of 5 and upwards most children will have started school and have become socialized to the company of strangers and are able to make a much more confident entry into the operating room. The choice of words is very important to ensure communication is congruent.

Concrete versus logical thinking

Children younger than 10 years tend to think in concrete rather than logical terms. Children will interpret '*going to sleep*' for their surgery as going to sleep in the way they do at home (see Case study 4 below). Children tend not to have the experience to be able to attribute different logical meanings to this phrase as adults would—for example, going to sleep meaning 'surgery' or 'night time' or 'euthanasia'. Some children will concretely think that they are being put to bed early if they are told they are going to sleep. Many children are told that they will be '*going to sleep*' for their operation so there tends to be an expectation of using this form of words to describe anaesthesia. It is helpful to accept this, and reassure the child and parents that the anaesthetist will be looking after the child during the operation, and that the child when awake enough will be returning to the parents as soon as possible.

Adolescents

For communicating with adolescents it is '*cool*' on occasions to slip into the vernacular in a '*really random*' way. This can be '*wickedly*' powerful '*stuff*'. The term '*neat*' can be a bit '*suss*' but there usually is an '*epic*' turn of phrase that can facilitate rapport. Although such language can be '*awesome*', continuing medical education in it is essential as adolescent communication changes with the seasons, fashion, culture and, sometimes the lunar cycle.

The child's journey and using 'GREAT'

The pre-operative visit and preparation of the child for surgery are more important than the choice of premedication[2]. The anaesthetist can take this opportunity not only to evaluate the medical and anaesthetic requirements of the planned surgical procedure but also to make an assessment of the communication styles of the child and family, explain possible approaches to the induction of anaesthesia and address any concerns. Reducing parental anxiety is associated with a reduction in child anxiety[3].

Greeting, Goals

A considerable amount of information can be gained as the anaesthetist approaches the patient. Is the baby or infant in a stroller or clutched to mum's chest? Is the older child clinging to their parent or off gluing stars on paper with the play leader or nurse? A systematic approach can help, similar to reading a chest X-ray. It is important to confirm the status of the child's carer so as to avoid calling the 'parent' '*Mum*' when in fact they are sister, aunt, grandmother or even a close friend or guardian!

First the parents' body postures. Are they 'open' or 'closed'—that is, legs crossed, arms folded? Are they looking around nervously, or idly leafing through a magazine?

Attention can be turned to the interactions between the various players—patient, sibling, carer or friend—in this unfolding drama. Closer connections often denote higher levels of anxiety—for example, a child burying their head in the mother's lap. Finally, any reaction to the anaesthetist's approach and engagement can be observed. Is this welcomed or perceived as an intrusion?

When approaching the child the anaesthetist should identify himself. It is frequently helpful to direct the first words towards the child, even a pre-verbal child. Perhaps, '*Hi, I'm Dave, I'm a sleep doctor*'. For infants and babies, making eye and verbal contact of any sort may be a useful first step—'*Hi, how are you doing*?' This initial contact will facilitate the developing rapport, as the child, parent and anaesthetist interact and establish trust in each other. The anaesthetist should avoid looking down on children while engaging with them. Kneeling on the floor, while younger children are seated or standing, can facilitate engagement at their level. Commenting in a positive way to children on what they are doing, wearing, etc., can be a useful first step—for example, '*Lovely pink shoes!*' The interview should be kept 'short and sweet' by asking the child some simple, direct questions: '*Can you tell me your name?*' and '*How old are you?*' followed by a request '*Do you know why you have come in to the hospital today?*' In this way, the development of rapport can begin with the child and indirectly the parent.

Important information is also established regarding the child's and parents' understanding of the procedure.

Rapport

The child's autonomy can be respected by stating: '*I am going to talk to your Mum and Dad for a few minutes and then I am going to talk to you. Is that OK?*' This facilitates engagement at several levels and begins to establish important baseline knowledge. No matter what the child's age or what activity they appear to be deeply engaged in, they will inevitably hear the anaesthetist–parent discussion about them and take on board everything that is said.

A funny hat or koala bear on the stethoscope may be useful distracters and focus the attention of the child. Casual clothes will put some parents at ease, while others may feel more confident if they see the doctor formally dressed. Theatre scrubs can be useful. They are sufficiently novel that the child is unlikely to have negative associations with them unless they are 'frequent fliers'. They also serve to prepare the child for how the anaesthetist will look in the operating theatre. With the simple addition of a name badge or stethoscope they can symbolize authority to the parent. A confident approach can increase rapport as patient safety and comfort is both explicitly and implicitly implied.

Sitting on a chair beside a standing child allows engagement at eye level and facilitates rapport. The child's response to some non-anaesthetic questions can provide valuable information that can increase rapport and be utilized later. For example: '*What is the favourite thing in the whole wide world you like doing?*' or '*What is your favourite colour?/food?/drink?*' For the older child '*Do you have any hobbies or sports that you like?*' or for adolescents '*Do you like shopping?*'

Evaluation, Examination and Expectations

Evaluation

In order to allow older children due recognition for their abilities and autonomy, it is useful to include them in the medical interview with questions they will easily be able to answer themselves; '*Do you need to take any medicines or inhalers?*', '*Are there any medicines you can't take for any reason such as allergy?*' This can also take the conversation in unexpected but informative directions, providing useful clues where to go next (see Case study 3 below). If a child appears pressured in any way it may be preferable to direct questions towards the parents (see above).

Examination

As the anaesthetist moves on to physical examination, they tend to learn more from the child's response to examination than the stethoscope tells them about cardiac status.

At this point the anaesthetist will have gathered a great deal of information. If the initial approach leads to a withdrawal response, it is time to reflect and change tack. Trust needs to be earned either directly or through the parent. Never just place a stethoscope on the child's chest, or otherwise examine him or her, without permission. The anaesthetist will frequently need to demonstrate that nothing will happen without warning. Many children, especially if they have been examined before, will simply lift up a T-shirt or dress for auscultation. Others will require a more subtle approach.

Pre-verbal children frequently find a direct approach unnecessarily distressing. Slow, careful, indirect movements will invariably succeed when more direct ones fail. For example, when examining the chest, start by placing the bell of the stethoscope on the mother's or carer's hand. This non-verbal communication shows indirectly the painless nature of the examination and that the carer is in agreement with what you are doing. It also is an indirect non-verbal communication to the child that this would be OK for him or her too. Then, with the stethoscope still on the mother's hand ask the mother to place her hand on the child's lap. At each step, the aim is to place the stethoscope a little nearer the child's chest such as his thigh, then his hand or forearm, then the abdomen and finally the chest. The child can be encouraged at each stage with simple reassurance or praise such as: '*Well done!*' '*That's right!*' '*Good!*' as each step in the process is accepted. Then if the child doesn't breathe in when requested to do so, ask the child to blow, as children nearly always are familiar with blowing out a birthday candle. An alternative approach is simply to give the child the stethoscope to play with, to listen to Mum's chest and then their own, and then ask for permission to let the anaesthetist listen too. Whatever the technique—and there are as many techniques as there are anaesthetists—providing the child is engaged in a friendly and playful way, the interaction is likely to be successful.

Expectations

The pre-anaesthesia consultation is the ideal place to seed positive expectancy in both children and their parents about the upcoming procedure and recovery. Understanding the reasons for surgery from the patient's and parents' perspectives allows the anaesthetist to utilize their response in a positive way. For example, if the child says that they are having adeno-tonsillectomy because of recurrent infection, the anaesthetist can emphasize how good it will feel knowing that the throat will be so much more comfortable in the future. Indirect suggestions are useful—for example, '*Most children find that they recover quickly after this procedure and can eat and drink as soon as they feel like it*'.

Children can be shown the T-piece and mask, and encouraged to handle and play with it, take it apart and put it back together, developing a sense of ownership. They can also be reassured that they can take their favourite toy, if they have one, into theatre.

Planting the seeds for induction can begin by enquiring about subjects which may be useful later as a focus of attention. '*What is your favourite colour?*' or '*What is your favourite flavour?*' The answer will give a starting point for conversation with which to engage the child in theatre. The response can confirm that the answer has been heard correctly and that the child knows that the anaesthetist has listened and understood. For example, in response to being asked a favourite colour:

Child: '*Pink*'
Anaesthetist: '*So your favourite colour is pink is it?*'

Child nods.

The anaesthetist is also building a focus of attention where dual choices of comparable alternatives can be offered, allowing the child to feel a sense of control (See 'double binds' in Chapter 4). For example, '*Would you like to breathe in the pink magic gas or blow it away?*' If one of these choices is made, the anaesthetist has been 'informed' that the child will probably cooperate with an inhalational induction. The older or more cooperative child can be offered a more cognitive choice—for example, '*There are two options for getting off to sleep; the "sleepy wind" or a "plastic straw" in the back of the hand*'. If the child cannot decide at the time, the anaesthetist can explain about the '*numbing cream*' and draw smiley faces on the back of the child's hands to indicate to the nurses where to put the cream—perhaps saying '*We can decide when you get to theatre*'.

Asking and Answering questions, Acknowledging and Addressing concerns

Listening, observing and accepting the parent's or child's expressions of anxiety are vital components in gaining rapport. It is then easier to ask about and address specific concerns as these are raised, being careful not to dismiss them even if they seem silly. For example, if a 9-year-old asks whether anything will be felt, the anaesthetist could say '*No!*' or '*Yes!*'. Alternatively the anaesthetist could use the child's words and acknowledge that something may be '***felt***' or whatever is '***felt***' will probably '***feel** OK*' or '***feel** as comfortable as possible*' (see Chapters 2–4 and 20).

If an IV induction is planned: '*Some children say they **feel** something as the plastic straw or "drip" is positioned*'. Or for inhalational: '*Some children **feel** the magic wind over the mouth or nose as they blow it away, but most find that once we get started, before they know it, they are waking up in the recovery room or waking up room, surprised things went a little bit easier than they thought*'.

For some children it is best to avoid the word 'brave'. In general children are told they are brave before, or after, something bad happens. However, on occasion the child will proudly claim to be '*the bravest person in the hospital*' and calmly hold out an arm for the drip or blood test.

A pharmacological premedication may be useful for some children who are unresponsive to attempts at gaining rapport—for example, those with autism (see Chapter 13). Others will have had a premedication previously and the parents and/or the child may be asking for the same thing again. If there are clinical reasons that indicate this might not be the best option, it can be suggested that, '*Now the child is getting older, we often find things go a lot smoother whether a premed is given or not*'. Studies show that the anaesthetic visit can be equally effective as premedication when concerns are addressed and questions answered[4,5].

The importance of avoiding negative suggestions where possible cannot be overemphasized, when communicating with both parents and children. If, following questions from parents, you go into detail about the rest of the anaesthetic, be aware that little ears will be listening. Sometimes it is easier to send the child off to play. Otherwise you can end up with a child declaring, '*I don't want a tube in my throat*'.

> '*You will be asleep. You won't know about it*'.
> '*I don't want to go to sleep*'... tears.

There are two common concerns that older children express with direct questions or lie hidden behind anxiety; that they may wake up during the anaesthetic, or they may not wake up at the end of the procedure. The anaesthetist can casually say to the parent, in earshot of the child, '*I will be with him at all times to make sure he is safely asleep, and wakes up safely at the end*'.

Tacit agreement, Thanks, Termination

A physical touch for some parents can be helpful. A firm handshake with the father or a gentle pat on the shoulder, or a touch on the forearm of an anxious Mum, can be reassuring, but only if the anaesthetist is comfortable with this. The pre-anaesthesia consultation in some countries concludes with a symbolic signing of papers—an acknowledgement of a bilateral exchange of information and a contract of care—that is 'informed consent' (see Chapter 7).

The journey to theatre

The anaesthetist may not have much involvement in the physical voyage to the operating room but has already been integral to the start of this metaphorical journey (see Chapter 5). The communication along this path is often more structured. When the patient arrives in the holding area or is on transfer to the operating room, identification procedures, allergies and fasting times will be checked and rechecked. This repetition can be comforting to some parents and irritating to others. The physical surroundings of the journey can be utilized to develop a focus of attention, engagement and the development of a 'yes set' (see Chapter 4). Children can be encouraged to walk or pedal to theatre. The anaesthetist can 'seed' what is expected when reaching the operating room along the way such as '*Do you want to climb on to the bed all by yourself or get Mum to lift you up?*'— another double bind (see Chapter 4). Also one can use the curiosity of the child to engage them on the way. '*Can you see the fish swimming towards the MRI submarine?*' '*We are in theatre number 5; can you see the signs and help us find the way?*' '*When you are ready you can press the magic button to open the doors*'. This engages the child further and facilitates cooperation when the child reaches the operating room. Although the primary focus is the child, humour may be helpful for the anxious parent.

Induction of anaesthesia

The primary concerns of comfort and safety will be accomplished by allowing parents and their child to gain a sense of control as much as possible during this stressful time. The management of the induction has as many possibilities as there are parents, children, anaesthetists and anaesthetic nurses. Minimizing the number of people talking can be helpful. The presence of only one parent may help the child focus their attention rather than splitting between the two. The patient, one parent, one anaesthetist and one anaesthetic nurse are part of a team of players where the patient is the focus of attention. Whatever happens, the need for flexibility is essential as the anaesthetist engages with patient and parent as induction of anaesthesia progresses. Avoid having this focus divided if at all possible.

When the patient arrives, the anaesthetist can re-establish the contact made at the pre-anaesthetic interaction. The child can be introduced to the theatre team. For example, '*Lizzie this is John, he goes to St Mary's school*', or '*Lizzie this is John, he has asked for the strawberry flavour in the mask*'. This also introduces your assistant to the parent and it shows you were listening and have made the effort to personalize the child's anaesthetic. Sometimes deliberately getting the favourite colour wrong can engage the child when other strategies aren't working, as this redevelops a focus of attention as the anaesthetist accepts being corrected by the child. The anaesthetist can then check in at each stage as the various steps during the induction process take place.

The following are possible communication strategies during induction that are performed in suggested age ranges. On occasion these techniques may be equally applicable to children outside these ranges. Flexibility at all times will stand the paediatric anaesthetist in good stead, whatever the situation[6].

Inducing the clinging 2–4 year old

Sometime the focus of attention is intensely physical, with the child 'glued' to the parent and head tucked down. This can be accepted by sitting the parent on a chair with the child facing them, one leg on either side of their waist. Alternatively the child sits laterally with back to the table to facilitate the parent lifting the child onto the operating table after the initial induction of anaesthesia. In either position the child is either in direct eye contact with the parent or snuggled into the parent's chest. The parent can use their free hands to hold their child's hands if necessary. For a mask induction the anaesthetist can stand or kneel behind the child, either facing or behind the parent depending on how the child is seated. From this position the anaesthetist can bring the mask around from behind the child's head. If the child leans forwards towards their parent they lean into the mask. If they throw their head back the anaesthetist can support it and apply the face mask. This is a non-verbal communication accepting that all responses, be they positive or negative, can then be utilized further.

For an intravenous induction one of the child's hands can go over the parent's shoulder or under a parent's arm. The anaesthetist is then positioned behind the parent where the IV can be placed, out of sight. In these approaches it is important that only one person (usually the anaesthetist) is verbalizing. The parent, an anaesthetic assistant or anaesthetist can be the primary communicator depending on circumstance, through touch, eye contact and soothing words. The anaesthetist can verbalize but it is best not to request a response from either parent or child during the induction as this can divide the focus between them.

Communication can signal the anaesthetist's position and encourage any useful responses. A quiet monotonous voice or simple song or story frequently helps to calm both parent and child, plus information can be provided at the point of IV cannula insertion, that the child may or may not feel something.

The inquisitive 3–5 year old

The child in this age group may walk into the theatre with toy in one hand and parent's hand in the other. Some will prefer to sit on their parent's lap while others will tolerate lying on the bed with the parent nearby. Children are in danger of being overwhelmed by 'helpful' staff who want to say '*Hello*'. An induction room can be invaluable in minimizing outside distractions. If inductions always occur in theatre, it can be explained politely—preferably before the patient enters the operating room—that it would be appreciated if other staff go quietly about their business in the background. ('Below ten'; see Chapter 16).

The child can fit the mask and T-piece together themselves or place the pulse oximeter probe on their finger to engage them while at the same time promoting a sense of autonomy and control. Some anaesthetists encourage the child to paint the inside of the mask with a lip gloss with a flavour of their choice. Others may apply the mask either to their own face and pretend to breathe in, or to the parent—'*Try this Mum*'—as they offer the mask to the parent. Unfortunately, some parents grimace at this, giving the child the subconscious cue something smelly and bad is in the mask. An alternative strategy is to offer, in order, the choice of anaesthetist, child or parent to hold the mask. Invariably the child will choose the parent and will thereby have indicated an intention to cooperate with the induction.

Many anaesthetists use the balloon blowing technique for inhalational induction—'*When you blow in the mask the balloon will get bigger and bigger and bigger*'. This can be demonstrated by occluding the gas in the mask and letting the bag inflate. '*Now let's see what you can do!*' Many children will happily help the anaesthetist by holding on to their own mask, with a little direction on how to obtain a good seal. With the mask in place, the anaesthetist engages the child, re-enforcing blowing up the balloon by encouraging suggestions—for example, '*Well done, that's a really good breath, that's the biggest balloon so far*'. Alternatively the focus can be away from breathing, allowing 'closet singer' anaesthetists to display their talents with a favourite nursery rhyme.

Counting as a focus of attention

One technique that usually works well without mentioning the smell is to focus the child's attention by explaining to the child that the anaesthetist '*Will count your breaths up to the number 20 as you blow the balloon up. When I get to the number 20 two things happen. First, the balloon will change to your favourite colour. The second thing that you will notice is waking up in the recovery room with the operation finished and soon back with Mum*'.

The implicit suggestion is that the child is focused on getting to the number 20. It is therefore important not to get to '20' before the child is unconscious as focus may be lost at this point. If for some reason the child is still awake at 16, then continue counting more slowly or in fractions, such as 16 and ¼, 16 and a ½. The actual number the child is asked to focus on—but not count, is not important as it is a symbolic representation of an end-point of focus for the patient's perceptual experience. The actual induction involves letting the child practise blowing for 30 seconds or so (with an N_2O/O_2 mixture), before starting the count and with each counted breath turning the inhalational agent up a notch until it is at maximum on approximately the eighth counted breath.

As mentioned previously, children don't particularly like being told to go to sleep and fear a loss of control, so rather than say '*You will start feeling sleepy*', one could say, '*if you feel a bit sleepy you can relax back into the pillow*'. Direct suggestion may enable reinterpretation of unknown sensations that may otherwise be interpreted as unpleasant. For example, '*This sleepy medicine may look like milk, but sometimes it feels cool, like snow. If you feel that, you know it is working well!*'. Alternatively the 'sleep' word can be avoided altogether and a child reassured that they will be back with Mum or Dad.

Once the child is anaesthetized, it should be remembered to reassure the parent. It is important to avoid saying '*would you like to kiss your child goodbye?*' as this can indirectly imply death[6–8]. An alternative statement at this point might be, '*Thank you for your help. Would you like to give him a kiss? We will take care of him and get him back to you as soon as he is awake*'. This implies that the child will wake up and soon be back with the parent. It can be helpful, if the child is a good colour and breathing well, to show this to the parent indicating the moving breathing bag and skin colour, as evidence that all is well with their child.

If an IV induction agent is preferred a similar range of focusing techniques can be used such as story-telling, or singing a nursery rhyme. A 'lived in imagination' technique—guided imagery—can be used, such as asking the child to pretend to draw a picture. Asking what colour crayon the child ***is*** using, what part of the animal the child ***is*** colouring in and so on. If the child responds as if actually doing the activity, it is very likely the insertion of the drip cannula will not be noticed. It is still important to inform children that they may or may not feel something and, if it bothers them, to take a deep breath, without suggesting what to feel.

Children behaving badly

When things do not appear to be going well it is useful to stop whatever is happening and recognize that the situation is only temporary. A different approach can then be considered. Explanation and further encouragement usually facilitates cooperation, even if the tears continue. Children with previous anaesthetic experience can be provided with the control they need by holding the mask themselves or being allowed to tell the anaesthetist when they are ready—not for the IV cannula to be inserted—but for the insertion to be finished with!

The anaesthetist's expectations can sometimes get in the way of flexibility especially if the child has been labelled as 'difficult' or 'naughty' and does not accept a face mask or IV induction. Appreciating that there are always other choices and ways of doing things will usually avoid a battle of wills or an exercise in authority.

If the child is crying and fighting the mask before an inhalational induction has commenced, an IV cannula insertion can be offered as a less distressing alternative. Similarly, an apparently stoic adolescent who breaks into tears at the thought of a needle can be offered an inhalational induction. However, the anaesthetist should be aware that a good experience of having a painless IV cannulation can be an opportunity to build resilience rather than reinforce avoidance behaviours that may make future injections or anaesthetics even more stressful (see Chapter 14).

If the child refuses to allow the anaesthetist to proceed, a considered, flexible response is required. Sometimes, leaving the room to allow parent and child some space to discuss the situation resolves the difficulty. Oral or intranasal pharmacological support can also be offered. On occasion it may be appropriate to postpone or even cancel the procedure (see Case study 1).

The importance of talking directly to children regardless of their age cannot be overemphasized. Some clinical examples of how communicating effectively with children has enhanced their care are given below.

Case studies

Case study 1 The child refusing surgery—a lesson in competence, autonomy and control

An 8-year-old girl presented for adeno-tonsillectomy. She seemed cooperative and answered all the anaesthetist's questions appropriately and allowed auscultation of the chest without any particular persuasion. Her father was from former Yugoslavia and seemed to have an easy relationship with the child. On arrival at the anaesthetic room the child allowed an IV cannula to be inserted. As the anaesthetist picked up the syringe of propofol, the child stated that she did not want the surgery. The anaesthetist asked the child '*Why not?*' She replied that she had '*Not had an infection for the past three months and didn't need the operation any more*'. The father then insisted that the anaesthetist proceed. The child then stated to her father, '*Dad, you are not listening, look at me. I don't need the operation!*' On discussion with the surgeon it was decided not to proceed and the child was reviewed in outpatients six weeks later and no further surgery was thought to be indicated. This case emphasizes the importance of listening to young children who can, on occasion, demonstrate an ability to make logical, autonomous decisions regarding their care. Few children, however, can express it as well as the patient in this case.

Case study 2 The child with intellectual disability saying she didn't want the needle or the mask

This 10-year-old girl with Apert's syndrome presented to the anaesthetist in the pre-anaesthetic clinic for assessment prior to her MRI scan. Her mother stated that the anaesthetist '*Wouldn't get near her with a mask or needle*'. The anaesthetist asked the child what she liked doing and her favourite colour. She said, '*Watching Spongebob Squarepants*' and her chosen colour was '*green*'. The anaesthetist then stated that he had a magic balloon that could change colour to just the green that she wanted as he counted her breaths blowing up the 'magic balloon'. On arrival at the MRI suite the child was very apprehensive and initially was refusing to come in to the room. The anaesthetist then asked about Spongebob and whether there were any of Spongebob's friends that she liked. She was then given a 'double bind' (see Chapter 4) and asked whether she wanted to get Mum to lift her or whether she wanted to climb up all by herself now she was getting so grown up. She climbed on the bed and was pushing the mask away with both hands outstretched as the anaesthetist asked what Spongebob was doing, aiming to engage the child's imagination.

> **Patient:** '*He is cooking hamburgers*'.
> **Anaesthetist:** '*And is there any sauce while the hamburger is cooking?*'
> **Patient:** '*Tomato sauce*'.
> **Anaesthetist:** '*I wonder which hand is going to rest comfortably on your tummy first ... is it going to be this one or this one?*'

As the left hand relaxed its grip the anaesthetist encouraged its movement by saying '*That's right, well done, there it goes, well done, all on its own, all by itself resting comfortably on the tummy.... and I wonder when the next hand will follow its friend just like Spongebob's hands resting comfortably on his tummy or by his side while the hamburger is cooking*'.

Sevoflurane was then added to the gas mixture as the mask was moved in small increments nearer the face. As the mask was moved closer, the anaesthetist repeated how '*well the hamburger was cooking*' as the child blew the balloon up.

The child was induced smoothly, and during the induction it was emphasized to the child and mother how cooperative the child was, '*When Spongebob helped her blow the balloon up so it could change colour as she woke up in the recovery or waking up room*'.

In the above case, focus of attention was utilized initially by engaging with the child regarding her favourite TV character. Guided imagery was then utilized to encourage 'lived in imagination' where the child was asked what Spongebob was doing (see also Chapter 20). The child's response was that he was '*cooking hamburgers*'. This indicated that she was fully engaged in this fantasy. The anaesthetist then indirectly suggested that one or other of her arms could move to her abdomen in order to encourage the child's arm in a new direction away from pushing against the mask. The mask was reframed as something to blow in to, so that the balloon could change to her favourite colour (see also Chapters 2, 4 and 20).

Case study 3 The child left with a bad taste in her mouth

A 10-year-old girl weighing 39 kg presented for laparotomy and portocath CVC insertion under general anaesthesia, for translocation of the ovary prior to radiotherapy. When asked if she had any problems with her previous anaesthesia she replied that she didn't like them as she always woke up with a really bad taste in her mouth. She was then asked by the anaesthetist what her favourite food was and what she liked to eat when she was feeling well.

> **Patient:** '*Strawberries*'.
> **Anaesthetist:** '*Interestingly when children who like strawberries pretend to eat them before their operation they often wake up with a really pleasant delicious taste in their mouth*'.

This is an indirect suggestion (see Chapter 4) that if other children who like strawberries can wake up with a pleasant taste perhaps she can too.

> **Anaesthetist:** '*When I catch up with you later, I'll show you how you can look forward to having a really good taste and feel like eating and drinking as soon as you feel like it after the operation*'.

This statement creates a positive expectancy and seeds future communications that are likely to then function as positive suggestions.

In the operating theatre an hour later…

While the IV cannula was being inserted and the monitoring attached, the child was asked if it would be OK to start imagining eating some strawberries and ice cream. Following an affirmative response and a further 30 seconds she was asked whether she had eaten the whole strawberry or whether she had only had a bite.

> **Patient:** '*Just a bite*'.
> **Anaesthetist:** '*Is there any ice cream with it or is it just the strawberry on its own?*'

The anaesthetist encourages a 'lived in imagination' using the present tense '*Is there any ice cream?*' rather than asking whether the child is '*Imagining any ice cream?*'

> **Patient:** '*Both*'.
> **Anaesthetist:** '*How many strawberries are left in the bowl?*'
> **Patient:** '*10*'.
> **Anaesthetist:** '*You can carry on eating them throughout the surgery and wake up in recovery looking forward to eating and drinking as soon as you feel like it*'.

The anaesthetist gives an anti-emesis positive suggestion by suggesting that the child can eat and drink after surgery. Note, the anaesthetist did not say '*You won't feel sick or have a bad taste*'. As this would be a suggestion 'to be sick' and 'have a bad taste'.

The child woke up in the PACU and made an uneventful recovery. When questioned on the ward post-operatively, both parents and child voiced surprise at how well she had recovered and that she had had no unusual or unpleasant tastes after surgery unlike after her previous anaesthetics.

Case study 4 Utilizing 'concrete' thinking

Dr Marion Andrew provided the following case example.

A 7-year-old child on the operating table was asked by the anaesthetist as part of the pre-induction communication:

> **Anaesthetist:** '*Do you know how to go to sleep?*'
> **Child:** '*Close my eyes and stop talking*'

This is a 'concrete' interpretation of a previous communication from a parent.

> **Anaesthetist:** '*That's clever! Would you like to learn a different way of going to sleep?*'

This utilizes previously expressed ability, accepting that going to sleep is a skill. It also differentiates the sleep at home as something different from that here.

> **Child:** '*Yes*'.

The child appears pleased with being praised as clever and an uneventful inhalational induction follows.

Key points

1. There are numerous simple techniques that can help the anaesthetist care for children in ways that are likely to make their journey easier.
2. Difficult behaviours are usually temporary, and there is always another choice in the way communication can be used to engage the child.
3. Flexibility in approach is of the utmost importance.
4. The child's communication will guide the anaesthetist on how to communicate effectively.
5. A belief that the child can do more than he, his parents or the anaesthetist thinks he can, will frequently engender surprisingly useful responses that facilitate anaesthetic care.
6. Communicating in a way that respects the child's autonomy and need for control will usually facilitate cooperation and is well worth the effort.

References

1 Wood I (1997). Communicating with children in A & E: what skills does the nurse need? *Accid Emerg Nurs*, **5**(3), 137–41.

2 Cote CJ (1999). Preoperative preparation and premedication. *Br J Anaesth*, **83**(1), 16–28.

3 Yip P, Middleton P, Cyna AM, Carlyle AV (2009). Non-pharmacological interventions for assisting the induction of anaesthesia in children. *Cochrane Database Syst Rev* **3**:CD006447.

4 Calipel S, Lucas-Polomeni MM, Wodey E, Ecoffey C (2005). Premedication in children: hypnosis versus midazolam. *Paediatr Anaesth*, **15**, 275–81.

5 Egbert AM, Battit GE, Welch CE, Bartlett MK (1964). Reduction of postoperative pain by encouragement and instruction of patients. *N Engl J Med*, **270**, 825–7.

6 Carlyle AV, Ching PC, Cyna AM (2008). Communication during induction of paediatric anaesthesia: an observational study. *Anaesth Intensive Care*, **36**(2), 180–4.

7 Bjenke CJ (1996). Painful medical procedures. In: Barber J (ed.) *Hypnosis and suggestion in the treatment of pain: a clinical guide*. pp. 209–61. London: WW Norton.

8 Cyna AM, Andrew MI, Tan SGM (2009). Communication skills for the anaesthetist. *Anaesthesia*, **64**(6), 658–65.

Chapter 11

Critical care

Daniel Nethercott and Maire Shelly

'The problem with the world today is communication—too much communication!'
Homer Simpson

What this chapter is about

It is well recognized that errors of communication are associated with causing harm to patients on the Intensive Care Unit (ICU)[1]. By means of presenting a patient-based narrative, this chapter looks at communication in intensive care medicine focusing attention on styles of communication that are useful in different areas of common practice.

It must be accepted that communication needs to convey a message that sits within its own context. For instance, the way that proxy decisions are made for patients who lack capacity varies with both culture and region. Resources are variable, and this includes the time that can be allocated to communication. It is clearly beyond the scope of this chapter to offer guidance on exactly what information should be given to patients and their relatives, but we aim to highlight useful ways of making the communication of that information more effective.

Crisis situations

03:00 in a District General Hospital Emergency department. The on-call intensive care doctor is fast-bleeped to the resuscitation bay to see a 35-year-old man called Stephen who has been brought in by ambulance from a roadside accident. He is conscious but distressed, with significant injuries to both legs and thorax. A 'trauma team' of doctors is assembled, plus the delivering paramedics, accident and emergency-qualified nurses and healthcare assistants.

Communicating with teams in time-critical situations presents a clear challenge. Team members can be unknown to each other with an unknown skill mix, the clinical problems are undefined, different personnel have different—sometimes conflicting—motives, and goals, and clinical priorities can shift over time. The anaesthetist must be confident to communicate with authority in these circumstances. Under stress, most team members will respond well to someone else taking the lead. They will usually do what they are asked if they understand the instruction, are competent to undertake the task, and are not overloaded with other tasks.

Closed-loop communication is a good way to keep communication efficient: '*Someone get me a tube!*' can be misunderstood or ignored by most of the team.

'*Sarah, I want you to get a size 8 endotracheal tube from the trolley and test the cuff for me. Do you know how to do that?*' is specific, directed to a named individual and asks for confirmation of understanding and competence to complete the task.

'*Yes, I'll get you a size 8 tube*' closes the communication loop.

Some trauma teams use jackets which clearly identify the team members' roles, but this is not universal. It can save time and promote clarity to ask all members of the team to have their name badges visible during a resuscitation scenario.

Although the default should be to communicate to identified individuals, sometimes addressing the whole group is required. This needs authority expressed through tone of voice, clarity of speech and effective volume.

The anaesthetist may become aware of an impending crisis before the rest of the team. The aim is to re-focus the team to the acute change. Guidelines from the Difficult Airway Society (UK) for the management of failed direct laryngoscopy recommend that after three or four unsuccessful attempts, '*Failed direct laryngoscopy!*' should be announced to the assistant[2]. This allows the team to prepare to change strategy. Another example in a resuscitation scenario might be, '*I think he's about to arrest. Prepare for CPR!*' The situational awareness of the individual is thus spread to the team.

When leading a team, communication should be modulated to match the clinical situation. Keeping communication quiet, calm and encouraging whilst things are proceeding as expected allows for a contrast in volume and urgency when a crisis is encountered. Communication which is continuously at 'crisis pitch' quickly becomes background noise and loses impact. Similarly, a running commentary from the team leader can be successful in helping the team act cohesively with focused goals and priorities, but beware the commentary that becomes either repetitive or verbose. This style of communication can dominate the team and discourage other members from expressing themselves.

Debriefing teams is important after critical incidents. Unfortunately, it often only takes place after either an adverse incident or a bad patient outcome, but should be done more consistently. In a debrief, communication has to be changed from the authoritative, direct and specific style that suits the acute situation to being more open and gentle. Most medical debriefing happens informally. Unless there are serious concerns about a team member's performance (which might require further action) then debriefing is most successful when it is relaxed and chatty. It is more common to have to reassure team members that they did well, and that the poor outcome was not their personal fault, than to have to encourage insight into unseen failings.

Prioritizing communication

Emergency situations require tasks to be effectively prioritized, and this includes communication. No communication is wasted, but on occasions can distract from other more important tasks or generate damaging emotional responses in the clinician that, once recognized, can be stopped and re-directed.

A junior surgical trainee wants to insert a urinary catheter into the patient and asks the nurse to set up the equipment; however, the anaesthetist is preparing to intubate and decides that the catheter can wait.

Anaesthetist: '*I think the catheter can wait until we've got the airway sorted out*'.
Junior surgeon: '*But we need to assess his urine output*'.
Anaesthetist: '*That's important, and you can do it once we've got him asleep and his airway is secure*'.
Junior surgeon: '*We need to know how well we've resuscitated him. I think I should put in a catheter now*'.
Anaesthetist: '*You can do it after I've intubated*'.
Junior surgeon: '*It won't take long…*'
Anaesthetist: '*You can do it after I've intubated*'.
Junior surgeon: '*If we just get the trolley now…*'
Anaesthetist: '*You can do it after I've intubated*'.

This technique is called 'Broken Record'. It involves consistent repetition of the same phrase in the same tone of voice and meter using exactly the same words. Even though it should be conducted with a calm and neutral attitude it is in reality potentially aggressive as it presents a brick wall in terms of communication. It says, '*I'm not willing to communicate at the moment*'. The other party will often re-phrase what they are saying or shift subject to try to negotiate out of the cul-de-sac they find themselves in. 'Broken Record' is a technique that requires a certain degree of steeliness to carry through and also good judgement. In the wrong context it can escalate a situation inappropriately.

A softer approach is to show that the behaviour is unwanted by stressing the emotional effect it is having and then proposing an alternative, such as, '*Talking about the catheter with you like this makes me worried that I can't concentrate on drawing up the anaesthetic drugs. Shall we talk about it in a few minutes when I have finished?*'

An alternative communication utilizing the '**LAURS**' concept (see Chapter 2) might be as follows:

> **Anaesthetist:** '*I think the catheter can wait until we've got the airway sorted out*'.
> **Junior surgeon:** '*But we need to assess his urine output*'.
> **Anaesthetist:** '*That's important, and you can do it once we've got him asleep and his airway is secure*'.
> **Junior surgeon:** '*We need to know how well we've resuscitated him. I think I should put in a catheter now*'
> **Anaesthetist:** '*OK why don't you go and wash your hands and put some gloves on, by which time the patient's airway should be secure*'.
> **Junior surgeon:** '*OK*'.

Listening to the surgeon allows the anaesthetist to ***accept*** his reality even if not agreeing with it. It can then be ***utilized*** by giving the surgeon something to do that allows him to move towards his goal of catheterizing the patient, while, at the same time, allowing the anaesthetist to secure the airway uninterrupted.

Handover

Stephen is stabilized in the Emergency Department. Bilateral chest drains are inserted, he is intubated and ventilated and then taken to CT scan. This shows lung contusions and splenic injury. He is taken to theatre where he undergoes splenectomy and open reduction and internal fixation of a femoral fracture and compound tibial fracture. He requires a massive blood transfusion. He is admitted to the ICU post-operatively, ventilated and sedated, and the theatre team hand over to the intensive care team.

Handover should be considered as a risky procedure that poses a threat to the patient. The more handovers the patient has, the greater the likelihood of information being altered or omitted. Altered information can have serious consequences, and direct patient harm is not uncommon[1].

A hospital in the UK changed its handover process after an analysis conducted by a member of a Formula One motor racing team who specialized in training mechanics working under high pressure in the 'pit stop'[3]. The changes which reduced handover errors included: communication between matching professionals—that is, nurse to nurse, anaesthetist to anaesthetist, surgeon to surgeon; categorization of information—for instance, by body systems such as airway, breathing, circulation, microbiology, etc.; and a check of the success of the communication by the receiving team member repeating back the information.

The handover should be respected as an important but vulnerable process. There should be minimal interruptions or distractions, and it should not be cut short for the sake of expediency. Sometimes handovers between medical teams can lose focus and actually become debriefing sessions or 'story-telling'. Debriefing has an important role, but it should not subvert the function of the handover, which is to communicate the information needed to continue patient care.

Meetings with relatives

Stephen's family is waiting in the Intensive Care relatives' room to be spoken to by the on-call doctor. Present are his mother and father, his sister and three of his friends, one of whom was involved in the accident but was relatively unharmed.

There is very little advice from professional bodies on how much to say to the relatives of patients who lack the capacity to decide who they wish medical details to be disclosed to. In the UK the General Medical Council guidance on communicating medical information to relatives only states that '*consideration and sensitivity*' be used[4]. It is a fair assumption that in most cases critically ill patients would want their close relatives to be kept informed about their condition, and so communicating with relatives could be viewed as acting in the patient's interests. However, this assumption will not always be correct.

A discussion of whether the clinician has a duty of care to relatives is beyond the scope of this chapter, but an interesting development in this regard is a civil action against a UK hospital for post-traumatic stress disorder (PTSD) suffered by the husband of a patient and claimed to have been caused by inadequately communicated information. The case did not make it to court[5].

Judgements must be made in individual cases with regard to the principle of maintaining patient confidentiality. Particular care should be taken with information that is more likely to be sensitive or secret, but remember that issues which might objectively be considered trivial or non-sensitive may not be so to the patient or to their family. The overall seriousness of the clinical circumstances combined with closeness of the relative to the patient usually informs how much information should be given, but this will vary and must be adapted to culturally accepted norms.

A truly structured approach to these meetings can be difficult as the clinician has to respond to the unfolding communication fluently and instinctively, but these meetings often have a natural progression through distinct phases.

Using 'GREAT' to structure the interaction

Greeting, Goals

Be certain of who you are speaking to. Asking relatives to introduce themselves is not merely courteous, but also gives useful clues to their individual emotional state and to the dynamic of the group.

Rapport

This can be misinterpreted as meaning that the clinician is striving for popularity or friendliness with the relatives, but this is not always desirable and not unequivocally suited to all situations. Rapport is really about establishing a mutually agreeable 'tone' for the dialogue to progress in. The '**LAURS**' principles aid the development of rapport in that they help the clinician attune to the 'voice' of the relatives and modulate their own tone in response.

Evaluation, Expectations, Explanation

Decide on the degree of detail of the information you are imparting before you begin. Beware information overload during the first meeting. If the relatives seem not to understand, then repeat the same message in simpler terms. Avoid the temptation to respond to confusion by giving more and more information.

Asking and Answering questions, Acknowledging and Addressing concerns

See 'Do you have any questions?' in this chapter.

Tacit agreement, Thanks, Termination

Summing up the very essence of what has been said in one or two sentences aims at allowing the relatives to leave with at least a fundamental message. It is often stated that people only remember 5% of what they have been told. Let that 5% be an important element.

It is common to be faced with a room full of relatives, some of whom may not have a close relationship to the patient or to each other, and it is difficult—if not impossible—to tease out the exact nature of the relationship for every single person who might visit the unit. When faced with large groups, it is probably advisable to err on the side of non-disclosure of all but the most basic of information so as to respect patient confidentiality. The clinician should be confident to take an authoritative position and, if required, then make the group smaller. Establishing chosen representatives to receive information can resolve this issue. Close relatives can then make judgements on how best to disseminate information to the wider group.

Using 'SPIKES' to structure the interaction

Another template useful in these situations is called '**SPIKES**' (**S**etting, **P**erception, **I**nvitation, **K**nowledge, **E**motions, **S**ummary and plan) which has been developed for the breaking of bad news[6] (see Chapter 12), but is applicable to general consultations and can illustrate an approach to communicating with a group.

Setting

This applies to the physical environment of the meeting, the preparation (such as avoiding interruptions) and the introductions, with establishing rapport. As above, the introductions will give immediate clues to the overall dynamics. Often, individuals introduce themselves, but occasionally there is an introducer and, if so, then this is a useful sign that this person is appointing him or herself 'chairman' for the group.

Perception

This is the '*What do you know so far?*' stage. The first responder to this question often emerges as the primary 'information giver'. Others may then fill in details or even present an alternative story. This is an important stage for developing rapport and further establishing the group roles.

Invitation

This stage presents the answer to '*How much do you want to know?*' In groups, each member may have a different answer to this question and it is often easier to identify a start point at this stage and calibrate the amount of information in proceeding through the next stage. The primary 'information receiver' can often be identified at this point.

Knowledge

This is the information-giving stage. Information can be presented to the 'information receiver' though it is important to scan the entire group to check understanding. It is particularly important to check that the 'information giver' understands what is being said as it is most likely to be this person who disseminates information to others.

Emotions

Consultation is not just about giving information, but also about understanding and acknowledging the emotional response to the information. '*How do you feel about this?*' is a very direct way to elicit the emotional response. Less direct alternative statements such as '*I imagine this has come as a shock...*' perform the same function (also see 'Silence and empathy' below). Another important group member can become evident here—the 'emotional responder'—who will express emotion for the group. Often other group members will comfort, collude with or deny this individual. The group might find it difficult to move to the next stage until this person's emotions are under control.

Summary and plan

This is where the conversation is summarized and the next steps are explained. All group members should be involved in this, particularly the 'information receiver'. The final element is ending the conversation; at this point the 'chairman' should again be involved to ensure conversation structure is maintained.

Group dynamics can be highly variable: sometimes one member occupies all the roles, at other times each role is taken by a separate individual. Attending to a group dynamic in this way means that the clinician will be likely to be in rapport with the most effective member of the group at each stage and that communication is optimized. Talking to large groups can be a daunting prospect, but the needs of the whole group can be met by communicating with each 'role player' in turn as an individual, and thus the clinician feels less like a lecturer addressing an audience.

Recording and relaying communication

Good medical records are as vital to good continuing communication as they are to continuing patient care. The medico-legal importance of full contemporaneous records of communication is well illustrated by the case of PTSD mentioned above, where the quality of documentation of the communication formed a central part of the case for the defence. Communicating important issues with families is more effective if it is longer and allows more time for them to talk[7], and so full transcripts would be impossible in normal clinical practice. However, all key messages should be recorded. The level of understanding should be assessed and recorded. Verbatim quotes are helpful.

Continuity of message is important. This can be achieved through careful and comprehensive handover of what has been communicated. Some ICUs use specific communication forms in the patient notes with spaces for separate themes or

Intensive Care Unit Communication Sheet

Date: 11/4/09 Time: 08:30

Patient Name: Stephen Smith Hospital number: 234567

Present:

M. Smith (mother), D. Smith (father), F. Smith (sister), J. ?Clements (friend, in the car), 2 other friends (?names), R. Pandit (Nurse, ICU). Dr Evans (Cons), Dr Hussein (Registrar).

Information given:

Punctured lung, damaged spleen, broken leg, long/combined operation. Now sedated, try to wake up later depending on lungs/oxygen levels.

Level of understanding:

Good understanding of injuries and operation.
Probably underestimating extent of injury/speed of recovery.
Friend also involved upset++

Conclusions/Comments/Problems:

Updates PRN, No major issues.

Signed: R. Evans, 11/4/9

Fig. 11.1 Intensive Care Unit communication sheet.

messages, equivalent to system-based daily intensive care review forms for patients. These forms can prompt the recording of information which might be forgotten such as exactly who was spoken to and what their subjective level of understanding was. Different messages from different members of staff increase stress in family members[8]. Figure 11.1 shows an example of an ICU communication template that can be used as an aid to continuity and consistency of message when communicating with patients and their relatives. Note that the notation of non-technical language used serves to aid congruence.

In situations where communication becomes very difficult between staff and relatives, such as conflict over plans of management with major clinical consequences, then it can be useful to have one clinician to act as lead communicator. The perception '*they don't know what they are doing*' that results from discordant inter-physician messages can thus be decreased.

It is also useful to pre-empt confusion about the fact that the clinical condition of critically ill patients can change very quickly and that a different message from one moment to the next does not mean a difference of opinion amongst staff.

Silence and empathy

Silence can feel uncomfortable to the lead communicator in a dialogue, but families need time to absorb messages. Critical illness is neither planned for nor welcome.

What they are hearing usually represents a cardinal life event, something shocking and tragic that they are likely never to forget. For the clinician, however, the same meeting is a part of the working day. Most doctors will have experienced some family encounters that affected them emotionally more than others, but there is always an 'emotion gap' between the relatives and the doctor.

Expressions of empathy are important to relatives, but must be well judged to avoid inappropriate intimacy and maintain professionalism. A well-observed silence after the communication of serious, life-changing news is a good way to express empathy without risking insincerity. It marks the gravity of what has just been said and it can be an effective way to draw speech from others. Remember that the perception of time is altered in states of high emotion, and what the doctor feels to be a long silence will feel shorter to the relatives (see Chapter 4).

When actively expressing empathy many doctors fear appearing glib and so might tend toward a very clinical manner to avoid this. Of course, it is important to be true to one's own nature; a forced or sentimental statement will be at best awkward and at worst insulting.

One method to strike an acceptable balance is to use empathic words, but to use them in an indirect context. Rather than, '*I'm sorry for what has happened to Stephen*', which is a direct expression of empathy, '*I'm sorry to have to be so blunt with the facts of what has happened*', contains the subtext '*I'm sorry*', but is slightly more oblique.

'Do you have any questions?'

Consider the following paraphrased communication:

> '*Hello, I am Dr Evans... information, information, information, percentage, information, ratio, information, information, uncertainty, information, likelihood, unknown word, confusing metaphor, information, information... Do you have any questions?*'

The answer invariably is '*No*', probably because what has just been said is quite a challenging phrase. It carries the undertone of being a test of the listener. The answer '*Yes, I do have a question*' is either an accusation that the message has been poorly communicated or that the listener has failed to listen properly, neither of which wants to be admitted. '*Do you have any questions?*' is also heard as a conclusion and implies that the process of information giving has finished.

It is important to check the understanding of listeners in some way to find out what has been heard and so correct any misinterpretation. This can be done more effectively by a phrase simply designed to let them speak. Rather than the challenge of '*Do you have any questions?*', eliciting an emotional response to the information and acknowledging that the information itself is complex gives a more welcome space for them to articulate themselves:

> '*This must be a terrible shock*',
> '*I'm sure this is all very confusing*',
> '*That's a lot of information to take in, isn't it?*'
> '*I can see that what I've said is not what you expected*',
> '*Were you expecting me to say something different?*'

'*Do you have any questions?*' can work as part of the conclusion or summary of the conversation, but it is not likely to be fruitful whilst an emotional reaction is still forthcoming.

The ICU patient with a tracheostomy

Stephen has been on the ICU for eleven days. He has developed an acute lung injury after his initial operation and associated blood transfusion. Respiratory weaning has been slow and his progress has been hampered by poor tolerance of the oro-tracheal tube. A tracheostomy tube is sited, allowing the sedation to be stopped and consciousness to return fully.

One of the advantages of tracheostomies in the management of intensive care patients is to allow for sedation to be reduced and thus communication will be more likely. However, the tracheostomy itself is a barrier to communication in that it interferes with vocalization. There is a common subconscious bias that means when someone cannot speak they are less likely to be spoken to. Perhaps communication is avoided when it is known that it will be difficult. Not being able to verbalize is tremendously frustrating, and writing messages down, using communication boards or electronic systems are poor substitutes for speech. A sad but common sight is the patient who gives up after the clinician, who is trying to lip-read, has repeatedly mistaken their words. In this situation a closed question will often get to the point more quickly than an open one. '*Is the pain worse when you're being turned?*' allows a nod or a thumbs up, rather than '*Tell me about the pain*'.

The limiting effect on communication that tracheostomies have can be very burdensome for patients. It is important to emphasize that it will be removed as soon as possible and that it is performing a useful role in helping the patients get better. There is a risk that patients become de-motivated, and a downward spiral of non-communication develops. Change to a tube that allows speech as soon as possible. In the meantime acknowledge the frustration, use non-verbal adjuncts and avoid the bias that '*can't speak equals can't hear*' by making deliberate regular efforts to communicate simple and routine information about their progress.

Withdrawing life-prolonging treatment

Stephen has been on intensive care for 26 days. Weaning from the ventilator has been prolonged and he has lost much of his body mass. He develops pneumonia and, despite antibiotics, this progresses to severe sepsis. He soon becomes unresponsive to high doses of vasopressors. Oliguric renal failure and thrombocytopenia develop. The next day he is noted to have fixed and dilated pupils. A CT scan reveals haemorrhage in the midbrain. There is a consensus reached amongst the treating team that limitation of therapeutic effort and progression to end-of-life care is appropriate.

Communicating the withdrawal of therapeutic effort is not the only discussion that is important on the ICU, but it can be a complex message and so is a good example to take. The principles involved can be translated to meetings with other themes. Although this often takes the form of 'breaking bad news', one should recognize that it might not actually be perceived as bad news. Relatives *can* express great relief that the time has come for palliation.

The response to the message can vary greatly, which makes the 'check of understanding' or 'evaluation' phase paramount. Certainly it is a failure of the communication if the relatives don't understand that death is inevitable. A common misunderstanding is that the option being presented is between life and death, rather than the true option being the optimal management of inevitable progression toward the end of life.

Of course, limitation of therapeutic effort should only be decided on the patients' behalf when they cannot make that decision themselves and when there is enough certainty that death is indeed inevitable. The degree of certainty should be communicated. That all avenues have been explored and all opinions sought should be said explicitly. If the decision to withdraw therapy is made by the physicians, as is commonly the case in the UK model of decision making, then this should be conveyed. Relatives should not be left to believe that they alone are making a proxy decision on this issue.

Lack of understanding of even fundamental issues at the first consultation is common in the relatives of intensive care patients,[9] and the clinician should strive for absolute clarity on the underlying message. If the message is, '*He is going to die, regardless of what we are doing for him*', then this message should be made up of unequivocal words. A consultant in emergency medicine once told the friend of a man who had suffered an out-of-hospital cardiac arrest that the patient had '*passed away*' to then be immediately asked '*Do you think there's any hope for him, doctor?*'

'*Death*', '*die*' or '*dying*' are clear, and, once understood, the clinician can substitute softer or more sensitive phrases such as '*passed away*' or '*passed on*'.

Being positive in a bleak situation

Some clinicians feel it very important to be explicit on the details of withholding cardiopulmonary resuscitation (CPR) when explaining withdrawal of therapy, but this can be unhelpful and even confusing to relatives, and so great care should be taken.

'*If his heart stops then we don't think its right to jump up and down on his chest or give him any electric shocks*' was said by a senior trainee in intensive care to a patient's wife. She seemed to have no idea that this referred to the process of advanced life support and was clearly nonplussed. It was bizarre to have had described such a strange process with no reference to its aim, and then be told that this process *will not* be applied to your loved one.

Raising the potential for a therapy by explaining it and then snatching it away by telling the relatives that it is futile can lead the meeting into a very bleak landscape. Explaining that medical treatment is considered futile and that extreme measures are not appropriate should ***always*** pave the way for talk of what ***will*** be done. Withdrawal of treatment is often conveyed with a negative pitch, which is a natural gravitation in the context, but positive themes can still be brought to the fore when discussing death.

An unsolicited list of all the things that are sometimes done in the aim of organ support such as mechanical ventilation, haemofiltration, inotropic therapy, etc., but which are thought to be futile in this case, and which will not be continued or embarked upon, can build up a picture of impenetrable hopelessness. Very many relatives have no idea what such therapies involve or achieve. Clearly, some relatives have specific queries about specific treatments, and these should be addressed, but although the technicality of providing critical care is important and interesting to the practitioner, it is only uncommonly so to the relative.

Beware that the attempt to 'cover' oneself by explaining every possible option of medical management does not automatically result in a relative being 'informed'. Indeed, the opposite is more likely. Sometimes clinicians run through the options for medical management and the reasons why these will not be effective as a way to openly affirm the decision to withdraw. This can become a process of self-soothing for the doctor at the cost of leaving the relative confused.

Positivity and hope may seem perverse when death is deemed inevitable, but the communication can be done with positive language and hopeful messages. Hope in the face of calamity is a fundamental human quality. To completely crush the natural hope of the family in crisis threatens their trust and belief in the doctor. Honesty and clarity about the negligible chance of survival are vital, but hope can be re-directed. False hope for a miracle cure can be maladaptive and distract relatives from psychological preparation for the impending death.

If re-directed towards hoping for an achievable goal, then hope itself is maintained. Good quality palliative care is by no means universal on intensive care, but it is certainly an achievable goal. The negative instruction 'Do Not Resuscitate' is being replaced in some areas with the more neutral phrase 'Allow Natural Death'.

Non-abandonment is a crucial concept to convey to relatives. It means that although certain *treatments* might be withheld or withdrawn, *care* certainly is not. When this is turned into a positive aspect of the communication of withdrawal it serves as a good conclusion to the meeting.

The decision to withdraw life-sustaining therapy from Stephen is explained to his family by the intensive care consultant. The discussion is concluded:

> ***'This is a really important decision, but now that everyone who is caring for Stephen is clear that we can't get him better, we will be really focused on keeping him as comfortable as we can and letting his death be as dignified as possible, with whoever he might wish to be near him to be there if they want'.***

Again this emphasizes what ***can*** be done (comfort and dignity) and not what can't or won't. It suggests that care will still continue—*'we will be really focused'*, that everyone caring for him agrees, and that the family are an important part of our consideration. The decision to concentrate on the things that matter, and not be distracted by treatments that don't matter, or won't influence the outcome, is put in a good light. The decision in itself is important. It has been made on the patient's behalf and it will result in positive things happening.

The fear of abandonment is commonly expressed when approaching the end of life. Non-abandonment should be conveyed whether the relatives explicitly state it or not, and it can be done in different ways. Evidence from the analysis of recorded family conferences suggests doctors use three modes of expressing non-abandonment[10].

'*We will not abandon your relative*' is rarely stated explicitly. The description of maintaining comfort by treating pain and agitation properly implies that care will continue. The promise of continuing accessibility—for example, '*We're here 24 hours a day, there's always a nurse by the bed, and the doctors work only on the ICU so are close at hand*' said to the family implies that the patient is not being forgotten. The offer to make sure that relatives can be with the patient if they wish at either a point of deterioration or death—'*Have we got your contact details up to date, so we can call you if there's any change?*'—carries the message that the family is still valued and that they are not being abandoned either.

Patients from whom curative and supportive treatment is being withdrawn with the move to end-of-life care are sometimes discharged to ward areas rather than cared for on the ICU, usually for many clinical and organizational reasons. Regardless of the patient's destination these can both be given a positive presentation.

> '*Intensive care is a good place for him to be. He's got his own nurse and there are always doctors on hand to make sure he gets any medication he might need*'.
>
> '*He's got a bed on the ward, which will be quieter for the family; less noise and a bit more privacy, too. We'll hand over to the ward doctors, so they know how we've been treating his discomfort*'.

This might seem too much like 'political spin' on two opposing policies, but both statements can be true and delivered with sincerity. Although the message of non-abandonment is implicit, it is clear even with discharge from the ICU.

Personalizing communication

Patients should always be the centre of the communication. Referring to them by name or specific status (e.g. '*your son*') helps confirm this. The ICU is renowned for being a busy place with high demand on its resources, and families may easily be aware of 'bed-status' issues. The doctor should quickly and assuredly dissipate any misapprehension that the process of withdrawal is because of lack of beds or the rationing of any other resource, or indeed that subsequent organ donation has any influence on the decision. In fact, it is paramount that consideration of potential organ donation is clearly separated from issues such as withdrawal of care and resource management.

Active listening should be employed to allow the family to tell you about their loved one who is near death. The doctor is the expert on the condition of the patient and their treatment, but the relative is the expert regarding the patient before they became a patient. As well as seeking out narrow information, such as pre-existing attitudes to intensive care or pre-morbid exercise tolerance, it can be fruitful to ask open questions.

'*What was he like before all this happened?*' can open up a torrent of heartfelt anecdotes about the patient's sense of humour, kindness, free spirit and independence. The conclusion that '*This isn't what he would have wanted*' often spontaneously follows. Small insights into the patient's life can raise empathy in the doctor, and empathic body language is a common progenitor of rapport. A family that feels you've listened to them talk about their relative will have more faith in the strength of your judgement. Actively eliciting and listening to these stories is usually time well spent.

Bereavement interviews

Very often our contact with the relatives of our patients ends when the patient has been discharged or dies. Bereavement interviews should perhaps be considered part of the normal process of communication.

Although personal experience suggests that many relatives do not take up the offer of a bereavement interview, for those that do fundamental misunderstandings can be cleared up in a small amount of time. Explanations can be given, such as the details of the death certificate. Distressing concerns can be explored, such as perhaps that the patient could have survived if something else had been done, or that they died in pain. Those relatives that do attend often give good feedback on the care their loved one received, which is good for staff morale, and occasionally they recommend improvements that could be made in the future.

Interpreters

Communicating through a translator is fraught with potential for error. Although it is often recommended not to use family members to act as translators, this can be unavoidable in emergency situations. Independent, professional interpreters are not always readily available even in office hours. It should be accepted that using family members or friends as interpreters increases the potential for misunderstandings and may inadvertently precipitate family conflict. The translator may unwittingly misunderstand or mistranslate, and there always exists the potential for them willingly to attenuate or distort the message for personal motives, both benign (protecting the receiver of the translation from distress) and less benign (holding information as power). Ad hoc translators, such as relatives, nurses or social workers, are more likely to make errors than professional translators, and these errors have a high chance of clinical significance[11].

Translation is rarely a perfect process. Consider this extreme example of a translation that completely inverts the intended message:

A meeting is held between two diplomats to discuss trade between their countries. The first diplomat wants to convey his country's intention to cooperate fully with trade agreements: '*Our governments both think along parallel lines*', he says. The translator says: '*Our policy and your policy will never meet each other*'!

Good translation conveys not only the content of the message, but also the meaning and the tone. There are different cultural responses to issues commonly seen in intensive care, such as patient autonomy versus paternalism in the doctor–patient relationship, acceptance of death and palliation versus active treatment at all cost. As well as interpreting words, translators are likely to be acting as cultural buffers to some extent.

When using professional interpreters it is worth briefing the translator before the translation takes place as to the factual content of what is to be said and the ***meaning*** of what you want to convey. The bare facts must be communicated, but just as important are other non-factual themes, such as the severity and seriousness of the situation or the degree of uncertainty of a diagnosis or prognosis.

When breaking bad news, it helps the translator if they can prepare themselves to deliver it in a controlled way. A survey of professional medical interpreters showed a pre-translation briefing to be recommended, as well as an explicit instruction either to translate in a literal manner or to allow cultural brokering[12]. It is also worth considering a post-translation debrief to get an idea of the translator's view of the success of the translation, and potentially address their emotional response to having delivered serious news. The use of a translator uses up time, and the overall amount of clinical information may be smaller because of this. Clinicians have also been shown to provide less emotional support to the family when talking via an interpreter[13].

Despite the use of a professional interpreter, errors in communication are still commonplace. In a study of ten family meetings of relatives of ICU patients conducted through professional interpreters, an alteration occurred in 55% of passages of speech. Seventy-seven per cent of these alterations were deemed to be clinically significant in affecting the goals of the meeting, the majority having a potentially negative effect[14].

If no pre-translation meeting can be organized then speak slowly and in short sentences to give the translator time. Translating large portions of information in real time can lead to omissions which are clinically important. If it appears that the relative is responding in an unusual way to information given, such as not showing the expected emotional response, then strongly consider whether the message has been successfully conveyed or not. Equally, an unusual question or comment may be the result of an error of translation rather than representing a true concern.

Unintended communication

Although we often worry that patients and relatives aren't getting the message, too often they are getting messages, but messages we did not intend to give. An awake, agitated and mildly hypoxic patient is having a CVC placed by a doctor, with another doctor observing.

Doctor 1 (observing): '*… there has been a lot of staff sickness this week….*'
Doctor 2 (inserting line): '*I know, I was doing a vascular list yesterday and there was no trainee with me, which was a real shame*'.
Patient: '*You haven't had any vascular training! Do you know what you're doing?*'

Clearly there is misinterpretation of the conversation, and what is being said has no relevance to the patient. Acute psychological distress can result in hypervigilance with enhanced sensory sensitivity and heightened attention to environmental threats. This can lead to a state of paranoia—not paranoia in a persecutory sense, but in its true meaning of believing that everything in the world pertains to oneself. It would be natural to think that the doctor who is treating you is talking about you and, when further distorted through the fog of critical illness, an aberrant reception of what is being communicated is almost inevitable.

This phenomenon can also affect the family. The stress of having a critically ill relative is considerable, and it does not necessarily reduce over time. Watch the way that the relatives by the bedside react acutely to the persistently chiming alarms that are merrily ignored by staff. Anxiety correlates with cognitive biases such as tending to interpret neutral information as being negative and increasing attention toward threatening or negative perceptions. These biases occur at a subconscious level via an automatic evaluation mechanism that registers emotionally significant cues. Attentional vigilance increases exponentially in high anxiety states[15].

Staff members should always remember this. Relatives and awake patients often feel starved of information and they can pick up any scraps available. Messages which are objectively neutral or insignificant can be perceived as significant and negative. Body language and tone of voice are particularly important at the end of the bed. Communication cannot simply be delivered in neat aliquots when it suits staff who should consider themselves to be communicating all the time by the bedside.

Discussion of other patients, disparaging remarks about colleagues and dressing down of juniors within earshot erode trust and respect. An attitude of thoughtfulness, diligence and care provides indirect but positive communication, and these are basic components of professionalism. Actors are told that even though they may not be delivering their lines centre stage, even though they might be at the back in the shadows, someone in the audience will be watching them.

Key points

1. Emergency situations require tasks to be effectively prioritized and this includes communication.
2. Handovers are risky procedures and the more handovers the patient has the greater the likelihood of information being altered or omitted. There should be minimal interruptions or distractions, and they should not be cut short for the sake of expediency.
3. When talking to relatives on the ICU, beware of information overload. Repeat the same message in simpler terms. Avoid the temptation to respond to confusion by giving more and more information.
4. Different messages from different members of staff increase stress in family members. Specific communication forms can prompt the recording of information which might be forgotten, such as exactly who was spoken to and what their subjective level of understanding was.
5. A well-observed silence after the communication of serious news is a good way to express empathy without risking insincerity, marks the gravity of what has just been said and is an effective way to draw speech from others.
6. We should consider ourselves to be communicating all the time by the bedside. Discussion of other patients, disparaging remarks about colleagues and dressing down of juniors within earshot erodes trust and respect.

References

1 Reader T W, Flin R, Cuthbertson BH (2007). Communication skills and error in the intensive care unit. *Curr Opin Crit Care*, **13**, 732–6.

2 Henderson JJ, Popat MT, Latto IP, Pearce AC (2004). Difficult Airway Society guidelines for management of the unanticipated difficult intubation. *Anaesthesia*, **59**(7), 675–94.

3 Anon (2008). Improving safety of handovers. *Clin Serv J*, **7**(10), 52–4.

4 GMC (2006). *Good medical practice*. London: General Medical Council.

5 Bodenham AR, Bell D (2008). Communication with next-of-kin: a trigger for PTSD, a cause for compensation? *J Intensive Care Soc*, **9**(3), 255–8.

6 Baile WF, Buckman R, Lenzi R, Glober G, Beale EA, Kudelka AP (2000). SPIKES—a six-step protocol for delivering bad news: application to the patient with cancer. *Oncologist*, **5**(4), 302–11,

7 Curtis JR, White DB (2008). Practical guidance for evidence-based ICU family conferences. *Chest*, **134**, 835–43.

8 Pochard F, Azoulay E, Chevret S, Lemaire F, Hubert P, Canoui P et al (2001). Symptoms of anxiety and depression in family members of intensive care unit patients: ethical hypothesis regarding decision making capacity *Crit Care Med*, **29**(10), 1893–7.

9 Azoulay E, Chevret S, Leleu G, Pochard F, Barboteu M, Adrie C et al (2000). Half the families of intensive care unit patients experience inadequate communication with physicians. *Crit Care Med*, **28**(8), 3044–9.

10 West HF, Engelberg RA, Wenrich MD, Curtis JR (2005). Expressions of nonabandonment during the intensive care unit family conference. *J Palliat Med*, **8**(4), 797–807.

11 Flores G, Laws MB, Mayo SJ, Zuckerman B, Abreu M, Medina L et al (2003). Errors in medical interpretation and their potential clinical consequences. *Pediatrics*, **111**(1), 6–15.

12 Norris WM, Wenrich MD, Nielsen EL, Treece PD, Jackson JC, Curtis JR (2005). Communication about end of life care between language-discordant patients and clinicians: insights from medical interpreters. *J Palliat Med*, **8**(5), 1016–24.

13 Thornton JD, Pham K, Engelberg RA, Jackson JC, Curtis JR (2009). Families with limited English proficiency receive less information and support in interpreted intensive care unit family conferences. *Crit Care Med*, **37**(1), 89–95.

14 Pham K (2008). Alterations during medical interpretation of ICU Family Conferences that interfere with or enhance communication. *Chest*, **134**(1), 109–18.

15 Mathews A (1997). Cognitive biases in anxiety and attention to threat. *Trends Cogn Sci*, **1**(9), 340–5.

Chapter 12

When bad things happen

Diana C Strange Khursandi

'Though it be honest, it is never good to bring bad news'.
William Shakespeare

What this chapter is about

When bad things happen, good communication skills and honesty are of supreme importance. Breaking bad news to patients, relatives or staff is never easy. Anaesthetists are most familiar with imparting bad news when they are working in a critical care unit, where the possibility of bad news is implicit. The necessity to do so in anaesthetic practice arises relatively infrequently.

When patients are acutely unwell, elderly or frail prior to surgery, the patient and his or her family may be met with beforehand to signal a possible or probable unfavourable outcome related to natural disease processes. If the worst does happen, the patients and relatives will be somewhat prepared.

Adverse incidents following anaesthesia require anaesthetists to be skilled in communicating honestly to the patient and relatives. These incidents can range from an unanticipated but treatable complication—for example, dural puncture—to an unexpected major mishap in theatre resulting in a serious adverse outcome (disability or death).

Effective communication is as important when the issue is a more minor adverse outcome or side effect as it is when an adverse event has had disastrous consequences. Major mishaps in anaesthesia create stressful and difficult situations, since anaesthetists are required to communicate the bad news. Why is one anaesthetist's day in court another anaesthetist's invitation to dinner at a patient's home? The good news is that breaking bad news is a skill that can be learned and taught.

The initial 'breaking bad news' communication to the patient and/or relatives about the series of events in a serious adverse outcome will be more thoroughly followed up in the subsequent disclosure process. An investigation into the contributing factors in such events (root cause analysis) may need to occur, and staff members involved in the incident must be supported (critical incident support).

Each department or group of anaesthetists should consider designating one of their number to respond to major adverse events. The 'duty anaesthetist' may be caught up with other clinical duties, and additional senior support will be required. One anaesthetist will be needed to manage ongoing clinical work, while another will be required to manage the aftermath.

In the aftermath of an adverse or unexpected outcome, patients and/or relatives (depending on cultural background) may want to know:

- The truth—what, if anything, went wrong?
- Why did it happen? To understand the 'why?' results in the patient or relative regaining some control in the situation, and gives some meaning to the event.
- What's the diagnosis?
- Is the patient going to die?
- Will there be any pain or suffering?
- The consequences and social effects of the clinical diagnosis and treatment (e.g. colostomy, being on a ventilator).
- Will this happen again to anyone else?

Principles of breaking bad news ('SPIKES')

A mnemonic, '**SPIKES**'[1,2], has been proposed to provide a framework for the steps to be followed in breaking bad news—**S**etting, **P**atient **P**erception, **I**nvite patient to share **I**nformation, **K**nowledge transmission, **E**motions and **E**mpathy, **S**ummarize and **S**trategize (see also Chapter 11).

Setting

After a serious adverse event, the anaesthetist and other key staff involved, including, for example, the surgeon, should meet as soon as possible to plan the debrief interview with the patient and/or relatives. The first thing to consider is which staff member is going to do the talking. Then the team need to agree on the details so that the patient or relatives hear a consistent account of what has happened—the when, where, how, and why the adverse event occurred.

The 'breaking bad news' interview should take place at a time to be negotiated, but as close as possible to the incident. It is important that all staff members relay consistent information of known events. The interview should take place in private. The anaesthetist, even if not new to breaking bad news, will need to think about what will be said to the patient. The persons conducting the interview should ensure that their pagers and mobile phones are turned off. The number of people in the interview room may range from two to several. Frequently there will be at least four persons—the patient or relative, a support person, the doctor and the doctor's support person. It may be that the anaesthetist involved in the incident is too upset, in the immediate aftermath, to meet the patient or family. However, it is advisable that this anaesthetist does speak to the patient or relatives at some stage. This allows patients or relatives to talk directly to the person who was there at the time of the incident, as he or she can provide the most accurate factual information. This strategy will convey implicitly that an open process is occurring.

The presence of the whole team, as suggested by Bacon[3], may be overwhelming for the patient or relatives, or may be perceived as 'closing ranks'. The planning of the 'breaking bad news' interview must include weighing up these considerations with regard to individual circumstances, and choosing the most appropriate staff members for the interview. A senior anaesthetist should be present for advice and expertise, as well as offering support to the trainee if the incident involved a trainee.

If the patient has died or is in intensive care, it is the relatives who are receiving the bad news. An interview with these relatives should be arranged in consultation with the other healthcare workers involved with the patient. The relatives may also wish to have a support person present—perhaps the family doctor, social worker or religious representative. They should be asked, '*Is there someone you want to bring with you?*'

At the start of the interview, greetings and a simple introduction of the hospital staff in the room will help to increase rapport. This can be followed by identification of the patient or the relatives with whom it is intended to talk. Don't assume that the person by the patient's bed is the spouse, a parent or son/daughter.

Perception

The anaesthetist should check how much the patient or relative knows already. Even if the interview has been arranged as soon as possible, it is often unclear how much information they may have acquired before the breaking bad news interview. The patient and family members may have had discussion with nurses or other personnel to find out what has happened. The patient or relative may have no information, a little or incorrect information, or may have misinterpreted what others have said.

Important information about the patient's or relative's emotional state can be gained at this stage. Uninterrupted listening is important (see Chapter 2).

Invite patient to share Information

Checking what the person already knows or thinks will allow a better assessment of the situation, will gain some rapport and will gauge how much information the person may ***want*** to know. Some people will need every detail—others will need an outline, or very little information.

The anaesthetist can ask,

> '*Can you tell me what you know?*'
> '*What's your understanding of what's happened?*'
> '*Did you think something serious was going on?*'

Knowledge transmission

Communication of bad news to patients and relatives is about giving information in a caring, supportive and genuine way[1]. It is likely that the patients or relatives will be anticipating that there will be bad news communicated in the interview. Emotions will be running high. To expect bad news is different from actually hearing it! It is helpful for the anaesthetist to have thought about how to signal that bad news is coming before it is actually delivered. This tactic is called 'firing a warning shot'.

'I'm afraid I have bad news'.
'I am sad to have to tell you that X is seriously ill'.
'Unfortunately I am here to tell you about an accident'.
'I am very sad to tell you that something unexpected has happened in theatre'.
'I am really sad to have to tell you some bad news'.

Information is delivered or confirmed, and, not infrequently, misinformation corrected. The aim should be to build on what the patient or relative already knows, to deliver the information in small bites, and to ensure that no jargon is used. A check for understanding is necessary, as people vary in how much information they can take in, and in their ability to understand what is being said.

It is important to emphasize that the facts as communicated are those known at the time of the interview, to restrict the discussion of what happened to the facts currently known, and to avoid any speculation as to cause or blame directed towards the hospital and/or colleagues.

In situations where there has been a critical incident resulting in an adverse event, rather than a natural death or adverse outcome, patients and relatives often want to know whether changes in policies and procedures have been implemented that will reduce or abolish the chance of a similar incident happening again. This may be their primary concern. If the 'why?' is unknown, patients and relatives can be informed that the hospital is investigating the incident (outline the process of root cause analysis), and that they will be informed of the results of any enquiry as soon as these become available.

'We will look at our processes to see if anything can be changed to ensure that this accident will never happen to another patient'.

Since it is unlikely that all the answers will be available at the breaking bad news interview, the recipients can be informed that after further investigation, during the root cause analysis process, more information will be available.

The stress of hearing bad news can significantly reduce the ability to process information. Pauses should be allowed for the news to sink in. In many cases patients or relatives will be hearing the worst news they have ever had. Everyone takes time to digest momentous new information. So, giving too much information at once should be avoided (see also Chapter 11).

'Can you tell me if you have understood what I am saying, or would you like me to repeat something?

It is very important to allow time for the recipients to identify their feelings about the news, and then allow time for them to frame questions.

Emotions and Empathy

It is vitally important to communicate bad news with empathy.

'I am really sorry to have to be the bearer of such tragic news'.
'I know how upsetting this news must be for you'.
'Obviously this is terrible news for you'.

The hearer's emotional response to the grief of bad news can range from disbelief, anger, sadness, desolation and wailing, to resignation—the latter especially if the information has been expected for some time. It is important to acknowledge and encourage expressions of emotion.

'I can see you are really angry about this incident'.
'I can see that this is very upsetting for you'.

It is also helpful for the bearer of bad news to recognize the following:

1. Anger is a common response of the patient or relatives in these situations, and is the hardest one to deal with. It is important to recognize, acknowledge and validate this response.
2. Where an adverse event has occurred, an apology should be made for any harm incurred (without blaming an individual), and reassurance that the incident is being investigated so that it will not happen again; this may help to defuse the anger.
3. In response to the patient's or relative's hostility, the anaesthetist may be tempted to show frustration, irritation or defensiveness, or may blame others for what went wrong. Awareness and insight of these possible responses will allow unhelpful emotions and behaviours to be kept in check.
4. There is a natural tendency to plan what to say next, rather than listen to what the patient or relative is saying. This temptation also needs to be avoided where possible (ideally by prior planning of several statements), so that the patient or relatives feel and see that they are being taken seriously, being listened to, and that concerns are being heard, understood and addressed.
5. Attentive, uninterrupted listening is the most effective strategy to allow further useful discussion. Pauses can be used to advantage.
6. Even if emotions are running high, the anaesthetist should avoid calling hospital security in the first instance. Nevertheless, be mindful of your own safety.
7. Anger can resurface at any time—if so, return to attentive, uninterrupted listening, and acknowledge again the emotion with an empathic remark.

'I can understand that this makes you angry'.

When the bad news has been relayed, empathy expressed, and emotions acknowledged, it is then possible to move on to ask if there are any other concerns. It is particularly helpful for the anaesthetist to allow time for questions, and to avoid rushing the interview. If she or he appears to want to get things over with quickly, this attitude can be interpreted as uncaring.

The anaesthetist may have to ask for questions more than once during the breaking bad news interview, as new concerns may surface at any time. Useful statements might include:

'Have you any other particular concerns at the moment?'
'Can you tell me any of your thoughts or worries?'
'Is there anything else that is troubling you about the situation?'
'Do you feel I have covered all your concerns?'

Summarize and Strategize

There will be a need to check that the patient or relatives have understood the information they have been provided with—including follow-up arrangements. Receiving bad news can put all other thoughts out of their heads temporarily, so the topic may need to be returned to more than once.

An appointment with a psychologist, or a minister of religion, can be offered and arranged where appropriate:

'Would you like me to arrange an appointment with someone who can help you to deal with this tragic situation?'
'Would you like to talk to the social worker, or someone else who could help you?'

Ongoing support is frequently appreciated by patients and relatives, and demonstrates genuine concern and care on the part of the anaesthetist:

'Perhaps we should meet again, to answer any further questions you might have'.
'If you would like to come to talk to me any time in the future, please contact me on this phone number'.
'We can arrange another appointment at a mutually convenient time'.

Documentation

It is vital to document immediately afterwards what material was covered in the debriefing interview, as well as who was present. To enable this to happen, one of the interviewers should take notes at the time, or document the information at the earliest opportunity after the interview. It is important to document the ***facts*** only, regardless of one's own personal opinions, thoughts or feelings, and resist the temptation to opine on causation, assign blame to any member of the team concerned, or express judgements on an individual's actions.

The salient details should be documented in the patient's records. It may be necessary in the future to provide this account in court or to a medical defence organization (MDO); therefore, it is wise to retain a personal copy of the document as well, and to supply another copy to the MDO if required.

During the crisis it is often impossible to document what happened. The account in the patient's record of what happened must often be written after the episode has been brought under control. The record must clearly indicate that it has been written following the acute episode. Any subsequent comments about the crisis in the patient's record must also be signed, dated and the time of writing indicated.

Breaking bad news needs to be done well for many reasons

Patient perceptions

In these difficult communication situations, hospital staff are likely to feel uncomfortable, edgy or embarrassed, and may want to get the whole process over with quickly. Such feelings tend to translate into behaviour that may be perceived by the patient or relatives as uncaring or insensitive. Creating this perception must be strenuously avoided, as it may cause mistrust in the recipient. It can also generate unnecessary distress, interfere with good communication and may increase the likelihood of long-term adverse consequences. Recognition, acceptance and even admission of these uncomfortable feelings may allow the anaesthetist to behave in a more authentic way.

Stress/burn-out

Anaesthesia is, by its nature, a specialty where the need to break bad news is infrequent. Therefore, no matter how experienced the individual, the process is always stressful to some degree. Knowledge, training, practice, and shared experiences of the skills required when breaking bad news, can reduce stress to the doctor and may be a factor in minimizing the development of 'burn-out'.

If concerns are not addressed or emotions acknowledged, the patient or relative may suffer long-term distress, especially if the amount of information is not tailored specifically to each occasion—that is, too much or too little information. Time taken to ensure that emotions are recognized and validated is time well spent.

Litigation

Patients and relatives are more likely to proceed to litigation if they feel that:

- the breaking bad news interview has gone badly and/or the doctor was uncaring or insensitive;
- they were not given enough information;
- they were not being told the truth in a timely fashion;
- concerns were not being heard and dealt with.

Critical incidents and open disclosure

What is a critical incident?

- An incident in which a patient or staff member has experienced an adverse event or an incident in which a patient or staff member has just avoided an adverse event—a'near miss'.
- An incident which has caused distress to patients or staff.

What might constitute an adverse event?

- Death
  - A young male Jehovah's Witness dies after a motor vehicle accident because he refused a blood transfusion.

- Paraplegia
  - A young mother becomes paraplegic due to an abscess resulting from an epidural provided for analgesia in labour.
- Loss of limb
  - An older man whose left leg was amputated in error.
- Trauma or anaesthetic incident resulting in brain death
  - A patient who had been told 'never to have a GA again' at his last operation, becomes brain-dead from hypoxia after a failed intubation.
- Staff suicide or drug overdose
  - A colleague is found on the floor of the theatre toilet, apnoeic and blue, with a needle attached to her arm.

What processes need to be followed after one of these events?

- **Breaking bad news** to the patient and/or the family (see above).
- **Critical incident support** involves providing support for the anaesthetist(s) and other staff involved. There may be a need to support the 'second victim', the person or persons directly involved with the adverse event—for example, the young anaesthetist whose patient has died on the operating table—as well as support for all other staff involved.
- **Root cause analysis.** This process is an investigation to examine possible causes or contributing factors leading to the incident. It is important for relatives to know that an investigation has been started. Whatever the institution, there should always be a risk management process initiated after serious adverse events. Root cause analysis examines and analyses all the likely factors (root causes) which have contributed to a serious adverse event, and culminates in a report highlighting what can be done to avoid or mitigate future errors in similar circumstances. Implementation of the recommendations arising from the root cause analysis will result in improvements in the health care process.
- **Open disclosure** is defined as the frank discussion of incidents that result in unintended harm to a patient while receiving healthcare, as well as the associated investigation and recommendations for improvement of practice. The definition of open disclosure in different countries is not exactly the same, but most emphasize open and honest communication with patients and their families after an adverse incident[4,5]. The initial breaking bad news interview, which needs to occur immediately after the incident, is the start of an open disclosure process.

Critical incident support —'the second victim'

The second victim is the anaesthetist or other person involved in the adverse event. Many doctors feel that they are directly to blame for an adverse incident occurring to one of their patients, even when the causes are not the doctor's fault in any way. More often than not it is a team responsibility, and system errors are frequently uncovered.

The *perception* of self-blame by the doctor involved 'at the sharp end', even when no fault can be attributed, may result in major personal stress. It can cause depression or other mental illness, including the potential for adjustment disorder and PTSD. Tragically it has occasionally resulted in suicide. It is thus of extreme importance to offer practical and emotional support to those involved.

The guilt felt by the individuals involved is worse if:

- the incident was potentially avoidable;
- the patient is young;
- the anaesthetist is inexperienced;
- the anaesthetist thinks the case was mishandled;
- the case was an emergency;
- a junior anaesthetist was unsupervised;
- there was no support from colleagues;
- the anaesthetist was not working in the usual team or a familiar environment (e.g. when acting as a locum);
- a member of staff is the patient.

The stages of distress at the event experienced by the 'second victim' can be likened to the stages of bereavement or other traumatic event—denial, isolation, anger, bargaining, depression and, finally, acceptance[6].

If litigation follows from the adverse event, then these feelings are likely to be exaggerated, and the stress can continue for several years. The chances of doctor suicide are greatly increased by the inevitably prolonged medico-legal process[7–10].

In the immediate post-incident period, the person responsible for critical incident support (perhaps a designated senior anaesthetist, as suggested above) should contact the 'second victim' to offer comfort, support and relief from duties[11]. A confidential interview in private should be suggested.

> *'I've just heard what happened, would you like to come to talk about it with me? I have arranged for someone else to take over your list. If you need time off work, this will be arranged'.*

The individual involved should be encouraged to reflect on the episode and talk about it. Any expression of blame should be avoided. At a later stage, when the doctor is ready to write down the facts, a mentor can offer help with this document.

Empathy for the person involved can be shown by validating the experience—perhaps with examples from personal experience: '*I had a similar thing happen to me some years ago—and I found it very difficult to come to terms with—I was enormously helped by...*'

In some centres the 'second victim' will be informed that a root cause analysis will take place. The support person should emphasize that there are usually several contributing factors in any adverse incident, and that system errors are frequently uncovered. Knowing that deficiencies in the system may be identified can help the anaesthetist come to terms with what has happened. It is appropriate to ask if the second victim would like access to professional help—for example, a psychologist, counsellor or a religious representative.

'Would you like me to contact anyone to help you? For instance, someone to talk it through with you?'
'Would you like me to let your partner or family know what's happened?'

Ongoing support can be offered,

'My door is always open if you need to talk further, or explore anything else you might be feeling later down the track'.

Where a trainee is involved and is to rotate to another anaesthetic department or hospital, it is essential that there is communication of the incident to the trainee's supervisor in the new environment to ensure ongoing support.

Some individuals can deal with adverse events without external support, although this may depend on the nature of the incident and indeed the individual concerned. If the anaesthetist initially refuses help, or says '*I'm OK—I can deal with it*', the support person will need to continue to check with the person involved on a daily basis. This will be particularly important during the root cause analysis or medico-legal processes, which will continue for some time after the incident, and are sources of continued stress for the doctor(s) concerned.

What should the 'second victim' do?

The 'second victim' should expect to be offered support. If this does not happen, he or she should contact the department head, the on-duty anaesthetist or a mentor for this to occur. It is often hard to persuade young doctors to seek outside help—the stigma of 'mental health' problems remains strong. Some may be able to cope alone with the help of family and friends[11], although the capacity to deal with all their feelings may depend on the nature and severity of the incident.

The need for outside professional help from, for example, a psychologist or another appropriate person, may not be recognized initially. However, the mentor can emphasize that these professionals are better able to give impartial and supportive advice.

If litigation is a possibility, the incident has the potential to cause distress for several years and there is an increased danger of consequences as noted above—that is, depression, PTSD (post-traumatic stress disorder), adjustment disorder, or at the very worst, suicide.

Case studies

The following case studies serve to demonstrate the practical aspects of communicating in clinical situations that have been discussed in this chapter.

Case study 1

Dr X is an international medical graduate. He lives alone, as his wife and child have remained in his country of origin. Three months before he obtained any support, he was involved in an adverse incident as one member of the team responsible for a patient. There was a delay in diagnosing an epidural abscess in a post-partum patient, resulting in paraplegia. His performance began to deteriorate. He had several sick leave days, and had refused to come into work when asked. In addition he had been upset about registration issues with the medical board. After the critical incident both his supervisor and the director of medical services had talked to him and suggested ongoing contact, but his reaction to the actual incident had not been discussed.

At a later interview Dr X was crying. He related the story of the incident, and said '*It didn't hit me hard until later*'. He had been at home alone, contemplating suicide. He also disclosed other issues he was concerned about. These included financial and family matters, as well as disparaging remarks made about his part in the incident by another senior doctor in public. He was taken off work for 3 weeks on sick leave with full pay, referred to his general practitioner, and later to a psychologist. A gradual return to work was planned, with several follow-up interviews, which showed that he had made progress in resolving his reactions to the adverse event.

Case study 2

A middle-aged man having an excision of a lesion under local anaesthetic was inadvertently given 50 mg suxamethonium instead of the intended fentanyl. Resuscitative and sedative measures were immediately instituted and the operation cancelled. The anaesthetist attended the patient immediately afterwards when he was again conscious.

A follow-up interview was arranged with the patient and his wife. At this interview the anaesthetist was accompanied by a senior colleague. The patient felt that the anaesthetist had done all that could have been done, but the patient's wife was angry.

> **Wife:** '*How could this happen to my husband? You have paralysing drugs in theatre?*'
> **Anaesthetist** (pause): '*Yes we use them every day; unfortunately we think that a small dose of one of these drugs was given to your husband in error—we are extremely sorry that he had such a bad experience. We are looking into how we organize these drugs to ensure that this accident will not happen again*'.

After further careful ***listening*** and ***acceptance*** of the anger as valid, and a repeated, detailed explanation by the anaesthetist, the patient's wife's anger dissipated. She acknowledged that the anaesthetist had admitted the error, had empathized with the patient's feelings of terror of being awake and paralysed, and had apologized.

Case study 3 (see also Chapter 15)

How to respond when a patient in pre-anaesthetic clinic indicates that she might have been 'aware' (when asked about previous anaesthetics):

> **Patient:** '*I had a **frightening** dream last time—I dreamt I died*'.
> Several responses could be made:
> **Hostile response:** '*I'm sure you must have been mistaken!*'
> **Closed question:** '*Who was your previous anaesthetist?*'
> **Open question:** '*How did you feel about that experience?*'
> **Empathic response:** '*You must have been very **frightened** by that*'.

The first two responses are implicitly blaming firstly the patient and secondly another anaesthetist. The empathic response is recommended, to be followed by some open questions to allow the patient to express her feelings about the episode.

Case study 4

The anaesthetist is the registrar in intensive care. Mrs Smith has been on a ventilator for four days, following a massive subarachnoid haemorrhage. Tests of brain function have shown no activity on two occasions. The anaesthetist has met the family before, and now it is your job to discuss turning off the ventilator and the possibility of organ donation.

> **Anaesthetist:** '*Mr Smith, is it OK to talk now—Please come in to this room. Would you like to bring your son in? This is Dr X, and Nurse Y, who are looking after your mother. I am sad to tell you again that things have not improved. I think you know what has happened—that she has had a big bleed inside her head*'. (Pause for questions)
> '*You remember that this blood clot has been pressing on her brain* (pause) *unfortunately this has resulted in her brain not working properly*'. (pause)
> '*You remember that yesterday and the day before I discussed with you the tests for brain function that we have done? Well, both sets of tests show that your wife has lost all her brain activity; although her heart is still beating she can no longer breathe for herself and she is on a machine that is doing the breathing for her*'.

The anaesthetist allows more pauses for questions, and for grief to be expressed. This might be the third or fourth conversation with Mr Smith, and the relatives can now be introduced to the possibility of organ donation.

Author's note: The case studies have been taken from real life cases; details have been changed to safeguard anonymity.

Key points

Breaking bad news and the management of critical incidents require:

1. acceptance that 'bad things happen', through disease processes, system factors and the inevitably of human error;
2. anaesthetists to communicate with patients and relatives with empathy and care in a planned interview, including attentive uninterrupted listening;
3. follow-up to be offered to patient and relatives;
4. support to those involved in the incident (critical incident support).

References

1 Buckman R (1992). *How to break bad news: a guide for health professionals.* Baltimore, MD: The Johns Hopkins University Press.

2 Baile WF, Buckman R, Lenzi R, Glober G, Beale EA, Kudelka AP (2000). SPIKES—a six-step protocol for delivering bad news: application to the patient with cancer. *Oncologist*, **5**, 302–11.

3 Bacon AK (1989). Death on the table. *Anaesthesia*, **44**, 245–8.

4 Allan A, Munro B (2008). *Open disclosure: a review of the literature.* Western Australia: Edith Cowan University, Joondalup, Available at: http://www.psychology.ecu.edu.au/staff/documents/allanA/86_Allan_OD_Literature_Review.pdf (Accessed 15 March, 2010)

5 Iedema RA, Mallock NA, Sorensen RJ, Manias E, Tuckett AG, Williams AF, et al. (2008). The National Open Disclosure Pilot: evaluation of a policy implementation initiative. *Med J Aust*, **188**(7), 397–400.

6 Kubler-Ross E (1997). *On death and dying*. New York, NY: Scribner.

7 Martin CA, Wilson JF, Fiebelman ND 3rd, Gurley DN, Miller TW (1991). Physicians' psychologic reactions to malpractice litigation. *South Med J*, **84**(11), 1300–4.

8 Charles SC, Wilbert JR, Franke KJ (1985). Sued and non-sued physicians' self-reported reactions to malpractice litigation. *Am J Psychiatry*, **142**, 437–40.

9 Birmingham PK, Ward RJ (1985). A high-risk suicide group: the anesthesiologist involved in litigation. *Am J Psychiatry*, **142**(10), 1225–6.

10 Wilbert JR, Charles SC, Warnecke RB, Lichtenberg R (1987). Coping with the stress of malpractice litigation. *Ill Med J*, **171**(1), 23–7.

11 Raphael B, Meldrum L, McFarlane AC (1995). Does debriefing after psychological trauma work? *BMJ*, **310**, 1479–80.

Chapter 13

Patients with special needs

Gillian M Hood and Suyin GM Tan

'A man has the right to look down on somebody, only when he is helping him to get up'.
Gabriel Garcia Marquez

What this chapter is about

Patients with communication difficulties

Most anaesthetists recognize that there are specific groups of patients with whom communication is especially difficult due to issues relating to language. These groups are patients in whom a disease process interferes with communication—for example intellectual disability or hearing impairment, those with whom we do not share a common tongue, and those patients whose cultural background differs from ours.

Patients with communication difficulties are disproportionately represented in the hospital population for a variety of reasons. The elderly form the bulk of hospital inpatients and are much more likely to have problems such as dementia, confusion, sedation and dysphasia.

It is important to be cognisant of the issues that may arise with patients who have communication problems and, in addition to being aware of these problems, it helps to have a structured way of approaching the issue.

Recognize and define the communication issue

Reading the patients' notes prior to consultation gives advance warning of issues such as dementia or hearing impairment and allows communication to be tailored to the patients' needs. Sometimes the patients' understanding of language may be difficult to assess on first meeting—anaesthetists have all encountered patients who answer questions with a smiling 'yes' or 'no', only to subsequently discover their comprehension has been minimal. Enquiring of relatives, friends and staff helps to give a picture of a patient's ability to communicate in the chosen language. Similarly, enquiring of the patient how communication can be facilitated, is helpful.

> '*It says in your notes that you have trouble finding words since your stroke—is there anything I can do to make it easier for you to speak?*'

Once the communication problem has been delineated it makes it easier to move on to the next step.

Orientation

Having orientated oneself to the patient's particular problems with communication, it is also important to orientate the staff with whom one is working.

> '*Rob, we are going to see Mr Smith now. He's had problems with alcohol withdrawal over the last few days and he is still a bit confused. It is probably best if just one of us does the talking—are you happy to do that?*'
> **Not**: '*I wish you wouldn't contradict me when I'm talking to patients...*'

Having made an effort to identify the barriers to communication in the patient, anaesthetists need to be mindful of the barriers to communication in themselves. Is the mind focused on the conversation or are thoughts straying to the 'difficult' patient on the afternoon list? Are we becoming irritated, angry, frustrated or simply bored by the patient's concerns or demands?

Recognizing their own emotional responses can help anaesthetists recognize that patients have emotional responses too, and that acknowledging and accepting these are key elements in improving communication skills. For example, the anaesthetist may become increasingly annoyed by the ex IV drug user who is angry, sarcastic and demanding, whenever he is visited on the pain round. Recognizing that the patient has poorly controlled pain, is scared of the disfigurement caused by his accident, and lacks social skills to communicate appropriately, helps the anaesthetist to view the patient dispassionately and to acknowledge any frustrations over the lack of progress, or prejudices about patients with drug use issues.

Using 'GREAT' to structure the interaction

Greeting, Goals

Anaesthetists should ensure that they are close enough to be seen and heard. It may be useful to show patients an ID badge so that the name and position of the anaesthetist can be read, especially if the patients are hearing impaired. Patients who are confused or demented may need to be reminded if they have met you before—for example,

> '*I'm Dr Thompson—I looked after you when you had your hip operation last Tuesday*'.

It is important to have in your own mind the essence of what you want the interaction to achieve, be it pre-operative assessment or a discussion with the patient about weaning their PCA.

The goal of the interaction can then be explained.

> '*I have come to talk to you about the anaesthetic for your operation tomorrow*'.

Rapport

Establishing rapport with these patients usually requires some lateral thinking and being mindful of particular patient needs. Reducing background noise is a valuable asset. Turning the TV off helps to focus attention and reinforces the importance of the interaction between anaesthetist and patient. Other helpful tactics include, where necessary, ensuring hearing aids are on and working, or organizing an interpreter to be present, or finding the patient's false teeth. Sitting on a chair sends a strong non-verbal signal that the anaesthetist is interested and engaged with the patient; folding the arms or staring out of the window does not!

The anaesthetist should be mindful that women from some cultures may feel intimidated by the close proximity of a strange male. It may be useful to consult colleagues who share a similar cultural background to glean further knowledge. An awareness of the medical issues affecting the patient aids effective communication. For example, patients who have recently been sedated for a procedure are unlikely to be able to communicate. It may be appropriate to return at a later time.

The presence of a nurse or relative who is familiar with the patient is useful in facilitating communication and provides the opportunity for the message to be conveyed in a way that works for the patient, and can be reinforced by repetition later. If the issue to be discussed is complex or sensitive, or an extended therapeutic intervention is intended, it may not be appropriate to have a huge entourage of medical students and trainees. Whilst it is entirely appropriate that trainees are exposed to difficult communication scenarios, this is often best done as a one-to-one teaching session rather than as a group, to avoid embarrassment, distress or confusion.

Evaluation, Examination, Explanation

The main content of the consultation should be as short and simple as possible whilst allowing the patient the opportunity to express any concerns or queries. This is especially true when a patient has very marked cognitive impairment—for example, severe dementia or the inability to verbalize. Rather than a technical discussion of post-operative complications, the use of metaphor, analogy or story-telling is often helpful in assisting patients' understanding as it allows meaning to be conveyed in simple language which is easy to recall—for example,

> '*Recovering from an operation is like a journey—sometimes it is short and easy, sometimes we end up taking a more twisting, turning route but in the end we reach the same destination. Sometimes we hit a bump in the road—for example a wound infection ...*'

Patients with memory problems, or from a non-English-speaking background, often benefit from written information that they or their relatives can refer to after the consultation—for instance, a list of their medications and their indications.

Asking and Answering questions, Addressing and Acknowledging concerns

Allow time for the patients and their relatives to absorb the meaning of what is being said, and check understanding by asking questions. Open questions requiring an extended answer rather than closed questions are a better way of ensuring patients have understood the issues. '*Tell me how you use the PCA button*', rather than '*Do you understand how to use it?*'

At the end of the interaction offer the opportunity for patients to ask questions. Often the type and quality of questions give an indication of the patients' understanding of the issues and highlights their particular concerns.

Tacit agreement, Thanks, Termination

The interaction is terminated with thanks and often explicit or tacit agreement as to the next stage of treatment.

Patients with intellectual and behavioural disability

This section looks at the issues of caring for children and adults whose communication abilities may be compromised by intellectual disability or by social and language development difficulties. The discussion focuses on patients with Down's syndrome and those with an autistic spectrum disorder, to provide some ideas as to possible interpretations of responses and behaviours seen in this complex group of patients.

Trisomy 21 and other conditions with developmental delay

Down's syndrome or trisomy 21 is the most commonly encountered congenital syndrome of intellectual disability, occurring in approximately 1 in 800 births[1]. Along with the characteristic physical features, people with this syndrome have a higher incidence of a wide range of medical conditions[2,3]. Extensive health supervision of people with this condition is recommended[4]. With improved healthcare people with Down's syndrome are living longer[5] and are likely to be 'frequent flyers' in primary and specialist healthcare areas.

Communication issues

Cooperation may be severely affected by multiple previous bad experiences, and it is highly desirable for patients and carers that effective communication creates a positive experience. Up to 10% of children and adults with Down's syndrome may also have a diagnosis of autism, necessitating a different communication style (see below). For most people with Down's syndrome, receptive language development follows a 'normal'[6], if slower, course than normally developing children. Almost all children with Down's syndrome have an impairment of verbal expressive language development. Many have poor articulation[7] and a number will have speech motor mapping problems with dyspraxia[8]. Thus, the gulf between receptive and verbal expressive language may be large. Hearing loss is common. Auditory processing may be impaired and short-term memory poor, especially with advancing age. Between the ages of 50 and 59 years, around one-third of patients with Down's syndrome may have an additional diagnosis of dementia[9].

Pre-operative consultation and transfer to the operating theatre

Prior to anaesthesia, speaking with a carer or parent of the patient is invariably helpful. Other than obtaining a medical history and a history of communication abilities, likes and dislikes can also be noted. Information about past experiences from patients themselves, their carers, or from the case-notes, can assist with planning and utilization.

Parents and carers of people with handicaps or rare syndromes or diseases may often be extremely knowledgeable about their wards' conditions. The rarer the syndrome, the more likely parents' or carers' knowledge will exceed that of the anaesthesia team looking after them. That well-worn cliché, '*Right or wrong, the customer is always right*' is worth bearing in mind under these circumstances. An open question such as, '*Can you tell me about your child's communication skills?*' is more likely to bring forth good information than, '*Can he talk?*'

It is vital to ensure that patients are not bypassed because there may be communication difficulties, and patients ought not to be talked about as if they are not present.

Comprehension is often better than expressive language. All initial greetings should be directed first to the patient, accompanied by an appropriate welcoming gesture—the ubiquitous '*High Five*' appears to work well in a wide age range. An additional amount of time should also be allowed for a response before repeating a statement or question. Listening to and observing the responses will give good clues for induction planning. Only if there is no response or an inadequate response should redirecting the communication to the carer be considered. Asking permission by way of, '*Is it OK if I ask your Mum some questions?*' is more respectful of the patient's autonomy than just turning away.

The pre-operative discussion with the patient can follow similar pathways to those described in Chapters 6 and 10, with age-appropriate utilization of the person's imagination skills. Unless volunteered by the carer or parent it may be ill advised to state the child's mental age. Anecdotally, this age-labelling of people with intellectual handicap is disliked by parents, particularly if the gap is large between this and the chronological age.

As children with Down's syndrome may also have hearing deficits and are good visual learners[8], the additional use of picture communication devices and sign language or gestures may be helpful.

Transferring the patient to the operating theatre should be conducted in such a way as to allow for a maximum sense of control by the patient.

Case study 1 A suboptimal transfer to theatre

A 15-year-old girl with Down's syndrome attended a day-procedure hospital for elective dental treatment under general anaesthesia. Although nervous, she was absorbed in drawing some pictures, and her mother said that it was one of the girl's favourite activities. The pre-anaesthetic consultation ended with an agreement that she could '*keep on drawing*' up to the time she would blow up some balloons in theatre. Some time was spent with the patient's mother rehearsing this plan so that she would remember the sequence of events. However, when the patient was brought to theatre she was very distressed. Her paper and crayons had been left in the admission area. An offer to get them was refused by the patient but, following renegotiations, she agreed to show the anaesthetist how good she was at blowing up balloons, and eventually peace and calm were restored. In a short debrief, the nurse that brought her to theatre reported that she had gone to collect the patient and had told her '*Put your crayons down now, we're going to theatre!*'

The lesson to be learned from this experience was that inadequate communication between the anaesthetist and ward staff led to the anaesthetic plan not being executed. Although the anaesthetist had spent time orientating the patient to a future successful outcome, the plan had failed by a simple lack of communication.

A double bind (see Chapter 4) at the time of transfer, '*Would you like to take your crayons and paper with you or leave them here while we go to theatre?*' might have been more effective. Interrupting what the patient was enjoying, and removing control from her, was poor utilization of her coping strategy—the drawing of pictures. Even when plans are derailed it is always possible to restore the patient's perception of control by redirecting the conversation back to a new modified plan—in this case one of balloon blowing. Regaining control can also include the use of double binds,

> '*Would you like to climb up on the bed from this side or that side?*'

A debrief with other team members can provide valuable education for future encounters.

Case study 2 Optimizing cooperation by promoting autonomy

A 13-year-old girl presented for examination of ears under anaesthesia. Her surgeon had been unable to examine her in his rooms due to poor cooperation. She was filling in a dot-to-dot puzzle so some numeracy skills were presumed. A chat with her mother revealed she loved helping at home. She chose '*banana sleepy gas*' (Sevoflurane) for an inhalational induction. A discussion about what she was going to listen to when her ears were clear and what she was going to have to eat after the operation created a positive expectancy for recovery.

The way to theatre was assisted with questions like '*Which one is theatre 3?... Thank you you're very helpful*',—utilization of her 'helpful' nature. Once in theatre, she chose which side of the bed Mum would sit while she lay down on the bed. She also decided which finger the oximeter probe fitted best (both double bind and maintaining control). The mask was placed near her mouth....

> **Anaesthetist:** '*Now it was banana flavour, wasn't it? ... Isn't that the best banana you have ever had?* (Girl nodded) *That's 1% banana, what's next?*'
> **Patient:** '*2!*' (Meanwhile, the anaesthetic assistant took this as his cue to increase the percentage of sevoflurane!)
> **Anaesthetist:** '*That's right, 2% banana, I'm so glad you're here to help me ... and what's next?*'
> **Patient:** '3!'
> **Anaesthetist:** '*That's right, 3% banana, I'm so glad you're here to help me... and what's next?*'

Utilization and repetition until the girl was anaesthetized.

Autism and related pervasive developmental disorders

This is a diverse group of conditions with a reported incidence ranging from 0.2 to 6 per 1,000[10]. As well as those children and adults who have a diagnosis of autism, a number may also present with other conditions associated with autism and autism-like behaviours and symptoms, including Asperger's syndrome, pervasive developmental disorder-not otherwise specified (PDD-NOS), 22q13 deletion syndrome (Phelan–McDermid syndrome), childhood disintegrative disorder and fragile X syndrome. None of the linguistic or behaviour characteristics is unique to, or diagnostic of, autism and may also be present in others with developmental delay.

Patients' development, including language development, may be affected in a wide range of ways and to varying degrees. Around 50% of people with a diagnosis on the autistic spectrum may have no verbal expressive language[11]. People with Asperger's syndrome may have little or no obvious language impairment but may have difficulty with idioms, sarcasm and humour. At the other end of the scale, a person with severe autism may have no verbal language development and little comprehension of spoken language. As with others with developmental delays and difficulties, they may use other communication devices such as PECS (picture exchange communication system) cards and sign language. Those with savant skills may have distinct abilities in one or more areas—for instance, musical ability.

Those who do talk may produce a bewildering array of words and phrases with many possible interpretations. Echolalia, or the repetition of vocalizations heard immediately or in the past, may be present. There may be other communication impairments (both receptive and expressive), and difficulty in relating to people, objects and events. Emotional responses may be non-existent or inappropriate—for example, laughing when a sad event occurs.

Immediate echolalia is the repeating back of a phrase just spoken. Echoic speech is normal in young children up to around 2–3 years of age and may continue a little later in people with intellectual handicap. The more pathological form, echolalia, persists in children and into adulthood in those with autism. Phrases repeated by the patient may appear to be inappropriate and out of context. For some the immediate repetition may be due to failure to comprehend[12]. For example, saying '*Can you take off your shoes, please?*' is likely to elicit a response, whereas '*Can you remove your footwear, please?*' is likely to be repeated back to the person. The anaesthetist should use immediate echolalia as both an indication of level of comprehension and a cue to modify or simplify their language.

Delayed echolalia, the term used when the person repeats a statement heard in the past, anything from a few minutes to many years ago, can be an indication of high emotions—either negative or positive[11]. Phrases uttered may have scant or no obvious relevance to current events, although a parent or carer may be able to explain a connection. When echolalia is accompanied by some acceleration of maladaptive behaviours, the likelihood is that it's time to reduce sensory input to the patient (see below).

An important communication skill, joint attention[13], may be poorly developed in children and adults with autism. Its development may also be delayed in others with intellectual disability. It is a pre-verbal mechanism for directing the listener and for being directed to an object or other person. Statements, for example indicating moving to another location, should be specific.

'*We're going to theatre through the sliding doors next to the elephant picture*' may be more effective than, '*We're going to theatre through that door*' and pointing.

In people with intellectual delay and in children with autism, the use of multiple adjectives may be confusing. Asking '*Would you like to blow up the big balloon or the little balloon?*' may be understood better than '*Would you like to blow up the big green balloon or the little blue balloon?*'

People with a diagnosis on the autistic spectrum may have a narrow range of interests sometimes to an obsessive level and to the exclusion of other subjects. They may demonstrate unusual play with toys and other objects. Sensory responses may also be very variable. A person with autism may appear to be completely unresponsive or hypersensitive to sounds. Certain colours may be highly desirable or despised. An inability to tolerate close contact with others may also be present. Repetitive body movements or behaviour patterns ('stimming' or 'stereotypy') may be present. Self-stimulating behaviours—hand flapping, rocking, head slapping and head banging are seen as maladaptive responses to stress and attempts at self-control.

The patient may have difficulty coping with changes to routine and unfamiliar environments, and may also have difficulty coping with loud and unusual noises. An inability to cope with a stressful event may result in an exaggeration in the manifestations of these behaviours and may culminate in a 'meltdown' (see below).

Pre-operative preparation

The parent or carer may provide valuable insights into communication strategies. Particular likes and dislikes can be identified and stressors that may trigger out of control behaviours can be noted. The parent should be encouraged to bring with them whatever they think may help to calm the patient. On arrival, it may be more calming for all to conduct the interview with the patient in a private room, away from excessive stimulation. At all times, the anaesthetist should look for increased frequency of maladaptive behaviours and use these indications to change or modify the direction the communication is taking. For example, a person, who initially seems to be coping with a story being told, starts to cover his ears. This is a cue to stop, modify or finish the narrative.

As mentioned, people with Asperger's syndrome and high functioning autism, despite superficially demonstrating good language skills, may have difficulty with humour and idioms. For example, a statement like '*Let's get the ball rolling*' is likely to have the person looking around the room for the ball! Similarly, '*Can you take off your shoes, please?*' may be met with '*But I'm wearing sandals*'. A delightful example of the literal interpretation of language is described by Schreibman in 'The Science and Fiction of Autism'[11]. The story is about a psychology student working with a child with autism. The child insisted on referring to the student as '*Poster*' despite many corrections. The student became frustrated with the boy and eventually told the boy '*My name is NOT POSTER*'. Thereafter the boy referred to the student as '*Not Poster*'. Thinking up and practising different ways of saying the same thing, as unambiguously as possible, is a worthwhile exercise.

People with autism and those with other disabilities often have difficulties with changing tasks or changing locations. Time should always be taken, and permission should always be obtained, before proceeding to the next phase of the process of anaesthesia. People with autism may struggle with making choices, thus increasing their stress levels. This may limit the use of the 'double bind' strategy which works well in many other areas.

Case study 3 Utilization of patient skills and motivations

A 28-year-old man, who attended for a colonoscopy under sedation, had a diagnosis of autism with savant skills. His carer described his skill as his '*party piece*' and '*obsession*'. This was the ability to calculate the day of the week that an event had occurred—for example, the day of the week that a person was born. He disliked being touched or having his personal space invaded.

During the pre-anaesthetic consultation he repeatedly asked the anaesthetist: '*When were you born?*' Having already established via the carer that this was his skill, it was then utilized with the phrase '*OK, I'll tell you once the drip is in*'—something he was reluctant to accept initially. In theatre he continued to ask all the nurses the same question but, with the staff educated about the bargaining tool, they all repeated the anaesthetist's plan. He was so motivated to perform his party piece that he allowed all the necessary monitoring devices to be applied as well as the intravenous line. Each time he allowed something to happen he was 'rewarded' with a team member's date of birth. The speed of his responses was astonishing. The transition from pre-anaesthetic consultation to induction was greatly facilitated by the bargaining and by seeking permission at all stages.

Anaesthetist: '*OK, now that you know I was born on a Tuesday, it's time to put the drip in*'.
Patient: '*Yup, OK, Dr Tuesday*'.

Minimizing and managing maladaptive responses

Temper tantrums are frequently seen in normally developing children from around age 9 months and can persist until age 3–4 years. Behaviours include screaming, hitting, throwing, breath-holding and head banging. Most children grow out of these as they develop communication and coping skills. Tantrums have several qualities that distinguish them from meltdowns. In a tantrum, the child will intermittently check to see if the behaviour is getting a response and does not usually self-harm. The tantrum will be extinguished when the child achieves his/her goal and may end as suddenly as it began. A meltdown in a person with autism can be of sudden onset, may be triggered by a seemingly trivial event and to the observer will manifest as an extreme version of a toddler tantrum. It may be preceded by acceleration in self-stimulating behaviours such as rocking or hand flapping. A person covering his ears may be indicating sensory overload. Self-injurious behaviour, such as head slapping, head banging or self-biting may also precede a meltdown. In contrast to a toddler tantrum, the person will not necessarily look for or care about a reaction to the behaviour. As there appears to be no clear age limit to this behaviour in people with autism, there are risks of injury to the patient, carers, onlookers and property. Such extreme behaviours are most likely to occur when these patients are under stress, while feeling unwell and out of their normal routines[14]. It would seem, therefore, that the hospital environment is the perfect location to trigger a meltdown!

Strategies to defuse a meltdown include the following:

- Identify the triggers beforehand.
- Reduce the sensory input by decreasing the number of people in the room, dimming the lights and speaking quietly.

- Distract—if the patient really wants to pull all the rubber gloves out of the boxes there may be something equally distracting but less destructive. Nevertheless pick your battles! The carer or parent may also have a 'calming toy' with them.
- If all else fails and meltdown occurs, move the person out of harm's way and ride it out. Continue to use a controlled voice and continue to use language suggesting '*calm*', '*time-out*' and '*control*'.

Communicating with children and adults with a diagnosis on the autistic spectrum can be as rewarding as it is exhausting. As with other fields of practice within anaesthesia, it is important to build a repertoire of skills—for example, finding different ways to say a single phrase when at first you are not understood.

Listen and look for triggers to both calming and heightening behavioural responses. Avoid idioms and complex syntax. Double binds may be ineffective as making choices may heighten stress. Environmental stimuli should be minimized to match the person's coping strategies. Finally, sometimes things will not go to plan and this should be accepted. To paraphrase Rudyard Kipling, 'Keep your head even when all about you are losing theirs'[15].

Key points

1. People with intellectual disabilities have diverse needs and may be challenging to look after.
2. Key strategies are to listen, observe, investigate likes and dislikes, enlist the help of the parents or carers, and to focus on abilities and utilize them.
3. The potential gulf between receptive and verbal expressive language should be remembered. The anaesthetist needs to be prepared to allow extra time for communication.

References

1 Irving C, Basu A, Richmond S, Burn J, Wren C (2008). Twenty-year trends in prevalence and survival of Down syndrome. *Eur J Hum Genet*, **16**, 1336–40.

2 Hasle H, Clemmensen IH, Mikkelsen M (2000). Risks of leukaemia and solid tumours in individuals with Down's syndrome. *Lancet*, **355**(9199), 165–9.

3 Zachor DA, Mroczek-Musulman E, Brown P (2000). Prevalence of celiac disease in Down syndrome in the United States. *J Pediatr Gastroenterol Nutr*, **31**(3), 275–9.

4 American Academy of Pediatrics Committee on Genetics (2001). Health supervision for children with Down syndrome. *Pediatrics*, **107**(2), 442–49. http://aappolicy.aappublications.org/cgi/content/full/pediatrics;107/2/442 (Accessed 15 March 2010)

5 Glasson EJ, Sullivan SG, Hussain R, Petterson BA, Montgomery PD, Bittles AH (2002). The changing survival of people with Down's syndrome: implications for genetic counselling. *Clin. Genet*, **62**, 390–3.

6 Bowen C (1998). *Speech and language development in infants and young children.* http://www.speech-language-therapy.com/devel1.htm/ (Accessed 15 March 2010)

7 Bray M. *Speech production in people with Down syndrome.* http://www.down-syndrome.org/reviews/2075/reviews-2075.pdf (Accessed 15 March 2010)

8 Buckley SJ (1999). Improving the speech and language skills of children and teenagers with Down syndrome. *Down Syndrome News and Update*, **1**(3), 111–12.

9 Coppus A, Evenhuis H, Verberne GJ, Visser F, van Gool P, Eikelenboom P, van Duijin C (2006). Dementia and mortality in persons with Down's syndrome. *J Intell Dis Res*, **50**(10), 768–77.

10 Wing L, Potter D (2002). The epidemiology of autistic spectrum disorder: is the prevalence rising? *Ment Retard Dev Disabil Res Rev*, **8**(3), 151–61.

11 Schreibman L (2005). *The science and fiction of autism.* Harvard, MA: Harvard University Press.

12 Prizant BM, Duchan JF (1981). The functions of immediate echolalia in autistic children. *J Speech Hear Disord*, **46**, 241–9.

13 Charman T (2003). Why is joint attention a pivotal skill in autism? *Philos Trans R Soc B*, **358**(1430), 315–24.

14 Groden J, Cautela J, Prince S, Berryman J (1994). The impact of stress and anxiety on individuals with autism and developmental disabilities. In: Schopler E, Mesibov GB (eds) *Behavioural issues in autism.* pp. 178–85. New York: Plenum Press.

15 Kipling, Rudyard, (1896). *If…* http://www.kipling.org.uk/poems_if.htm (Accessed 19 July 2010)

Chapter 14

Needle phobia

Allan M Cyna and Marion I Andrew

'Every problem has a gift for you in its hands'.
Richard Bach

What this chapter is about

Setting the scene

Needle phobia describes an anticipatory fear of needle insertion[1], and is a well-recognized clinical entity of particular relevance to the anaesthetist[2,3]. It may affect up to 10% of the general population, is more common in the young[4], and can prevent patients from seeking medical care[5] by avoiding immunizations, necessary blood tests or hospital procedures. The development of trust, a perception of control and an understanding of the conscious–subconscious aspects of the problem can help patients[6]. In addition, patience, time and recognized communication skills are frequently needed if this distressing problem is to be managed effectively[7].

Needle phobia is usually a learned response. Trust, control and perceptions rather than the pain itself are the key issues in needle phobia. Nevertheless pain reduction strategies such as EMLA, ice[8], premedication such as dexometomidine[9], stress-reducing medical devices[10,11] and hypnosis, may have a role in management[12–14].

Anaesthetists have traditionally used reassurance, EMLA and avoidance of needle insertion in the awake patient by giving inhalational inductions. However, this approach tends to reinforce the avoidance behaviour of both anaesthetist and patient! In addition, it wastes a valuable opportunity to educate patients in ways that can provide them with the necessary skills to manage future blood tests, drips and the like more easily. In some cases avoiding IV access prior to inducing anaesthesia—for example, at a Caesarean section—can put patients at increased risk of complications[5,15].

Understanding the conscious–subconscious aspects of needle phobia

Patients with needle phobia are like all patients only more so! At one level they function consciously and logically and are amenable to reason. However, in the context of hospital procedures such as blood tests and IV cannulation, subconscious responses take over. These patients often recognize that their behaviour is silly or even stupid, but find that they just can't help themselves. They may describe their predicament as being in '*two minds about it*' or '*beside themselves*'. This mind set illustrates, probably more clearly than any other, the conscious–subconscious basis of the problem.

To help engage with sufferers of needle phobia it is helpful to consider the anxiety response of the patient to needles as the ***subconscious*** response, and the desire to be able to have a drip or blood test as the logical ***conscious*** decision to obtain optimal medical care. The inability to comply with the treatment, despite logically recognizing the need for it, is brought about by the subconsciously generated fear. This anxiety response is typically expressed as sweating, cold and clammy hands, shaking, '*knots in the stomach*', hyperventilation, tachycardia and, on occasion, vaso-vagal episodes.

Patients often describe the needle in emotive language using kinaesthetic or visual terms—for example, as a '*horse needle*' or a '*knitting needle piercing the skin like a red hot poker*' or a '*molten sword*'. Sometimes it is difficult to empathize with these patients, especially if they present with tongue studs, nipple rings and the like. However, the fears are very real. Context is everything, as even patients with severe needle phobia may be able to tolerate body piercing with little difficulty, and yet generate a huge anxiety response to a blood test. The patient's 'reality' usually has nothing to do with the sensation of an injection, but everything to do with the perception, meaning, context and imagery associated with that perception. Needle-phobic patients are usually highly responsive to suggestion (see Chapters 3, 4 and 20)—if they weren't, they wouldn't be needle phobic in the first place!

Appreciating the origin of the problem

Some practitioners believe the source of the problem needs to be known and dealt with, but in practice this is usually unnecessary. Many patients are unaware of the origin of the problem. The initial sensitizing event could be something experienced by the person or by others that has led to the emotional response, and this may have had nothing to do with needles, but has subsequently become associated with them at a subconscious level. This emotional response is often reinforced by repeated bad experiences in hospital and avoidance behaviour. Irrespective of the source of the problem, the phobia needs to be accepted as a very real experience before it can be managed. Dismissive belittling attitudes such as '*It's only a small needle what's the fuss*'. or '*Look—you are behaving like a baby!*' only serve to escalate the problem at hand.

The '**LAURS**' concept and the use of metaphor can be used to help manage needle phobia (see Chapter 2).

Listen reflectively: this is always of value as the patient's description of symptoms can be utilized later.

Acceptance: the development of trust and rapport is facilitated when the patient's behaviour and perceptions are accepted dispassionately no matter how bizarre these may appear.

Utilization: the anaesthetist can utilize the patient's language to communicate in a way that implicitly and explicitly recognizes that the patient is in control. The anaesthetist reinforces trust and builds confidence, by checking in at each stage and asking permission frequently as each step in the process is achieved.

Reframing: this may be useful on occasion, although suggestion is usually of far more value in these patients.

Suggestion: positive expectancy can be seeded by using positive suggestion.

Utilizing metaphor to promote patient rapport

Patient rapport and trust can be established by accepting the patient's reality and demonstrating to the patient that the anaesthetist understands that the problem is real. Metaphor can be a useful way of conveying acceptance and understanding of the patient's difficulty, thus further facilitating patient rapport.

The 'plank of wood' metaphor involves asking the patient if there would be any problem walking across a plank of wood lying on the floor when it is 1 metre wide and 6 metres in length. The patient usually responds with a '*No!*'

The question can then be asked,

> '*What if exactly the same plank of wood was over a precipice with a 300 metre drop and you had to walk across it? It is identical in every other way to the plank of wood lying on the floor. How would you feel?*'

Patients frequently respond with words such as '*Terrified!*' or '*Anxious!*' The anaesthetist's response to this could be:

> '*That is good because if you didn't have that response to dangerous situations you would constantly be putting your life and well-being at unnecessary risk. Anxiety regarding walking across the plank in this situation is not only useful but, potentially, lifesaving*'.

This normalizes the anxiety response to needles as it is accepted that the patient is experiencing the needle as if walking across a precipice even though consciously the plank is known to be on the floor.

> '*Unfortunately people with needle phobia have a part of their mind that thinks that they need protecting.... It is as if the plank is over a 300 metre precipice, even though it is consciously recognized as being on the floor*'.

The use of this metaphor frequently facilitates rapid patient rapport, as it usually becomes clear that the matter is being taken seriously and the problem is not being dismissed as trivial. The patient's reality is being accepted in a non-judgemental way. Patients normally smile spontaneously and acknowledge being understood. If this does not happen, alternative metaphors can be used, as may the use of suggestions.

Using repetition frequently brings home, and reinforces, the message.

> '*It is very common to be in two minds about this. You know in one part of your mind at some level that the plank of wood is on the floor, yet another part of your mind still thinks you need protecting for some reason*'.

Useful suggestions

1 '*Fortunately there are lots of well-recognized strategies that people can learn that allow them to have blood tests and drips much more easily than they might think*'. '*Lots of well-recognized strategies....*' tells the patient that there are a range of solutions that could be helpful to them. '*People can learn ...*' is an indirect suggestion that implies that the patient too can learn.

2 '*... we usually show people with needle phobia how they can feel more in control and feel more comfortable than they might have thought*' is an indirect suggestion that the patient too can experience this.

3 '*Patients with needle phobia can usually gain a sense of control by focusing their gaze on that spot on the ceiling. They can then notice that each time they take a deep breath they feel stronger and more in control and each time they breathe out they feel themselves relax. As they relax, the arm relaxes outstretched too. This allows the drip to be placed much more comfortably than previously thought*'. This is an indirect suggestion for relaxation, control and 'arm anaesthesia'.

It should be remembered that one of the most effective ways of promoting a sense of control is by obtaining the patient's permission at each stage, thereby letting the patient know that they are in the driving seat.

Using 'GREAT' for needle phobia

Greeting, Goal

Following an initial greeting, the goal is to allow the treatment that patients have come in for, to be as safe and as comfortable as possible. The goal of placing an IV cannula is facilitated in the extremely anxious patient by communicating in a way that involves a series of steps starting with the least threatening.

> '*Hello I'm Dr Sharpe, I'm told you like to be called Tyson. I've come to help you get your cannula placed as comfortably as possible*'.

Rapport

> '*I show a lot of people who are nervous about drips and injections strategies that they can use to experience things in an easier way than they might have thought*'.

'Is it OK to talk about how we usually show people how to feel more in control and more comfortable?'

During this phase, the '**LAURS**' concept and the use of metaphor as described above are invaluable tools to assist the anaesthetist.

Evaluation, Expectations, Explanation

The evaluation usually takes a few seconds and determines the pace and type of strategies that may be needed to manage the problem successfully. It involves an assessment of the patient's readiness to undergo the procedure. More anxious patients will need more time to develop trust and a perception of control. In the case of mild needle phobia it may be simply a matter of acknowledging the problem and suggesting confidence, calm and competence in performing the task comfortably.

In very anxious patients it may be advisable initially to wait at the door of the room when greeting the patient and begin developing rapport there, asking for permission to approach when the patient is ready.

'Is it OK if I come over to the bed to talk...?'

The anaesthetist emphasizes that the patient can say when they are ready for the next step in the process.

'I normally tell patients that I will not do anything without their permission, is that OK?'

Asking and Answering questions, Addressing and Acknowledging concerns

This involves managing any other concerns not yet addressed and how these can be resolved when the patient is ready.

Patient: *'Can you only go where the cream is?'* or *'Don't do it without letting me know!'*
Anaesthetist: *'I'll only go where its going to be most comfortable for you and will only start when you are ready, is that OK?'*

Tacit agreement, Thanks, Termination

Anaesthetist: *'You can let me know when you are ready for it to be finished'.*

After the cannulation, *'Thanks for allowing me to show how you can do this more easily in the future'.*

Strategies to consider

The anaesthetist can ask a series of questions 'checking in' with the patient at each stage. For example: *'Is it OK to come a little closer?' 'Is it OK to stand next to the bed?' 'Is it OK to look at the arm?' 'Is it OK to look at the back of the hand?' 'Is it OK to place the tourniquet around the arm?' 'Is it OK to tap the back of the hand to allow things to be more comfortable for you?' 'Is it OK to wipe away some of the sensations with some antiseptic to clean the skin?'*

It is not uncommon to have to wait before a request is accepted. It is important that the patient has the necessary time to comply with each request. Suggestions can be useful. For example,

'*In a moment the arm can straighten as if it is relaxing all on its own without you thinking about it*'.

Immediately prior to needle insertion it is important to inform the patient—but not to give a negative suggestion. For example,

'*If you feel anything at all that bothers you, a cough, wriggling the toes, or a deep breath can all help this to be completed as comfortably and as safely as possible for you*'.

Not

'*Sharp* ***needle*** *and a* ***BEE STING*** *coming now!*'

Very anxious patients find it easier to communicate non-verbally. This can be utilized by the anaesthetist to gain final permission from the patient for cannula placement. For example, '*You can nod your head when you are ready for us to finish*'.

Not infrequently, at this stage the severely phobic patient is either highly focused and quiet, or very anxious, trembling and crying.

If the patient is trembling, this can be utilized. '*You can shake off some of those concerns and worries just now. In a moment, as you shake off those unwanted feelings, things will just seem to settle down as you start to feel more comfortable*'.

Use of the words 'Try' and 'Not' therapeutically and a double bind may be useful here,

'*If you prefer, you can* ***try not to relax*** *and then* ***find yourself relaxing*** *all on your own without you thinking about it*'.

The procedure can be completed with a double bind and a focus on success—that is finishing the cannula insertion rather than starting the procedure.

'*When you are ready for this to finish you will find that you can just nod your head or let me know with an "OK" as soon as you are ready!*'

Reinforcing success

At the end of the procedure it is very important not to waste any success that has been achieved. Each step that went well can be re-enforced and it can be suggested that in future any time a blood test or a drip is needed, it will be easier to achieve success now the patient knows what to do.

'*As with anything—for instance, learning to drive—when we practise new skills things become easier, and seem more in control*'.

'*Most people find that before very long they are surprised that things that would previously bother them for some reason are no longer a concern and we don't even have to know why. In the future any time a blood test or drip is required people find that once they have achieved the success that you have had today they build on that much more easily than they thought. You can look forward to it all being much easier should anything similar be required in future*'.

This statement combines the use of positive suggestion, re-enforcement and repetition.

Emergency management

A 35-year-old woman presenting for emergency surgery started shouting at the anaesthetist as she approached her with an 18G IV cannula for IV access to facilitate a rapid sequence induction of anaesthesia.

Patient: '*If you come near me with that needle, I'll* ***die!***'
Anaesthetist: '*Well that's* ***OK.*** *Just let* ***the arm die*** *for a* ***moment***'.

The patient's left arm rapidly became limp and relaxed allowing the anaesthetist to insert an 18G cannula without local anaesthetic. A second or two later the patient realized the drip was in place. She had experienced this quite comfortably and was surprised how straightforward it had been.

The explanation of how '**LAURS**' was utilized in this case is detailed below:

Listening—the anaesthetist listened to the words the patient used; '***I'll die!***'

Acceptance of the patient's reality involved accepting her belief by saying '*OK*'. This was essential to engage with the patient and develop rapid rapport; no attempt was made to contradict the patient's irrational belief, for example, by saying, '***Of course you are not going to die***—*it's just a little needle!*'

Utilization involved using the patient's words to facilitate the subconscious response to the suggestion that only the arm can '***die***' and for only a '***moment***'.

Reframe—the patient's own words were reframed in a new context so that the 'dying' can be for just '***the arm***' and only for '***a moment***'.

Suggestion—a direct, rather than indirect, suggestion was used, that only 'the arm' rather than the whole body can die, as the patient was extremely anxious and was unlikely to reject a useful way out of her predicament. Using the words '*the* arm' rather than '*your* arm' also encouraged dissociation of the arm from the rest of the body. '*Just let* ***the*** *arm* ***die*** *for a* ***moment***'.

Key points

1. The specific conscious and subconscious aspects of the problem need to be recognized.
2. The '**LAURS**' concept can be used effectively to establish patient rapport and trust.
3. Metaphor may help the anaesthetist to express empathy with the patient's predicament.
4. Positive expectancy is generated by a confident, calm approach with a clear expectation of success.
5. It is vital to ask permission at each stage as control and trust are critical.
6. It is important to reinforce any success achieved.

References

1 Thurgate C, Heppell S (2005). Needle phobia—changing venepuncture practice in ambulatory care. *Paediatr Nurs*, **17**(9), 15–8.

2 Rice LJ (1993). Needle phobia: an anesthesiologist's perspective. *J Pediatr*, **122**(5Pt 2), S9–13.

3 Bamgbade OA (2007). Severe needle phobia in the perianesthesia setting. *J Perianesth Nurs*, **22**(5), 322–9.

4 Veerkamp JS, Majstorovic M (2006). [Dental anxiety and needle phobia in children. A relationship?] *Ned Tijdschr Tandheelkd*, **113**(6), 226–9.

5 Simon GR, Wilkins CJ, Smith I (2002). Sevoflurane induction for emergency Caesarean section: two case reports in women with needle phobia. *Int J Obstet Anesth* **11**(4), 296–300.

6 Searing K, Baukus M, Stark MA, Morin KH, Rudell B (2006). Needle phobia during pregnancy. *J Obstet Gynecol Neonatal Nurs*, **35**(5), 592–8.

7 Cyna AM, Andrew MI, Tan SG (2009). Communication skills for the anaesthetist. *Anaesthesia*, **64**(6), 658–65.

8 Sarifakioglu N, Sarifakioglu E (2004). Evaluating the effects of ice application on the pain felt during botulinum toxin type-a injections: a prospective, randomized, single-blind controlled trial. *Ann Plast Surg*, **53**(6), 543–6.

9 Nafiu OO, Srinivasan A, Ravanbakht J, Wu B, Lau WC (2008). Dexmedetomidine sedation in a patient with superior vena cava syndrome and extreme needle phobia. *J Cardiothorac Vasc Anesth*, **22**(4), 581–3.

10 Kettwich SC, Sibbitt WL Jr, Brandt JR, Johnson CR, Wong CS, Bankhurst AD (2007). Needle phobia and stress-reducing medical devices in pediatric and adult chemotherapy patients. *J Pediatr Oncol Nurs*, **24**(1), 20–8.

11 Kettwich SC, Sibbett WL, Kettwich LG, Palmer CJ, Draeger HT, Bankhurst AD (2006). Patients with needle phobia? Try stress-reducing medical devices. *J Fam Pract*, **55**(8), 697–700.

12 Morse DR, Cohen BB (1983). Desensitization using meditation–hypnosis to control 'needle' phobia in two dental patients. *Anesth Prog*, **30**(3), 83–5.

13 Dash J (1981). Rapid hypno-behavioral treatment of a needle phobia in a five-year-old cardiac patient. *J Pediatr Psychol*, **6**(1), 37–42.

14 Cyna AM, Tomkins D, Maddock T, Barker D (2007). Brief hypnosis for severe needle phobia using switch-wire imagery in a 5-year old. *Paediatr Anaesth*, **17**(8), 800–4.

15 Sehgal A, Mendonca C, Stacey MR (2001). Needle phobia in a patient for urgent caesarean section. *Int J Obst Anesth*, **10**(4), 333–4.

Chapter 15

Intraoperative awareness

Christel J Bejenke

'...To sleep perchance to dream: ay, there's the rub, ...'.
William Shakespeare

What this chapter is about

Intraoperative awareness (IOA) represents a range of heterogeneous experiences and is a topic of considerable relevance, not only to anaesthetists, but to all theatre staff. This chapter focuses on communications that the anaesthetist may find helpful in ameliorating or preventing adverse sequelae associated with IOA. This is a well-described, infrequent complication of general anaesthesia[1–4] which can have serious long-term psychological consequences[5–9].

First recognized as a medical complication in 1846, there have been numerous reports since the 1950s[10–21]. Considerable research has been devoted to its understanding and prevention over the past two decades[1,22,23]. IOA has increasingly come to the attention of clinicians, patients and the media. It is also a medico-legal issue and high compensation awards have been made[24].

Definition

The ASA practice advisory for anaesthesiologists states that, 'Intraoperative awareness occurs when a patient becomes conscious during a procedure performed under general anaesthesia and subsequently has recall of these events.'[7] This may include: sensations of weakness; inability to communicate, move or scream; auditory and tactile perceptions; feelings of helplessness; acute fear, panic and pain; believing to have been abandoned and betrayed; and being dead, or about to die[1,5–13,22,25–27].

Explicit awareness (declarative memory) permits ***conscious recall*** of intraoperative events such as auditory, visual and tactile experiences, paralysis and pain. There is a striking similarity of experiences among patients, but only a minority (35%) may inform their anaesthetists[23,25]. Explicit awareness has been the subject of the majority of investigations related to IOA and is the main topic of this chapter.

Implicit awareness (non-declarative memory): information can be recollected but cannot be recalled[2,23,28] or consciously retrieved. There is strong evidence for auditory information-processing of material relevant to the patient's well-being, whether beneficial or threatening[19–21,29,30].

Incidence

The overall incidence of IOA varies, but has been reported to be between 0.1 and 0.9% with 30 000–40 000 cases annually in the USA[1,7–9,31]. However, the true incidence of recall is probably underestimated. According to a 2010 report by the ASA closed claims project, IOA occurs in less than 1 in 700 cases. Causes were largely attributed to light anaesthesia and anaesthetic delivery problems[8].

Risk factors

Risk factors include light anaesthesia, cardiac and severe trauma surgery, haemodynamically unstable patients, emergency Caesarean sections, ASA status IV, a history of awareness, chronic use of central nervous system depressants, younger age, obesity, inadequate or misused anaesthesia delivery systems, insufficient knowledge about awareness, and total intravenous anaesthesia (TIVA).

Adverse sequelae of awareness

The trauma experienced by some patients has been well documented[5,9,21–23,25] and '*may lead to ... intense emotional states which interfere with the ability to develop a narrative of the events... memories may gradually emerge over time*'[21]. Moerman found that 70% of patients report sleep disturbances, nightmares, fear of future anaesthetics or daytime anxiety. Symptoms may be aggravated when patients are not taken seriously by physicians or family and told that they were '*making it up*' or '*are crazy*'[23]. Late psychological symptoms may lead to PTSD[5,9,16,25,26,32] a seriously debilitating psychiatric condition which may require decades of treatment. PTSD is characterized by re-experiencing the traumatic event, hyperarousal, sleep disturbances, nightmares, intrusive memories ('flashbacks') and avoidance behaviour. Patients often cannot will themselves to set foot in hospitals, even to visit family. Those with the most severe symptoms often claim to be '*OK*', avoid healthcare providers, decline to take part in studies and panic when surgical procedures are contemplated[1,5,9,22,25–27,32]. However, simply suffering pain and hearing voices or noises does not cause late psychological symptoms. In fact, wide-awake patients who suffer greatly during the procedure may have fewer traumatic symptoms afterward than obtunded patients, perhaps because what happens is not in doubt when awake[33].

Recommended preventive measures

BIS (bispectral index) monitoring—considered the standard of care by the ASA[7,8] and by most researchers—was expected to reliably identify the depth of anaesthesia, function as an index of consciousness and ensure the prevention of awareness. However, recently Avidan reported that '*awareness occurred even when BIS values were within the target ranges*', and that BIS '*could give anesthesiologists a false sense of security*'[34].

Recommended clinical measures are[6,7,35,36]:

1. Use of multiple modalities to monitor depth of anaesthesia, including clinical techniques (checking for purposeful or reflex movement), and conventional monitoring systems (electrocardiogram, blood pressure, heart rate and capnography).
2. Avoiding total paralysis by limiting the use of neuromuscular blocking drugs, as they may mask purposeful or reflex movement and responses to painful stimuli.
3. Avoiding TIVA.

Neither scopolamine nor benzodiazepines reliably reduce the incidence of recall[4].

Mitigating the adverse effects of awareness

While the anaesthetist usually does not consider communication skills to be a part of the management and prevention of the serious consequences of IOA, specific approaches are proposed below[36]. The goal is to ameliorate the acute experience of awareness; to lessen or prevent long-term sequelae; to facilitate the short- and long-term management of patients who have experienced awareness in the past and now suffer its consequences; and to facilitate the often extremely difficult pre-operative preparation of panic-stricken patients who previously experienced IOA. Finally, effective communication may obviate litigation.

Aspects of communication to consider include:

- Pre-operative preparation.
- Intraoperative communication.
- Management of patients who report having just experienced awareness.
- Management of patients who have previously experienced awareness and may suffer from PTSD.

Pre-operative preparation

Information is essential. It establishes rapport and confidence in the anaesthetist's competence and commitment. A description of the sequence of events from admission through to the recovery room is an essential part of anaesthesia care in general. Specific issues are the induction, emergence and extubation. Reasons for and benefits of endotracheal intubation, ventilation and paralysis can be included, as well as what takes place during presumed unconsciousness—and that the first priority, as always, is ***safety***[37–39].

The impression that unconsciousness is an absolutely necessary component of successful, safe anaesthesia should be corrected. Instead, patients can be reassured that, while complete unconsciousness cannot always be guaranteed, every effort will be made to provide effective analgesia, and that becoming aware of touch, lights, sounds, etc. does not necessarily mean that 'something went terribly wrong'. In cases where awareness and pain may occur for reasons of safety such as Caesarean sections, major trauma, cardiac surgery and high-risk patients, appropriate explanations should be given pre-operatively.

By using a metaphor of '*...the surface of water*' the anaesthetist can explain that '*depth of anaesthesia*' varies, '*Sometimes patients come up slightly above the surface... that's when they may hear or feel something... and then drift down again....*'

Strategies for communicating with the anaesthetist in the event of awareness can be discussed.

> '*... from time to time you may feel me squeezing your hand ... and if you feel like it ... you can squeeze back ....*'

Pre-operatively this simple statement conveys a sense of control to the patient, and is perceived as empowering. Even during muscle relaxation, residual muscle power may allow the patient 'to squeeze back' and an aware patient is apt to do so. For it serves his own best interest to provide such information to the anaesthetist. A 'hand squeeze' by the anaesthetist, together with a reassuring communication, may calm the patient. If appropriate, anaesthesia can be deepened, if it is contra-indicated, the anaesthetist can explain that,'*... it will be just another few moments ... before it is the right time ... to give you more medicine ....*' Even when experiencing pain, just hearing such a statement can be comforting to the patient.

How detailed the descriptions of possible sensations should be can only be decided by the anaesthetist after assessing the patient and the situation. However, knowledge of the facts, as well as verbal and tactile contact with the anaesthetist, can significantly mitigate the patient's fear during an awareness episode (see case below). It therefore makes sense to inform those patients who are at increased risk for IOA that this is a slight possibility. While such information could function as a negative suggestion[37,38] (see Chapter 20), whether it actually does or not depends upon how this information is communicated. If IOA is addressed, it should be done without being defensive or apologetic in advance.

Because the induction of anaesthesia is one of the most likely periods for awareness, explaining intubation and the endotracheal tube as '*normal, modern and safe*' may reduce the fear and psychological trauma of assuming that 'something went wrong', should the patient experience awareness and recall.

> '*Once you are relaxed, the anaesthetist will put a breathing tube through your mouth (nose) into your windpipe ... which makes breathing extra **safe** during the operation ... and is a part of **modern, safe** anaesthesia*'.

As with all patient–anaesthetist interactions, the anaesthetist should make only those promises which can realistically be kept. Patients should be reassured that the anaesthetist is committed to scrupulous vigilance in protecting them until their autonomy is re-established. Positive suggestions can be included with every item of information, during all interactions, including induction[37,38] (see also Chapter 4, 8 and 20). The patient can also be advised of the possibility that another anaesthetist may take over intraoperatively.

An example of information provided during pre-operative preparation to a high-risk patient for cardiac surgery is given:

> '*As you know,* ***anaesthesia has to do with comfort and safety****—and most of the time we can provide both. But, every once in a while we must decide which is more important ... and you will probably agree that right now* ***safety*** *is most important. We, both you and I, are concerned about your heart. There may be a time when we want to* (**not** '***have*** *to*') *be extra careful ... and extra gentle... to keep your heart as strong ... and working as well as possible. Sometimes it is best to have as little anaesthesia medicine get to your heart as possible ... to keep it working at its best... I will be watching you very, very closely. When it looks like it is better that I hold off a little, that's what I will do. And that may be a time when you might hear or feel some of the work going on .... And just as soon as I know ... that your heart is strong enough ... to take a little more anaesthesia medicine. ... I will give it to you right away*'.

The administration of muscle relaxant effects can also be addressed.

> '*It is also important that your surgeons have the best possible conditions to work under .... So, I will give you a special medicine that makes you very, very relaxed, ... that all your muscles are completely loose and limp .... That will make it much easier for your surgeons ... to do the best possible job .... This feeling will be very different from anything you felt before ... but you will know that I am watching everything very closely ... and taking good care of you ... so that* ***you will be completely safe***'.

The patient has been given factual information with positive connotations. Possible awareness and paralysis is equated with '*doing the best for your heart*'. The anaesthetist should note that:

1. The patient acts as a 'partner in care', rather than a passive recipient of medical technology, which can be very empowering.
2. Statements such as those above can be reassuring both pre-operatively and intraoperatively should consciousness, pain, and/or paralysis be experienced.
3. Explaining the beneficial purpose of paralysis and preparing the patient for this foreign and otherwise frightening sensation is helpful.
4. '*You are safe*' is one of the most important statements a patient can hear pre-, intra- and post-operatively.

Intraoperative communication[36,37]

It is important that the anaesthetist is cognisant that awareness can occur and treats patients as if they are awake under regional or nerve block. Signs of pain or distress should be looked for: movement, hypertension, tachycardia, tearing, pupil size changes or sweating. As always, optimal analgesia is desirable pre-emptively and intraoperatively. Apart from pharmacotherapy, speaking to patients in simple language—avoiding the use of technical terms and 'jargon'—may be helpful when clinical observations suggest they might be 'light': '*I am giving you a little more medicine right now to make you more comfortable*'. Word choice is important as patients tend to interpret communications literally under these conditions.

Reassuring, situation-specific comments, and occasional 'progress reports', can reduce patients' fear, if aware, and enhance recovery. The surgical and theatre team can be educated to avoid careless comments. When negative comments occur, corrective statements can be made with realistic positive connotations.

> **Surgeon:** *'He's full of cancer!'*
> **Anaesthetist:** '*Well—now that we know what the problem is ... the most effective treatment can be instigated!*'

This is not a false promise, nor an empty platitude like '*you're going to be OK*'.

Touch reassures the patient that someone is there—watching. Arms or blankets can be readjusted, a hand placed on the patient's shoulder, hands or feet—whatever happens to be accessible.

Communicating with the theatre team (see also Chapter 17)

Theatre staff have a strong expectation that general anaesthesia involves complete unconsciousness from start to finish. They may find direct communications to patients under general anaesthesia challenging and may question the anaesthetist's competence for providing adequate anaesthesia. This presents the anaesthetist with an opportunity to inform the operating team of current research on awareness and the role their speech may play. It may improve operating room decorum and etiquette for the patient's protection, particularly avoidance of conversations with negative connotations or content—even when referring to other patients.

Patients who report having just experienced awareness

Practice will vary as to whether to check routinely for awareness during the post-operative review. When awareness is suspected (intraoperative inadvertent TIVA disconnection or post-operative patient reports) a careful 'debrief' usually clarifies what was experienced or recalled. Care must be taken not to imply or suggest awareness[36,37]. The timing and frequency of the interviews may be important, more than one interview may be needed to clarify events and credibility of reports should always be verified. Awareness may be missed in some patients[4], especially when discharged from the hospital before an adequate assessment has been made.

Five questions are recommended[4] that do not suggest awareness:

1. What was the last thing you remember before you went to sleep?
2. What was the first thing you remember when you woke up?
3. Can you remember anything in between these periods?
4. Did you dream during your operation?
5. What was the worst thing about your operation?

The author proposes a modification of the last question, as 'worst' implies that something was actually 'bad'.

'*Was there anything that could have been better?*' or '*Was there something that you did not quite like?*' immediately followed by the positive qualification '*...so we can do better next time*'. Such a question will garner the same information, but it changes the tone of the inquiry by avoiding a negative connotation[36,37].

The following clinical example is provided by the editors (SGMT, AMC).

A 35-year-old electrician has had a partial lung resection for recurrent bullae. A thoracic epidural had been placed pre-operatively and TIVA used for induction and maintenance of anaesthesia. During the procedure the TIVA was inadvertently disconnected for approximately 30 minutes. The patient was reviewed post-operatively to check for awareness.

Using 'GREAT' in awareness

Greeting, Goal

Dr A: '*Hello Mr Wake, I am Dr A. I was your anaesthetist yesterday and I am here to check that everything is OK with you*'.

This is an open question without automatically suggesting that anything untoward has happened.

Mr W: '*Well, I was wondering what a "rib spreader" was, Doc...?*'

Rapport

Dr A: '*Where did you hear about a rib spreader?*'
Mr W: '*Well yesterday during my operation after the surgeon had talked about his golf lesson he asked for a rib spreader and I was a bit unsure what that might be*'.
Dr A: '*So you remember some discussion during the operation is that right?*'
Mr W: '*Yes, but I think I must have nodded off at some point 'cos I can't remember much else apart from someone telling me that they were going to give me some more sleeping medicine*'.
Dr A: '*How did you feel about that?*'
Mr W: '*Well I didn't feel any pain if that's what you mean*'.

The first thing Dr A does is to listen to the patient and confirm whether awareness is a possibility or likely. The anaesthetist accepts the report by the patient and acknowledges the episode. The patient seems to have perceived awareness, and this needs to be dealt with honestly, objectively, conveying concern and empathy as appropriate.

The anaesthetist can ensure that the patient realizes that his account is being taken seriously by documenting the account while explaining this to the patient. The anaesthetist's perspective of what happened can be discussed in the presence of the patient and explanations given, as appropriate. It is extremely important to avoid dismissing patient's concerns, even if they seem irrelevant.

Evaluation, Expectations, Explanation

Dr A: '*It sounds like you were awake for some of your operation is that right?*'
Mr W: '*Yes Doc*'.

Dr A: '*We know for a period of time during your surgery that the anaesthetic wasn't getting to you properly but we were unsure whether you would remember anything or not. We did give you extra anaesthetic as soon as we realized what had happened*'.
Mr W: '*Oh .... That's why I got off to sleep then*'.

The anaesthetist confirms that the patient was aware during his operation and offers an explanation to the patient as to how this has happened (see Chapter 12). Also during the procedure the anaesthetist mitigated the potential for a negative experience by appropriate calm, confident communication that more anaesthetic was being administered.

Asking and Answering questions, Acknowledging and Addressing concerns

Dr A: '*Do you have any concerns over what has happened?*'
Mr W: '*Yes, the surgeon says that I will probably need the other side done sometime soon—is this going to* ***happen*** *again?*'
Dr A: '*What has* ***happened*** *to you is a very uncommon event and for this to* ***happen*** *again with you is extremely unlikely. We will make a special note in your medical records so that any future anaesthetist will take particular care to stop this* ***happening****. Have you any other issues you wish me to address?*'
Mr W: '*No, I think I'm OK with that!*'

The anaesthetist uses the patient's own words in response to queries and, as the patient has not voiced the experience in a negative way, neither has the anaesthetist (see Chapters 3 and 4).

Tacit agreement, Thanks, Termination

Dr A: '*I will pop back to see you in the next couple of days to see how you are going. Is that OK?*'
Mr W: '*Thanks Doc—I'm hoping to get out by Friday!*'

The above case demonstrates that patients can be quite accepting of awareness providing they trust their doctors and have not had a painful or emotionally distressing experience. If awareness with pain and/or emotional distress has occurred, the principles of listening and acceptance are equally applicable (see also Chapter 12).

Patients benefit from a clear explanation of what has happened, and why—if this is known. If appropriate, an apology can be made. A frank discussion by the anaesthetist whom the patient might view as the '*perpetrator of his suffering*' can be therapeutic but challenging. Effective communication in these circumstances can obviate the development of persistent psychopathology (such as PTSD), and legal action.

If patients appear traumatized, they should be referred early to a knowledgeable and skilled psychologist. Maintaining contact with the patient and therapist demonstrates concern and allows the anaesthetist to participate or intervene as appropriate.

Patients who have previously experienced awareness

Most anaesthetists will encounter patients who are nearly unmanageable due to extreme fear of anaesthesia or of hospitals. They have often postponed necessary operations for weeks, months or even years. Normally rational and competent, they may not understand why they have been unsuccessful in willing themselves to set foot in a hospital. Many are even unable to visit hospitalized relatives or friends. These patients may have previously experienced explicit or implicit IOA, although they are often unaware of it as a cause of their fears and simply identify themselves as 'phobic'.

Possible approaches include: empathic listening; acknowledgment of the occurrence, and of any subsequent or continued suffering. If records are available these should be reviewed thoroughly with the patient. These patients yearn for information and every effort should be made to respond comprehensively to their numerous questions. Most important to the patient is trust, and ongoing support until resolution.

Natalie, scheduled for multi-level spinal fusions had had '*horrible experiences*' during two preceding operations a few days earlier. A 7-hour emergency surgery after a car crash (abdominal, thoracic and orthopaedic injuries) was followed by an equally long second operation. During both operations she experienced full consciousness and '*excruciating pain*'.

> '*I felt exactly what they were doing .... I tried to let them know ... but I couldn't move. Then I figured out that I was paralysed ... I screamed inside ... but they didn't hear me .... I thought I was dying ... and they had no idea ... I panicked .... I was completely powerless ... and there was nobody to protect me ... to help me*'.

She also recounted detailed conversations, comments and exclamations by individuals whom she identified by name. '*Many words I didn't know*'. Later, while being ventilated in ICU, she again reported being fully awake, paralysed and in excruciating pain '*For days... I didn't know what was going on—I thought I was dying there too. That tube in my throat was killing me... but nobody talked to me*'.

She was petrified of the upcoming operation, and had hardly slept since the previous surgeries.

The anaesthetist (who had not been involved in her previous care) communicated with her as described earlier, after which Natalie commented '*For the first time, I am not afraid*'. In the morning she reported excitedly that she had slept soundly.

During the operation in the prone position, she suddenly lifted up her head, pulled an arm from the securing straps, and reached for the endotracheal tube. The anaesthetist restrained her arm and spoke calmly: '*Everything is going well for you ...* ***and you are safe.*** *You are feeling the tube in your mouth and windpipe—exactly as we had talked about ... and you know that this tube is helping you breathe* ***safely****... so you* ***can feel very safe*** *... I already gave you more medicine .... So you can go back into a deeper sleep*'.

After the completion of the procedure, she awoke immediately after being transferred to her bed, then opened her mouth for suctioning and extubation, and immediately thanked the anaesthetist, repeating over and over '*How wonderful this has been!*'

Later on that day ...

> **Anaesthetist:** '*Do you remember anything about this operation* (making sure NOT to suggest awareness) *... you told me so much about your last ones?*'
> **Natalie:** '*No, it was just so different and ... so nice*'.

Anaesthetist: '*Do you remember me speaking to you?*'
Natalie: '*Oh that! You mean when you were telling me about the tube in my throat? I was so glad you were there, I felt so safe. It all was so different from the other two operations…*'.

This patient illustrates that awareness can be perceived and remembered differently. Awareness does not have to be a traumatic experience even when the patient is already 'primed' to expect it. Instead, effective preparation and intraoperative communication may have benefits.

Key points

1. Intraoperative awareness may occur in any patient during general anaesthesia.
2. Implicit awareness deserves greater attention.
3. The patient can be educated pre-operatively that '*modern, safe*' anaesthesia does not necessarily mean or require profound unconsciousness at all times.
4. Optimal analgesia should always be provided and, where possible, complete muscle relaxation avoided.
5. Signs of awareness should be looked for.
6. Theatre team education regarding awareness, being mindful of conversations in the operating theatre, is important.
7. Reassuring verbal and non-verbal communications to the patient pre- and intraoperatively may mitigate the adverse effects of awareness.
8. After an event, the patient needs to be believed and the evaluation discussed with the patient. Communications need to be genuine and empathic with early referral for psychological counselling and treatment if appropriate.
9. It is advisable that the anaesthetist remain in contact with the patient and his therapist until symptomatology is under adequate care and control.
10. Possible benefits of effective communication include:
    - pre-operatively-reduced anxiety, enhanced trust;
    - during an episode of awareness: amelioration of feelings of abandonment; reduced intraoperative 'terror';
    - post-operatively: faciltating the anaesthetist's review of the episode with the patient; reduction of symptoms; earlier treatment;
    - long-term-reduced severety of symptoms; prevention of PTSD;
    - for PTSD patients who require additional surgery: easier preparation, management and care by the anaesthetist.

References

1 Ghoneim M (2007). Incidence of and risk factors for awareness during anaesthesia. *Best Pract Res Clin Anaesthesiol*, **21**(30), 327–43.

2 Sebel P (1995). Memory during anesthesia: gone but not forgotten? *Anesth Analg*, **81**(4), 668–70.

3 Goldmann L (1988). Information-processing under general anaesthesia. *J R Soc Med*, **81**(4), 224–7.

4 Sandin RH, Enlund G, Samuelsson P, Lennmarken C (2000). Awareness during anaesthesia: a prospective case study. *Lancet*, **355**(9205), 707–11.

5 Lennmarken C, Bildfors K, Enlund G, Samuelsson C, Sandin R (2002). Victims of awareness. *Acta Anaesthesiol Scand*, **46**, 229–31.

6 Joint Commission on Accreditation of Healthcare Organizations (2004). *Preventing, and managing the impact of, anesthesia awareness. Sentinel Event Alert* (*32*), http://www.jointcommission.org/SentinelEvents/SentinelEventAlert/sea_32.htm (Accessed 12 March 2010)

7 American Society of Anesthesiologists (2006). Practice advisory for intraoperative awareness and brain function monitoring: a report by the American Society of Anesthesiologists Task Force on Intraoperative Awareness. *Anesthesiology*, **104**, 847–64.

8 American Society of Anesthesiologists (2010). *ASA Newsletter*, **74**(2), 14–6.

9 Ghoneim M (2010). The trauma of awareness: history, clinical features, risk factors, and cost. *Anesth Analg*, **110**(3), 666–7.

10 Winterbottom EH (1950). Insufficient anesthesia. *BMJ*, **1**, 247–8.

11 Graff TD, Pillips OC (1959). Consciousness and pain during apparent surgical anesthesia. *JAMA*, **170**, 2069–71.

12 Hutchinson R (1960). Awareness during surgery: a study of its incidence. *Br J Anaesth*, **33**, 463–9.

13 McIntyre JWR (1966). Awareness during general anesthesia: preliminary observations. *Can Anaesth Soc J*, **13**, 495–9.

14 Cheek DB (1959). Unconscious perception of meaningful sounds during surgical anesthesia as revealed under hypnosis. *Am J Clin Hypn*, **1**, 101–13.

15 Cheek DB (1960). What does the surgically anesthetized patient hear? *Rocky Mountains Med J*, **57**, 49.

16 Meyer BC, Blacher RS (1961). A traumatic neurotic reaction induced by succinyl-choline chloride *N Y State J Med*, **61**, 1255–61.

17 Cheek DB (1962). The anesthetized patient can hear and remember. *Am J Proctol*, **13**, 287–90.

18 Cheek DB (1964). Surgical memory and reaction to careless conversation. *Am J Clin Hypn*, **6**, 237–40.

19 Cheek DB (1964). Further evidence of persistence of hearing under chemo-anesthesia: detailed case report. *Am J Clin Hypn*, **7**, 55–9.

20 Cheek, DB (1966). The meaning of continued hearing sense under general chemo-anesthesia: a progress report and report of a case. *Am J Clin Hypn*, **8**, 275.

21 Levinson BW (1965). States of awareness during general anaesthesia. *Br J Anaesth*, **37**, 544–6.

22 Ghoneim MM, Block RI, Haffarnan M, Mathews MJ (2009). Awareness during anesthesia: risk factors, causes and sequelae: a review of reported cases in the literature. *Anesth Analg*, **108**(2), 527–35.

23 Moerman N, Bonke B, Oosting J (1993). Awareness and recall during general anesthesia. *Anesthesiology*, **79**, 454–64.

24 Domino, K.B. and Aitkenhead, A.R (2001). Medicolegal consequences of awareness during anesthesia. In: Ghoneim MM (ed.) *Awareness during anesthesia*. pp. 155–72. Woburn, MA: Butterworth Heinemann.

25 Wang M (2001). The psychological consequences of explicit and implicit memories of events during surgery. In: Ghoneim MM (ed.) *Awareness during anesthesia.* pp. 145–8. Butterworth Heinemann, Woburn, MA.

26 Samuelsson P, Brudin L, Sandin RH (2007). Late psychological symptoms after awareness among consecutively included surgical patients. *Anesthesiology,* **106**, 26.

27 Sebel PS (1997). Awareness during general anesthesia. *Can J Anaesth,* **44**(5 Pt 2), R124–30

28 Kihlstrom JF, Barnhardt TM, Tataryn DJ (1992). Implicit perception. In: Bornstein R, Pittman T (eds) *Perception without awareness: cognitive, clinical, and social perspectives.* pp. 17–54. New York: Guilford Press.

29 Howard JF (1987). Incidents of auditory perception during general anaesthesia with traumatic sequelae. *Med J Aust,* **146**, 44–6.

30 Schwender D, Kaiser A, Klasing S, Peter K, Pöppel E (1994). Midlatencey auditory evoked potentials and explicit and implicit memory in patients undergoing cardiac surgery *Anesthesiology,* **80**, 493–501.

31 Sebel PS, Bowdle TA, Ghoneim MM, Rampil IJ. Padilla RE, Gan TJ, et al (2004). The incidence of awareness during anesthesia: a multicenter United States study. *Anesth Analg,* **99**(3), 833–9.

32 Mashour G (2010). Posttraumatic stress disorder after intraoperative awareness and high-risk surgery. *Anesth Analg,* **110**(3), 668–70.

33 Blacher RS (1987). General surgery and anesthesia: the emotional experiences. In: Blacher RS, ed. *The psychological experience of surgery.* pp. 1–25. New York: John Wiley.

34 Avidan MS, Zhang L, Burnside BA, Finkel KJ, Searleman AC, Selvidge JA et al (2008). Anesthesia awareness and the bispectral index. *N Engl J Med,* **358**(11), 1097–108.

35 Lennmarken C, Sandin R (2004). Neuromonitoring for awareness during surgery. *Lancet,* **363**, 1747–8.

36 Bejenke CJ (1996). Can patients be protected from the detrimental consequences of intra-operative awareness in the absence of effective technology? In: Bonke B, Bovill JG, Moerman N (eds) *Memory and awareness in anaesthesia.* pp. 125–33. The Netherlands: van Gorcum & Co.

37 Bejenke CJ (1996). Painful medical procedures. In: Barber J (ed.) *Hypnosis and suggestion in the treatment of pain. A clinical guide.* pp. 209–66. New York: WW Norton.

38 Bejenke CJ (1996). Preparation of patients for stressful medical interventions: some very simple approaches. In: Peter B, Trenkle FC, Kinzel C, Duffner A, Iost-Peter A (eds) *Munich lectures on hypnosis and psychotherapy. Hypnosis International Monographs,* **2**, 27–36.

39 Bejenke CJ (1993). Hypnosis for surgical interventions. *Hypnosis,* **20**(4), 214–20.

Section 4

Communication with colleagues

Chapter 16

Safety-critical communication

Stavros Prineas

'Houston, we have a problem …'.
Apollo 13 crew

What this chapter is about

Communication errors—the mammoth in the room

In Chapter 1 we highlighted an example of failed handover in a tragic case report[1]. This example underscores the difficulty that doctors, as a craft group, often have when we try to talk about *communication* problems. When trying to explain why an adverse event has occurred, we frequently invoke 'poor communication' as a contributing factor. Deeper discussion, however, often proves to be a woollier beast, and we often retreat to the comforting realm of the technical, where the landscape is reassuringly familiar and the outlines are, for us, more clearly defined.

Unfortunately the mammoth in the room cannot be ignored; under systematic scrutiny, 'communication failure' consistently represents one of the lead contributors to serious adverse events[2–4]. Most recently, analysis of AIMS report data in an Australian area health service revealed that communication problems were the largest single contributing factor to severe and/or life-threatening clinical incidents over a 2-year period (2007–2009)[5]. Perhaps if we develop a better vocabulary of the types of communication errors that occur commonly in the workplace, we can be more articulate about them and develop more focused strategies to overcome them.

Communication can be defined as the ***transfer of meaning*** from one person to another. For the purposes of developing practical communication tools, communication can be broken down into a package of signals sent from one person—the transmitter—to another—the receiver[6]. These signals are both verbal and non-verbal.

It is essential to realize that as social beings we are all constantly 'transmitting' signals—not just in the content of our words, but the types of words we use, the tone of our voice, our facial expressions, our body language, our physical proximity to others, the way we dress, the material possessions we display, etc. At any one time most of us are only partly conscious of the total package of what we are 'saying' to others. At the same time we are constantly receiving signals and, to a greater or lesser extent, trying to read meaning into and 'make sense' of these perceptions. Again often we are only partly conscious of the meaning of the 'vibes' we receive; yet they can have a profound impact on what we hear from others.

The goal of good communication is to arrive at an ***effective, shared understanding*** of a situation. This involves a dynamic exchange of signals between transmitter and receiver. We don't communicate ***at*** people—we communicate ***with*** them—so good communication is as much about ***listening*** as it is about ***talking***, and as much about the dynamic conventions we use to arrive at an equilibrium of understanding—how we check that what was 'heard' matches what was 'said' as closely as possible.

In this chapter, a number of practical tools are offered to improve the fidelity of transfer of meaning between members of clinical teams. Communication skills need to be seen in the context of other 'non-technical' or 'paratechnical'* skills, such as situation awareness, task preparedness, team-working and decision making[7].

Communication styles

The way we say things often reveals what is important to us. Even when it doesn't, others will try intuitively to infer this (rightly or wrongly) from the way we say things. In a workplace, some communication styles are more constructive than others. Trainee pilots are taught a useful matrix for categorizing communication styles[8] according

* Author's note: while the term *non-technical skills* has become entrenched in prevailing literature, it is the author's contention that, as our understanding of and expertise in these important skills increases, this term may become a misnomer. Much research is being directed at developing practical tools, protocols and techniques to hone communication and team-work skills, supported by validated data—in other words, to 'technify' the 'non-technical'. One can foresee a time when communication techniques such as SBAR and graded assertiveness are as well-defined a part of an anaesthetist's technical armamentarium as the rapid sequence induction technique for emergency anaesthesia, or the primary survey technique for assessing trauma patients. Furthermore, there is a danger in assuming that these skills can be taught in isolation of (or, dread the thought, *instead* of) the technical skills with which they are meant to operate; rather they should be seen as operating alongside these skills, and indeed intertwined with them. In this sense the term *paratechnical* (from the Greek *para-* meaning 'alongside' or 'accompanying') may better reflect their true relationship.

to whether the person communicating is more focused on who will dominate in a conversation rather than the task at hand, and whether they are electing to lead—'stepping up'—or follow—'stepping back' (see Figure 16.1)[9].

With an ***aggressive*** style, a person elects to dominate a conversation irrespective of whether or not this is in the interests of the task. This style is typified by a range of readily identifiable behaviours— from the use of demeaning and intimidating language, put-downs, snide remarks, intrusive body language and stand-over tactics, to overt acts of violence and abuse.

A ***submissive*** style is one where a person elects to submit to intimidation irrespective of whether this is in the best interests of the patient. This style is typified by remaining silent even when a situation is deteriorating, not speaking up, not escalating concern, apologizing where no apology is required, etc.

In a ***cooperative*** style, a person elects to follow the lead of another and to actively support another's plan, believing it to be the right plan for the situation in the best interests of the patient. This style is typified by active feedback toward the achievement of the common goal, encouragement—'*Good idea!*', and acknowledgement—'*Thank you*', '*Well done!*', and offering assistance.

An ***assertive*** style is one where a person elects to articulate concerns in the best interest of the task, even in the face of a contrary point of view. This style differs from the aggressive style in that the language is not directed at intimidating others but framed purely around the task itself or the patient's interest, and around whatever actions need to be taken. In effect it's about articulating clearly a person's view of '***what***' is right, rather than '***who***' is right. Elements of this style are detailed in greater depth later in this chapter.

In the vast majority of situations a cooperative communication style—actively supporting and following an agreed plan—is all that is required. However, when a plan goes astray, or the plan seems unclear or wrong, staff must know when and how to speak up.

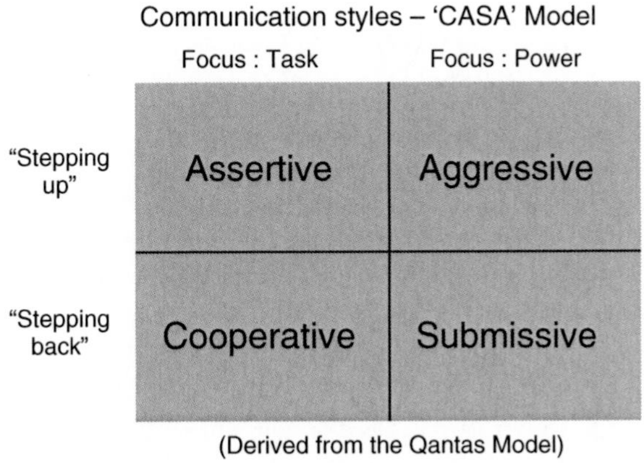

Communication styles – 'CASA' Model
Focus : Task
Focus : Power
"Stepping up"
Assertive
Aggressive
"Stepping back"
Cooperative
Submissive
(Derived from the Qantas Model)

Fig. 16.1 Communication styles[10].

In healthcare environments, aggressive communication styles are commonplace, and they significantly impair team function[11,12]. They tend to polarize others into reacting in an aggressive or submissive way, and set the cultural tone for how others are expected to behave in order to survive in their workplace. However it may well be the prevalence of ***submissive*** communication styles that poses the more serious threat to patient safety, as it directly subverts the 'duty of care' to our patients. If we don't speak up when we see things going wrong, who will?

In any hierarchical training environment, there are significant implicit barriers to speaking up[13]—the assumption that someone else will fix the problem, a reluctance to state the obvious, lack of confidence, fear of being wrong, fear of humiliation, fear of conflict, fear of reprisal, and so on. Thus, rather than assuming that staff will know when and how to assert themselves, healthcare organizations have an obligation to monitor and cultivate actively a work environment where personnel feel comfortable, safe and supported when they wish to clarify instructions and escalate concern, and to provide adequate ongoing assertiveness training for all staff. This can be done through a range of tools.

Graded assertiveness

Graded assertiveness[14] (GrA) is a technique for escalating concern in a graduated fashion until the 'asserter' (the person asserting) is either dissuaded, put on hold, or overruled by the 'assertee' (the person being asserted to). The technique was developed as a formal protocol by the aviation industry to help junior pilots articulate concern in situations where they believed a senior colleague was acting in error. Senior nursing staff will recognize this as a formalized variation of 'the doctor–nurse game'[15,16].

The protocol has four levels.

Level 1: Observation The asserter makes a neutral statement that relates to the concern. The statement could be as simple as stating a vital sign—for example, '*Her blood pressure is 80 systolic*' or '*Sats are 89%*'—or stating a relevant fact—for example, '*I've never used remifentanil before*'.

Level 2: Suggestion The asserter makes a positive alternative suggestion using a cooperative communication style. This can be in the form of a statement e.g., '*Perhaps I can check the pharmacopoeia for the correct dose*' or a question e.g., '*Would you like me to give some IV fluid?*'

Level 3: Challenge The asserter directly questions the plan or decision, requesting a clarification or explanation. The name of the person and the word 'you' are usually included to secure the attention of the listener. '*John, are you sure you want to give 40mg of vitamin K?*' or '*Excuse me, Sarah, but why don't you want to call your consultant?*'

Level 4: Emergency The asserter gives a direct order to deal with an emergency situation. It is used only when there is an immediate threat to life and limb. In aviation, the coded phrase always used in Level 4 assertions is '*Captain, you must listen*'. In healthcare, we can use the title of our colleague, followed by a coded phrase, followed by a direct instruction, and usually with some expression of the consequences of failing to follow the instruction. The actual words used are less important than having a standardized and readily recognizable phrase that is used throughout the organization. For example, '***Doctor, in the interests of this patient you must listen.*** *I will not give the drug as you've prescribed it. Please revise the dose*'.

What happens after Level 4?

In aviation, '*Captain you must listen*' is code for the equivalent of '*Captain, if you don't return the plane to a safe condition now, I'm taking over control of the plane*'. This is because the person asserting is almost always a co-pilot, and therefore trained to take over. In emergency situations, where a person is empowered to take over in a clinical situation, they should do so (however, see 'Prerequisites' below). Unfortunately in healthcare the person asserting is often not in a position to assume the task they're concerned about. There are nevertheless a number of alternative actions staff can take:

- The most important action wherever possible is to get help—a senior supervisor, a colleague of the same rank or indeed anyone that can help resolve the situation.
- Refuse to participate in the intervention, or to administer a prescribed drug.
- Withhold access to drugs or equipment.
- Document the Level 4 interaction in the patient record.

Refining GrA—entry level, escalation

It is recommended that where the situation allows, GrA is started at the lowest level of assertion, and escalated in a stepwise fashion until there is a resolution. In some situations, however—for example, in cardiac arrest resuscitation, there may be no time to step through the levels, and entry at Level 2, Level 3 or even Level 4 may be required. In other situations, there may not be an imminent threat to a patient's safety or there may be time to seek advice or a senior ruling outside the current conversation. In these cases, escalating beyond Level 2 may lead to needless confrontation. Like any skill, GrA requires practice to develop an intuition for when to step in and how far to step up.

Prerequisites to implementation of GrA training

Despite the absence of aggressive language, Level 3 and Level 4 assertions can be quite confronting, especially to senior personnel, who may feel that it is their authority overall which is being challenged, rather than their decision in this instance. Furthermore, it is not uncommon for the person asserting actually to be mistaken or misinformed, and that the other person has an entirely valid and appropriate explanation for their decision.

It is therefore important that certain conventions be in place to ensure the tool withstands the challenges posed by our work environment[17].

1. GrA requires formal ***managerial endorsement*** from the highest levels of the organization, encouraging junior personnel to speak up and also informing senior personnel that this language is being used not as a personal challenge to their authority but as an impersonal safety technique.

2 A ***standardized language*** and format should be taught throughout the organization, so that individuals, both junior and senior, can readily identify the tool and its intent when it is being deployed. Ideally training should be mandatory for all personnel.

3 One must be able to assume that people are ***acting in the best interests of the patient.*** Thus the use of the tool to pursue mischievous ends, personal agendas or 'point-scoring', undermines the credibility of the tool and must not be tolerated by the organization.

4 It follows from this that GrA works best in an environment where it is ***integrated into regular in-service training*** with other communication and team-work tools.

5 It must be understood that use of the assertiveness protocol is not rigid, but can and ***must be adapted according to the circumstances.*** Entry level, rate of escalation and the maximum assertiveness level will vary according to the situation and the people involved. Developing an intuition for this flexibility requires practice.

6 Finally, invoking higher levels of assertiveness (Levels 3 and 4) should be ***based on sound knowledge and awareness*** of the situation and on a clear and imminent threat to patient safety. Usually this means having clear evidence of concern. An exception to this is when it is evident that the team have not gathered the information needed to proceed safely with a critical task—for example, not knowing how a new drug might interact with a patient's concurrent medications. In this situation one can escalate concern not on the basis of facts, but based on the ***absence*** of requisite facts. The senior clinician can then decide whether there is time to get that information, consider alternatives or proceed on a calculated risk assessment.

In aviation the use of this tool has allowed both 'asserter' and 'assertee' to become sensitized to the various levels, so that all staff are attuned to responding to lower levels of assertiveness. This means that overt confrontation in day-to-day safety discussions is largely avoided, and that exchanges at higher, more confrontational, levels of assertiveness are less common. This cultural shift has occurred through application of and commitment to the tool over time.

Other assertiveness protocols exist. The Team STEPPS system advocates a three-step escalation process—'*I am concerned*'/'*I am uncomfortable*'/'*This is a safety issue*'[18]. Whatever system is employed, in-servicing of the technique should follow the prerequisite guidelines stated above, and it should be subject to ongoing audit and refinement.

Systematic handover and briefing techniques

Poor handovers and briefings prior to critical tasks are a well-recognized source of communication failures linked to adverse events[19]. Over the last decade a number of formalized handover and briefing tools have been developed for healthcare, derived loosely from models used in the military.

'SBAR'

SBAR is a simple tool for organizing and sharing information in a task-oriented way. The name is an abbreviation of its four basic elements—**S**ituation, **B**ackground, **A**ssessment and **R**ecommendation[20].

Situation

There are two parts to describing the situation. The first is a brief orientation—the person instigating the SBAR states who they are, where they're from and what their role is. They confirm the identity of the person they're talking to. The second part is a short, simple statement of the reason for the conversation, such as asking a person to come and help, asking for advice or simply notifying someone of results or events. If the discussion is about a particular patient, the identity of the patient is explicitly confirmed.

Background

The purpose of the background statement is to relay information needed to put the situation in context. Again there are two parts to this: first, a brief history of the patient's condition, medications, social/family issues, and clinical progress if they have been under care for any length of time; and second, anything about the staff member, the team or the facility that might influence their ability to respond to the situation—'*This is my first day here and I don't know where anything is*', or '*I've never used sodium nitroprusside before*'.

Assessment

This is a brief evaluation of what's happening now. This has three parts: first, a summary of recent examinations, investigations and interventions since the current situation began—vital signs, latest pathology results, etc.; second, the person's provisional diagnosis—what the person believes is causing or driving the current situation, even if that diagnosis is '*I don't know*'; and, third, a projection of where things are heading—is the situation stable, improving or deteriorating? In this respect the three parts of the assessment phase match the three levels of *situation awareness*—perception (eliciting signs), comprehension (forming a diagnosis), and projection (making a prognosis), described by Endsley[21].

Recommendation

The last statement is a summary of what needs to be done—this might be in the form of an itemized management plan, or something as simple as '*I need you to come in*'. In an ongoing critical situation, it may be useful to state what's been done already, and then lead on to what next needs to be done.

Using SBAR

Being an overview tool, SBAR works best if each element is kept as brief as possible initially. It is useful to think of SBAR not so much as an acronym or a checklist, but rather a way of organizing thoughts that is not that far removed from the traditional clinical model of presenting illness, history, examination, investigations, provisional diagnosis, prognosis and management plan. Given this, it is best where possible to take a little time to 'SBAR' in one's own mind before picking up the phone or walking into handover. By keeping things brief, and allowing the opportunity to spot (and fill) gaps in one's understanding of the situation before critical conversations, this tool would be appreciated by all time-pressured colleagues.

Variations on SBAR

A recent study of a pilot programme in West Australian hospitals revealed a number of practical issues with the use of SBAR[22]—first, it was not intuitively obvious to people that they should introduce themselves and confirm the identity of the other party or the patient during the *situation* phase; second, some critical situations remained unresolved whenever there was disagreement about what plan to follow; and, third, there were occasions where a plan was discussed but not clearly understood by all parties. As a result a variation of SBAR—iSoBAR—was developed to address these findings. iSoBAR is very similar to SBAR, the individual components being **I**ntroductions, **S**ituation, **O**bservations (equivalent to 'Assessment'), **B**ackground, **A**gree (on a plan) and **R**eadback. Further studies are awaited to determine how this paradigm improves the handover process.

Pre-operative briefings

In aviation and in the military, briefings before and after critical missions are standard operational requirements. Recently there has been a growing trend toward structured briefings before all surgical procedures to try to reduce the incidence of 'wrong patient' or 'wrong site' surgery. A popular version of this has been the 'Time-Out' procedure developed by the VA Hospital System in the USA and now used across many parts of Australia[23]. Most 'Time-Outs' constitute a brief period before surgical incision where all members of the operating theatre team go through an itemized checklist to confirm the patient's identity, the operative procedure, the surgical site, the presence of signed consent and other details such as the availability of X-rays and the use of antibiotics.

The World Health Organization has launched a Surgical Checklist aimed at reducing perioperative errors and adverse events[24]. Lingard *et al.*[25] have been developing a pre-operative checklist for theatre teams directed specifically at reducing specific types of communication error by using a validated assessment system. Initial studies suggest that use of the checklist halved the incidence of communication errors. This is an exciting field for future study.

A challenge to compliance with the 'Time-Out' tool is the differing cultural attitudes of nurses and doctors to the use of checklists. Generally nurses view checklists as an important and reassuring safety tool, while many doctors perceive them to be a bureaucratic intrusion[26]. The truth no doubt lies somewhere in between, and in any case will vary according to the situation. Anecdotally, in Australia at least, getting surgeons and anaesthetists to take responsibility for running the 'Time-Out' has proven difficult. It is the author's view that whatever its name, a 'Time-Out' is first and foremost a *briefing*—an opportunity for the whole team to join together for a moment in time to ensure they share the same mental model of what needs to be done, to whom and by whom.

No matter how many boxes get ticked, if the surgeon is not in the room then the fundamental purpose of the briefing is frustrated. Perhaps if the exercise were 'rebranded' as a briefing rather than a checklist, better compliance could be achieved. However, it is interesting to note that in their successful study Lingard *et al.* secured the *a priori* cooperation of local surgeons, who took responsibility for running the checklists.

The communication roles of leadership

Leadership styles can be defined according to the extent to which team leaders consult their subordinates and are prepared to accept questions, challenges or requests for clarification of their decisions. At one extreme, 'autocratic' leaders tend not to consult their juniors and expect their instructions to be followed without question[27], while 'consultative' leaders actively seek input, and encourage juniors to raise questions and concerns where appropriate. Finally there is the 'laissez-faire' style, where the 'leader' eschews any authority over others and effectively offers no guidance at all. Good leaders do not confine themselves to one leadership style, but rather adapt to the needs of the situation. For example, it may well be appropriate to lead autocratically during resuscitation, and equally to lead consultatively when assessing a complex patient for an elective procedure.

As stated earlier in this chapter, there are many cultural barriers to assertiveness; and while there are some generational differences, generally it is common for junior members of a team to feel unsure and insecure about speaking up, even on safety issues. Implicit within the duties of being a good team leader is to make explicit the ground rules of communication between team members, and to give permission to even the most junior member of the team to speak up respectfully on matters of safety. As one fighter-pilot would regularly say to his crew: '*You are my eyes and ears—if you see, hear or even intuit anything is wrong you must tell me, I'll only be angry if you don't*'[28].

Articulating who's in command: 'handing over/taking over'

It could be observed that the likelihood of an anaesthetic adverse event seems to increase in proportion to the number of anaesthetists present at the time. When two people are sharing a vigilance role, control of the mission (i.e. 'who's watching the patient?') is often *implicit*—it is assumed and not articulated. In aviation, control and transfer of control is always *explicit*. During handovers, the pilot flying says '*Handing over*' and does not let go of the steering column until the pilot monitoring says '*Taking over*'. When a consultant is supervising a trainee, it may be useful to adopt the aviation paradigm of nominating who has the controls, and to ensure, whenever a colleague hands over, goes on break, or needs to attend to an interruption, that control of the anaesthetic is transferred explicitly using a reciprocated code phrase.

Other communication tools

The 'Below Ten' rule

The aviation industry has a 'Sterile Cockpit' or 'Below Ten' rule[8]. This is based on the idea that whenever a passenger aircraft in flight is below 10 000 feet, it is either taking off, landing or crashing. Thus 'below ten', the crew should be focused exclusively on controlling the plane; they should not be discussing non-operational matters until the critical phase has passed. When the pilot states that '*We are below ten*', he or she is not necessarily declaring an emergency, merely that the crew need to focus on a critical task.

This technique can be used in any situation where you require the team to focus specifically—for example, during inhalational inductions of children in the operating theatre. It is useful, when dealing with an anxious child or parent, to have a neutral code phrase that is implicitly understood by the theatre team. When the anaesthetist says '*We're below ten*', the scrub nurse stops clattering instruments, and everyone stops talking, quietly preparing or standing ready to assist while the child is being anaesthetized. It is important to note that it is not the anaesthetist who is 'below ten'—it is ***the room and all the people in it***. The same rule can be invoked, for example, by the surgeon during a tricky dissection or by the scrub nurse if a surgical swab is still missing after a recount. This technique requires in-servicing of all operating theatre staff, as it only works well among well-established teams where all members are cognisant of the 'below ten' phrase and its meaning.

'Transparent' communication

In a team environment it is useful to make a habit of articulating one's intentions (*transparent communication* or what pilots call 'flying by mouth') for at least four important reasons. First, in general, conscious patients appreciate knowing in advance what is about to be done to them. Second, by making one's intentions explicit to the team, it improves the team's situation awareness of what is being done when, and by whom. The third reason is that it offers other team members the opportunity to notice and thereby trap an error in the making. Finally, since experts tend to perform most of their highly skilled actions on 'autopilot'—that is, intuitively and under minimal conscious monitoring[29]—making a habit of articulating one's intentions offers a final opportunity to bring a potentially erroneous action to one's own conscious attention before actually performing it.

There are exceptions where the overt or anticipated distress of a patient needs to be considered, but in most circumstances the routine use of transparent communication is reassuring and well tolerated. Personnel who have worked in medical air retrieval units, where medical teams and aircrew train together, are used to this style of communication.

English language traps

Pilots worldwide undergo formal telecommunications training. Part of this training involves learning specific ways to minimize ambiguity and error during all flight communications. This is because there are many language traps, particularly in English.

The most obvious is the ambiguity of 'right' which is used both as 'the opposite of left' and 'the opposite of wrong'. Another is the phonic similarity between the 'teen' numbers and their respective 'tens'—'thirteen' as opposed to 'thirty', 'fourteen' to 'forty', etc. Even the similarity between hypOtension and hypERtension demonstrates that we cannot rely on Greek or Latin pedantry to help us avoid ambiguity. Furthermore, this is compounded by a bewildering growth of acronyms, many with multiple meanings (e.g. RA, OA, NAD) and the lack of an internationally accepted standard for prescriber notation[30].

Specificity in communication training

There are a number of ways individuals can train to make their everyday language less ambiguous:

- Use the word 'right' only when referring to 'left' or 'right', and always use alternatives for its other meanings. '*The left knee is the correct knee, OK?*' as opposed to '*The left knee is the right knee, right?*'
- Learn the NATO phonetic alphabet '*Alpha*' '*Bravo*' '*Charlie*', etc. to clarify the spelling of names.
- When giving a verbal order for a drug dose involving 'teens' or 'tens', spell out the digits '*Please give 15—that's one-five—units of insulin subcutaneously stat*'.
- Take responsibility for the legibility of one's own handwriting.
- Get into the habit of following the 'five rights' of drug prescribing—the right ***drug*** in the right ***dose*** via the right ***route*** at the right ***time*** for the right ***patient***—when giving verbal or written medication orders. It is remarkable that this simple mnemonic is standard training for the nurses who administer drugs[31] but not for the doctors who prescribe them. Using the 'five rights' will not eliminate medication errors—the causes of medication errors are complex and multi-factorial—but it's a good foundation for reducing their incidence.

Using names and numbers

It is important to know and use the names of the patients, not only out of respect but also as a ready means of confirming identity. Do not accept a request to see '*a 19-year-old appendix*'—insist on the patient's name. Just as important is knowing the names of co-workers, and not just out of courtesy, but because it makes direction of instructions more effective during crises.

Many common pieces of anaesthetic equipment go by various names, and sometimes different staff use different names for the same object—for example, 'catheter mount' or 'liquorice stick', 'rosette clamp' or 'armboard knob'. It is useful over time to steer all staff, and any new staff, toward a common nomenclature for all objects, as this can minimize frustration and delay during crises.

A more difficult challenge is using 'context-independent' language. The use of pronouns ('it', 'them', 'you'), pronoun adjectives ('this', 'that') and temporal adverbs ('soon', 'in a moment') is useful shorthand in everyday conversation. However, these terms are 'context dependent': they rely on a person's mental context for their perceived meaning. This context changes from person to person, place to place and over time. Where precision is required, errors may arise when these convenient but non-specific terms are used. With training it is possible to learn to enter a mind set where one avoids context-dependent words, specifying the names of people, objects and drugs throughout a critical phase of a given procedure.

'*Fran, hand me the Yankauer sucker please*'

as opposed to

'*Somebody give me something, I can't see a bloody thing*'

or

'*I should be in theatre in 10 minutes, call me if you don't hear from me in 20*', as opposed to '*I'll get there soon*'.

Feedback and debriefing

Healthcare involves making management plans for patients, and often these plans are conveyed verbally. Complex instructions, including, drug names, dose regimens and operative sites, are passed from one caregiver to another. Sometimes a simple error—the transposition of a digit, mishearing a drug name, confusing an operative site—can have devastating consequences. Yet when a doctor discusses a patient's management plan with a colleague there is no current expectation that either party will formally ensure that what was said matches what was heard.

The military use a particular technique to ensure high-fidelity transfer of meaning from one soldier to another. While those outside the military may not be familiar with its name—***challenge–response protocol***—when the technique is used just about everyone would recognize it as a form of 'military-speak'. Soldiers are required to acknowledge that they have received an order, and for certain verbal instructions they are required to repeat the order itself.

A challenge–response protocol can be used during critical phases of a procedure, such as a MET (Medical Emergency Team) call or a difficult intubation. There is a convention commonly used by nurses receiving verbal orders over the telephone to ensure that the order is heard by a third person. This is done to verify that the first nurse has correctly heard the order that was given. Perhaps more important would be to read the order back to the person giving the order, so that they can verify that the order is actually what they intended.

A similar tool being used in North America is called 'Close the Loop'[32]. When a clinician gives an order or requests information, he or she is taught to seek an acknowledgement if they get no response by saying '*Close the loop*'. This is potentially a very useful way of engendering an appreciation of two-way communication during crises, and encourages staff not to assume, just because an instruction has been given, that it has been heard correctly, or even at all.

Mission debriefings are another important feedback mechanism for monitoring and improving team performance. Standard mission debriefs are conducted in three parts—what was done well, what could have been done better and a positive plan to improve future performance. This format, designed to cushion criticism between two layers of positive feedback, has become colloquially known as the 's*** sandwich'—'good news, bad news, good news'[33]. Indeed as a training aid, routine mission debriefing, perhaps over coffee after an operating list, is useful even when there have been no overt problems in performance. In contrast, in cases of repeatedly poor, vexatious or overtly dangerous performance, it is important to put patient safety first, and an assertive 'Level 3 or 4' approach may become a priority. Effective debriefing therefore is a subtle art that requires practice and reflection.

Key points

1. Anaesthetists cannot ignore the importance of communication skills in their practice.
2. Communication is the transfer of meaning from one person to another.
3. Good communication results from a dynamic two-way exchange between transmitter and receiver.
4. Some communication styles are more constructive than others.
5. Organizations that employ people to have a duty of care over patients have an obligation to provide assertiveness training to all staff.
6. Graded assertiveness is one such technique, but others are available.
7. Systematic handover and briefing techniques, such as SBAR or similar variants, are essential to patient safety.
8. Clinical leaders and managers have the power and the duty to set a constructive tone of communication for their teams and to articulate who is in control or command.
9. There are many English language traps that will lead to common communication errors—these can often be overcome by awareness and the use of specific techniques,
10. Feedback and debriefing techniques are important not only for training and pastoral care but also to trap errors and prevent them on future occasions.

References

1 Paul M, Dueck M, Kampe S, Petzke F, Ladra A (2003). Intracranial placement of a nasotracheal tube after transnasal trans-sphenoidal surgery. *Br J Anaesth*, **91**(4), 601–4.

2 Wilson RM, Runciman WB, Gibberd RW, Harrison BT, Newby L, Hamilton JD (1995). The Quality in Australian Health Care Study. *Med J Aust*, **163**, 458–71.

3 Agency for Healthcare Research and Quality (2003). *Interim Report to Senate Committee on Appropriations*. http://www.ahrq.gov/qual/pscongrpt/psini2.htm (Accessed 13 March 2010).

4 The Joint Commission (2008). *Physicians and the Joint Commission: the patient safety partnership*. Available through the Joint Commission website http://www.jointcommission.org/Physicians/md_tjc.htm (Accessed 13 March 2010).

5 Porteous J, MacIntosh W (2009). Western Australia Country Health Service. Personal communications drawn from internal AIMS report data 2007—2009–summary report available by contacting WACHS through http://www.wacountry.health.wa.gov.au/ (Accessed 21 March 2010).

6 DeVito JA (1988). *Human communication.* 2nd edn. New York, NY: Harper & Row.

7 Fletcher G, Flin R, McGeorge P, Glavin R, Maran N, Patey R (2003). Anaesthetists' non-technical skills (ANTS). Evaluation of a behavioural marker system. *Br J Anaesth*, **90**, 580–8.

8 Australian Airlines (1987). *Communication styles. Aircrew Team Management Handbook* pp. 73–86 (internal publication).

9 Prineas S, Wynne D. (2004). *The Caesar in Bed 12: facilitators' guide.* Sydney: ErroMed Publishers.

10 Prineas S (2005). *The Human Error and Patient Safety (HEAPS) training programme manual.* (Available through www.erromed.com).

11 Dunn H (2003). Horizontal violence among nurses in the operating room. *AORN J*, **78**(6), 977–88.

12 Inch J (2007). Horizontal violence: the silent destructive force. *Br J Anaest Recov Nurs*, **8**(2), 20–1.

13 Poroch D, McIntosh W (1995). Barriers to assertive skills in nurses. *Aust N Z Ment Health Nurs*, **4**(3), 113–23.

14 Qantas Airways Ltd (1989). *Managing upwards: flight operations crew resource management handbook.* pp. 4.25–4.28 (internal publication).

15 Stein LI (1967). The doctor–nurse game. *Arch Gen Psychiatry*, **16**(6), 699–703.

16 Stein LI (1990) The doctor-nurse game revisited. *N Engl J Med*, **323**(3), 201–3.

17 Prineas S, Wynne N (2006). *Bertha's fall—facilitators' guide.* Sydney: ErroMed Publishers.

18 US Department of Health and Human Services, AHRQ (2009). *TeamSTEPPS—national implementation.* Available through http://teamstepps.ahrq.gov/ (Accessed March 12 2010).

19 Wacther R, Shojania K (2004). *Internal bleeding.* New York: Rugged Land Publishers

20 Leonard M (2006). *Effective teamwork as a care strategy: SBAR and other tools for improving communication among caregivers.* On-demand presentation available through the Institute for Healthcare Improvement Website http://www.ihi.org/IHI/Programs/AudioAndWebPrograms/Effective+Teamwork+as+a+Care+Strategy+SBAR+and+Other+Tools+for+Improving+Communication+Between+Careg.htm (Accessed 12 March 2010).

21 Endsley M, Garland D (2001). *Situation awareness: analysis and measurement.* pp. 3–29. New Jersey: Lawrence Erlbaum Associates.

22 Porteous J, Stewart-Wynne EG, Connolly M, Crommelin PF (2009). iSoBAR—a concept and handover checklist: the National Clinical Handover Initiative. *Med J Aust*, **190**(11), S152–6.

23 NSW Health (2005). *Time out checklist for surgical procedures.* Available as downloadable pdf file from NSW Health website http://www.health.nsw.gov.au/resources/quality/correct/pdf/surgical_check_0208.pdf (Accessed 12 March 2010).

24 Heynes A, Weiser T, Berry W, Lipsitz SR, Breizat AH, Dellinger EP et al. (2009) A surgical safety checklist to reduce morbidity and mortality in a global population. *N Engl J Med*, **360**(5), 491–9.

25 Lingard L, Regehr G, Orser B, Reznick R, Baker GR, Doran D et al. (2008). Evaluation of a preoperative checklist and team briefing among surgeons, nurses and anaesthesiologists to reduce failures in communication. *Arch Surg*, **143**(1), 12–7.

26 Gawande A (2007). *The checklist. The New Yorker,* Dec. 10: 86-101. Also available via the New Yorker website http://www.newyorker.com/reporting/2007/12/10/071210fa_fact_gawande?currentPage=1 (Accessed 12 March 2010).

27 Sexton B, Thomas E, Helmreich R (2000). Error, stress and teamwork in medicine and aviation; cross-sectional surveys. *BMJ,* **320**, 745–9.

28 Nance JJ (2001). *Presentation for Institute for Healthcare Improvement.* Video available through IHI website www.ihi.org (Accessed 12 March 2010).

29 Reason J (1990). *Human error.* Cambridge: Cambridge University Press.

30 Davis NM (2003). Medical abbreviations: 24,000 conveniences at the expense of communications and safety.11th edn. Pennsylvania: Neil M Davis Associates.

31 ASHP (1993). ASHP guidelines on preventing medication errors in hospitals. *Am J Hosp Pharm,* **50**(5), 305–14.

32 Small S, Wuerz R, Simon R, Shapiro N, Conn A, Setnik G (2008). Demonstration of high-fidelity simulation training for emergency medicine.*Acad Emerg Med,* **6**(4): 312–23.

33 Adey P (2004) Professional development for cognitive acceleration: elaboration. In: *Professional development of teachers: practice and theory.* pp. 31–50. New York: Kluwer Academic Publishers.

Chapter 17

The theatre team

Suyin GM Tan and Andy McWilliam

'A good surgeon deserves a good anaesthetist. A bad surgeon needs one'.
Anon

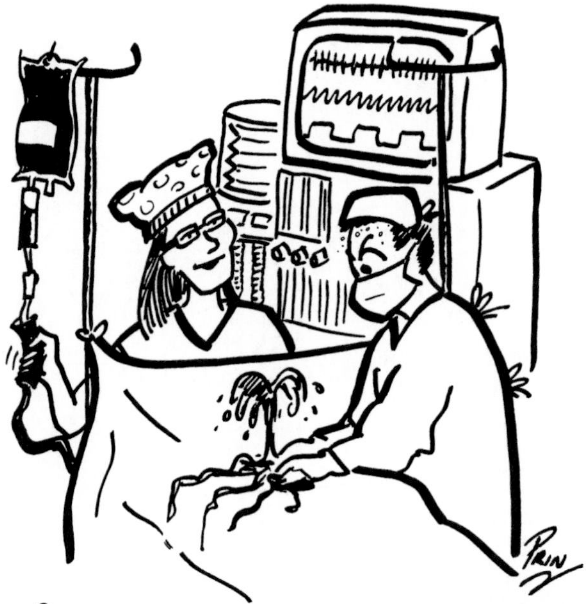

Sure I can do something about the @#?! bleeding, but who'll watch the patient while I scrub?

What this chapter is about

A core attribute of the anaesthetist is the ability to communicate effectively in a variety of difficult situations and contexts. During the course of a theatre list the anaesthetist may interact with literally dozens of people—surgeons, patients, nurses, wardspeople, radiographers, trainees, and so on. Many will be complete strangers while others may be old friends, or enemies! Virtually all of them will have some part, be it big or small, to play in achieving a safe and successful outcome for patients.

Operating theatres are often busy, stressful places. Events can unfold quickly and in unpredictable ways. Tension is frequently an integral part of the process of undertaking surgical procedures[1]. Observational studies[2] demonstrate that communication errors are common, and result in tension, delay, and wastage—as borne out by everyday experience. There is a tendency to view communication breakdowns as an inevitable fact of theatre life. However, evidence shows that behaviours and attitudes can be altered[3,4].

Improving teamwork and communication improves morale and has the potential to improve patient outcomes[5]. Most anaesthetists view themselves as good communicators, able to deal with virtually all communication problems, yet breakdown in communication is commonly cited as a root cause of medical error[6]. Interestingly most anaesthetists feel that their training in communication has been adequate and do not seek further education in communication skills despite the evidence that poor communication leads to adverse events[7,8].

Much of what follows is generic to all interactions with co-workers, and some aspects are of particular significance to particular disciplines. The evidence would indicate that everyone needs to improve their communication skills for the benefit of patients, and this chapter is written with the intention of providing tools to do this.

The nature of surgeon–anaesthetist interactions

The relationship between anaesthetist and surgeon is unique in medicine. In no other context, except possibly in the resuscitation room, do two or more specialists, from different disciplines, spend extended periods of time simultaneously treating a single patient. The quality of this relationship has important repercussions for patient safety and outcome, professional job satisfaction and the maintenance of good team-work in the theatre environment.

The anaesthetist–surgeon relationship has often been described as a 'marriage', and this may be the case, both figuratively and literally. However, in modern medicine, anaesthetist–surgeon interactions are more frequently a series of 'one-night stands'. Good communication is the key to a successful anaesthetist–surgeon interaction—be it a 'marriage' of 30 years or a single list.

Historically, surgeons have held the upper hand over anaesthetists. Initially anaesthetists were the most junior members of the surgical team, or even the medical student, who were given the job of administering the chloroform and, in many countries anaesthetics are routinely given by non-medical practitioners. Thus there has always been, and still is, a power and authority gradient between surgeons and anaesthetists. This is further exaggerated by differences in earnings, status and gender—there are many more female anaesthetists than female surgeons.

However, the development of anaesthesia as a specialty in its own right, and the formation of anaesthetic colleges across the world, has allowed anaesthetists to take their rightful place as the professional peers of surgeons. Anaesthetists can no longer be perceived as mere technicians whose job is to serve and service the demands of surgeons. They are equal partners whose expertise is indispensable to the care of the patient.

Understanding surgeons

Surgeons are people, and people are infinitely varied. However, most people would recognize that, as a group, surgeons differ from anaesthetists. They are often perceived as being more outspoken, confident and brash than their anaesthetist counterparts. The stereotype of the extrovert, bombastic surgeon and the introverted, unassuming anaesthetist still persists. Surgical training and culture tends to select individuals with no lack of self-esteem and with an ability to be the centre of attention.

The working practices of surgeons differ significantly from those of anaesthetists. Surgeons spend variable amounts of time in theatre, outpatient consultations and ward-based care of patients. In contrast, anaesthetists are essentially theatre-based unless they are involved in pre-operative assessment clinics, pain management or intensive care. Surgeons are often attempting to multi-task, supervising the care of patients scattered around or between hospitals and then switching to the sustained high-level focus of an operation. Anaesthetists likewise multi-task and perform high-level focused activities but are seldom in the position of having to care for more than one patient at a time.

Depending on surgical specialty, many surgeons work long hours with high stress levels. On a daily basis they deal with significantly higher levels of surgically related morbidity and mortality than anaesthetists. They are very often task-focused and less able to absorb the 'bigger picture'. Their lack of knowledge of the principles and practice of anaesthesia is a barrier to understanding just what it is that anaesthetists do, and this may lead to impatience with the time taken to perform anaesthetic tasks. These factors often underlie the tensions and conflicts that may occur in surgeon–anaesthetist interactions. It may be helpful to undertake a more detailed exploration of the factors influencing surgeons, their attitudes and behaviours.

Surgeons and anaesthetists typically have somewhat differing views of the quality of team-work and communication occurring in theatre[9,10], with surgeons having a somewhat rose-tinted view of how other disciplines perceive them. They believe that team-work and conflict resolution are good in their theatres, often contrary to the perceptions of the nurses and anaesthetists who work with them. Surgeons have a preference for steep hierarchies—that is, authority gradients[11]. They often consider themselves immune to the effects of fatigue and stress, and have a high level of confidence in their own judgement[12]. These factors combine to make surgeons often less sensitive to the nuances of communication happening in theatre and possibly less motivated towards improving matters. Anaesthetists are fortunately in an ideal position to facilitate team-working in the theatre for the benefit of all, especially the patient.

When one works in the theatre environment on an almost daily basis, it is sometimes difficult to recognize how abnormal or even surreal the surgical theatre setting is. To take a knife and cut a person open is an immensely challenging action requiring a great deal of skill and confidence, not always in equal measure. From the surgeons' point of view it places an enormous burden of responsibility on them to fulfil the implicit expectation that their actions will not kill the patient. In primitive societies, and even in modern ones until fairly recently, healers, doctors and, especially, surgeons were afforded a special status in recognition of the significance of their role. The erosion of that special status has been a mixed blessing for surgeons. To take a scalpel and cut a person open from xiphisternum to pubis requires the ability to dissociate oneself, at least momentarily, from the patient as a living individual.

When operating, particularly in difficult conditions, surgeons become very absorbed in the operation. They often fall silent, are intolerant or unresponsive to external stimuli such as background noise, and they often lose track of time. This dissociated state is what enables surgeons to do their job. This intense focus can be a barrier to communication if the anaesthetist does not recognize what is occurring and does not utilize the situation appropriately. Hence the importance of orientating oneself with the surgeon and the proposed surgery before the surgeon becomes engrossed in the task at hand. It is essential that the anaesthetist is, and remains, aware of the issues of 'in-flight' communication.

Using 'GREAT' with surgeons

Whether the anaesthetist is meeting a surgeon for the first time or starting a list with someone known for years, '**GREAT**' helps to ensure all the important communication aspects have been covered.

Greeting, Goals

Establishing and maintaining a good working relationship requires motivation, persistence and a degree of insight. Starting off on the 'right foot' is the beginning of this process. In the theatre environment, social 'short cuts' are often taken,—'*Hi there, I'm the anaesthetist*'. Fully introducing oneself engages the surgeon's attention and gives him, or her, an idea of what to expect, '*Hello, I'm Dr Jones. I'm a post-fellowship registrar on rotation from St Elsewhere—I'm here for the vascular list*'.

The importance of good eye contact, a smile and even a firm handshake should not be overlooked. If unsure of who the surgeon is, a brief enquiry such as, '*We've not met before, let me introduce myself..., and you are?*' may help ensure that when the bleeding gets out of hand you at least know their name!

Rapport

Surgeons respect anaesthetists who take an interest in the operation and have some knowledge of anatomy. It never fails to impress if the anaesthetist knows more about the anterior triangle of the neck than the surgical registrar! Looking at the scans, having a look at the surgical field, and enquiring about how previous patients have progressed reminds the surgeon that the anaesthetist is interested in patient management and outcome, and is not just a technician sitting by the machine doing the crossword. Doing crosswords or reading the newspaper sends a non-verbal message that the anaesthetist is either cool, calm and on top of everything, or completely oblivious to the four litres of blood in the sucker bottle!

An anaesthetist, as the only other doctor in theatre, is ideally placed to deal with page or phone enquiries, assuming this does not impinge on anaesthetic duties. It is far more sensible for the anaesthetist to take a message from a GP, decide if the surgeon needs to know immediately or not, and act appropriately, than a student nurse who has no experience or training to make that decision.

In facilitating the surgeon's work the anaesthetist must be assertive but not aggressive, cooperative but not submissive. It is not necessary to love or like our surgical colleagues, but anaesthetists must be able to communicate effectively with them and be able to show professional respect, and likewise be shown respect. A shared common interest in golf, fast cars, fishing or Ukrainian folk music is helpful, but it is not a prerequisite for a successful professional relationship.

Evaluation, Explanation, Expectations

Take the opportunity to let the surgeon know what your requirements are in advance. For example,

> '*Mrs Jacob has bad lung disease, so I'll be putting in a thoracic epidural for her. That'll take 30 minutes but as I have a senior registrar working with me today, we'll probably be able to do this in the anaesthetic room while the previous case is being transported to recovery*'.

Letting surgeons know at the beginning of the list what time or resource constraints there are enables them to manage their surgical time more efficiently.

> '*There's a department meeting at 6 pm which I'm chairing, so I will need to be out of here at 5.30 pm if at all possible*'.

Not

> '*Damn it's 5.45, I need to go now!*'

In many countries 'Time-Out' procedures have been adopted not only to confirm correct site and patient for surgery, but also to allow information exchange within the team, '*This is Mr Smith, he is having a right hernia repair. Please remember he has a mitral valve replacement and is usually on warfarin*'. (See also Chapter 16.)

Asking and Answering questions, Acknowledging and Addressing concerns

The process of orientating oneself to the list may be automatic if one regularly works with a surgeon and knows exactly how long it takes him or her to do, for instance, a hysterectomy. However, if the anaesthetist is unfamiliar with the surgeon or the procedure, it is vital to obtain the relevant information.

> '*Dr Smith, I've not anaesthetized for a Wiseman's craniotomy before. How long will the procedure take, do you anticipate much blood loss and are there any other specific requirements?*'

Not

> '*Is this going to bleed?—I hope you realize there's no cross-match*'.

Obviously information exchange should be a two-way event to ensure the surgeon has asked any questions he or she may have.

Thanks, Termination, Tacit agreement

Having confirmed who you are working with, what you are all planning to do and the special considerations of the patient, all that remains is to acknowledge that everyone is on 'the same page' and ready to start.

> '*OK so we are all clear that we are doing a lung biopsy on the left lung and Joe will call the technician once the specimen is out....*'

In-flight communication

The golden days of surgery, when all communication with the surgeon was conducted via the scrub nurse, are sadly gone, which leaves the anaesthetist with the sometimes thorny issue of when to interrupt a surgeon who may be deeply engrossed in the procedure or wrestling with a tricky dissection. Careful observation and an understanding of when a 'natural break' in the operation is likely to occur—for example, moving from one side of the patient to the other or adjusting their loupes, can provide an opportunity. Failing this, it is only polite to enquire if it is alright to interrupt for a second, but be specific about why you require information.

> '*I'm wondering if it is OK to call for the next patient*'.

Not

> '*How much longer?*' or, worse still, '*Are we there yet?*'

Recognize that a brusque or monosyllabic response from the other side of the drapes may be more a reflection of the fact that the surgeon is deeply engrossed rather than a reflection on the anaesthetist's personality!

Real-life approaches to resolving conflict

Why do surgeons get upset, angry or tetchy? Being a doctor is stressful, being a surgeon more so. Operating on a fit young person with a brain tumour, knowing that if you make a mistake, or even if you don't, the patient may die or end up hemiplegic and dysphasic, is bound to engender a degree of anxiety even in the most confident surgeon.

Paradoxically it is often elective surgery that worries surgeons more because they are playing for higher stakes. In an ideal world most surgeons want to be able to walk into theatre with a minimal amount of distraction and fuss and get on with the focused business of operating.

However, the reality is often delays with equipment, staffing issues and unexpected glitches. This is not helpful, and often the surgeon has no direct way to control these events. If the autoclave is broken it is not the surgeon who can fix it, so the frustration often manifests itself in a negative outburst. At a time when they are seeking to control themselves in the process of operating, surgeons are often faced with situations they cannot control and this leads to distress. Giving back a sense of control is often a helpful tactic:

> '*The endoscope you need will be ready in 40 minutes—maybe now is a good time to finish your ward round*'

or

> '*Would you like us to ring you ten minutes before we are ready to start?*'

Not

> '*No, we can't start yet*'.

Enlisting the surgeon's assistance is a useful way of occupying the impatient surgeon who is standing around breathing down the anaesthetist's neck keen to start operating.

> '*I am just going to scrub and put in a central line—perhaps you can do the arterial cannula to save time?*' (always assuming the surgeon knows how to put an arterial cannula in!)

Whilst any self-respecting anaesthetist would baulk at being a surgeon's handmaiden, there is a world of difference between being subservient and facilitating the surgeon's job to ensure an optimal outcome for the patient.

Although surgeons are rarely explicit in verbalizing their need for support, most will readily acknowledge that they seek and often receive the support of their theatre colleagues. This can take several forms: logistical, in terms of provision of staff and equipment to undertake operations; professional, in terms of medical advice and expertise offered by the anaesthetist and other theatre colleagues; and emotional, particularly when dealing with a difficult case or a bad outcome (see Chapter 12).

Anaesthetists are often focused on the logistical aspects of working with surgeons and can easily ignore the other important components of their relationship. Developing an appropriate professional relationship with a surgeon involves the provision of medical expertise to facilitate patient care so that the surgeon recognizes and values the anaesthetist's opinion and seeks input, especially with difficult cases. Inevitably the development of a good professional relationship will foster a greater degree of emotional support. Obviously this should be a two-way process, but inevitably there will be different degrees of support in different contexts. All of us work at our best when we feel we are being supported logistically, professionally and emotionally. In supporting our colleagues we generate support for ourselves.

In the stressful theatre environment it is inevitable that anaesthetist–surgeon conflicts will occur, and these are often perceived as personality clashes or just surgical personality! The problem frequently stems from poor communication and the failure to develop good rapport and working relationships. The issue may be chronic—for example, the surgeon recurrently arriving late or overbooking lists—or, acute—for example, the anaesthetist not sending for the next patient early enough.

There are some basic strategies which help to resolve conflicts:

1 Recognize the emotional component. If you feel angry, humiliated, offended etc. allow that emotion to pass before attempting to set things right. If the feeling won't go away, acknowledge it, '*I'm too angry to talk about this now*'.

2 Don't argue or fight in theatre or anywhere in the presence of patients. Anaesthetists in a high state of emotional arousal cannot care for patients properly.

3 Avoid the accusatory pronoun 'you' and take ownership of the problem using the pronoun 'I' or sometimes 'we'.

   '*I am concerned that the list is late starting and we are having problems with over-runs*'.
   '*We all want to get through the cases on the list and are dependent on each other to start the list on time so that unnecessary cancellations are avoided*'.

   Not

   '*You're always 20 minutes late!*'

4 Use facts, not accusations, to make a point.

   '*In the last two months 15 patients have been cancelled due to over-runs*'.

   Not

   '*You overbook your list*'.

Seeking to attribute blame is a common behaviour when faced with a problem. If a surgeon says something like: '*It's not my fault that you take 40 minutes to put in an epidural, no wonder the list over-runs...*' accept their reality either with a silence or by agreeing that it isn't the surgeon's fault, without taking it personally. Having the insight to appreciate that anger or frustration is a subconscious response allows the anaesthetist to avoid escalating the situation.

Focusing on identifying the problem and generating potential solutions enables all parties to feel that they are making progress and can be heard. Sometimes the intervention or support of a third party can be useful in helping to solve a problem, for instance the theatre manager or a senior colleague.

If there is conflict in theatre the most effective way of being constructive is to recognize and discard any unhelpful emotional responses and maintain logical thinking. This allows the anaesthetist to work out an effective strategy that can usefully be part of the solution. For example, the surgeon may be demanding that the theatre temperature be turned down as he is finding it too uncomfortable. The anaesthetist has the temperature up because of concern that the patient—a 3-month-old baby—be kept warm, so insists that the theatre temperature is maintained for patient safety. The focus of both parties is on the ***theatre*** temperature and tensions are escalating.

Interestingly, if the focus of the discussion were on the patient, it is more likely that a solution could be found. The temperature of the baby is, in fact, 37.1°C as measured by nasal probe. By agreeing to turn the room temperature down once the patient is draped and provided that the patient's temperature remains within normal limits, the focus is then on the patient rather than on the room. This sets a context for future dialogue concerning temperature. The anaesthetist may consider this strategy as 'giving in' or 'losing the argument'. However, this ability to be flexible both mentally and behaviourally is an essential requirement of the anaesthetist as a professional.

What if it just won't work?

As with marriages, not all anaesthetist–surgeon relationships work out. The frenetic workaholic, high-turnover anaesthetist will always struggle with the slow obsessive–compulsive surgeon, or vice versa. If the anaesthetist feels stuck with a surgeon that can't be reasoned with, rather than try and work out why, recognize that there are strategies available to deal with the situation, only they haven't yet been appreciated.

Often it is a conflict of perceived values. Surgeons often value fast turnover, acquiescent anaesthetists, whereas anaesthetists may value attention to detail and quality patient care in a stress-free environment.

Looking carefully and objectively at the quality of communication that is happening in the theatre may well give clues as to how best to address the issue. For example, does the surgeon lead the theatre team or sit back as a passive consumer of theatre services?

If the best efforts at initiating and maintaining rapport and good communication are failing, then it is almost invariably due to different realities and expectations on the part of the surgeon and the anaesthetist. These conflicting realities are often dismissed as purely due to personality problems. However, it is not enough to dismiss the surgeon as an 'arrogant psychopath', give up and make everybody else work with him or her. The '**LAURS**' concept can be usefully employed in this situation (see Chapter 2).

Systems issues such as poor staffing levels, inadequate theatre equipment or inept theatre management not infrequently contribute to the generation of a stressful environment that exacerbates communication problems. The solution often comes from a variety of approaches on both personal and institutional levels.

Crisis

The ultimate test of the quality of communication between anaesthetist and surgeon occurs in the context of crisis management. Surgeons who respect, trust and value their anaesthetic colleagues are more likely to communicate problems, explaining them in detail.

> '*I've just made a hole in the aorta—I think you'll need more blood*'.

Not

> "*Whoops!*"

Surgeons may well be inhibited from communicating in detail about the intraoperative problems they are encountering due to focusing intently on controlling haemorrhage, or a sense of pride or just sheer panic! However, encouraging dialogue helps to extract the necessary information and giving feedback helps surgeons to feel more relaxed.

> '*Things seem more stable at this end. Are you on top of the bleeding?*'

Likewise, when anaesthetists are having problems, 'thinking aloud' allows the surgeon to recognize a problem.

'*I can't see the larynx at all, we need the Fastrach*'.

Not

'*I knew I should have cancelled this one!*' (see also Safety-critical communication—Chapter 16).

When things start getting out of control, anaesthetists tend to function subconsciously and the capacity to think logically and purposefully is diminished; it is therefore important to take a step back to consider the important communication tasks involved.

In an on-table cardiac arrest situation, these might include:

- leading the resuscitation;
- calling for extra staff—for example, to take over at least every 3 minutes to give the massager a rest;
- delegating tasks to individuals by name;
- letting the surgeons know what is happening as they may not fully appreciate the severity of the situation.

The ability to communicate with others is strongly related to the ability to see others non-judgementally, to empathize and to recognize others' needs, motivations and emotional state—although 'putting ourselves in someone else's shoes' is not possible, it is possible to appreciate another's difficulty, and work on a strategy that might help them through it. These are high-level cognitive and social skills which, whilst they are innate in some, can be studied and acquired by others. In striving to improve our communication skills we inevitably improve ourselves by reflection on our own needs, motivation and emotional state.

Communicating with nurses

Much of what has been already written with respect to surgeon–anaesthetist communication is applicable to anaesthetist–nurse communication. Nurses often complain of the same failings in anaesthetists as anaesthetists do in surgeons. Unfortunately very few anaesthetists are telepathic, so are condemned to communicate by the usual methods.

Being aware of the capabilities of our anaesthetic nurse is the first step to establishing a safe, professional relationship.

'*Hello, I'm Dr Jim. We've not worked together before—have you done many leg re-implantations before? I'll need a size 8 tube*'.

Letting nursing staff know the anaesthetist's requirements well in advance, and sometimes by means of a 'shopping list', is always helpful. Recognizing that a fellow team member is overloaded with work is an important skill, as is helping out in a busy theatre. Clear and concise instructions avoid misinterpretation, as does the use of the correct, or at least generally accepted, name.

'*Pass me the size 8 ET tube with the gum elastic bougie please*'.

Not

'I need the white (brown or blue) thingy thing quick!'

Nurses, being often female, are sensitive to tone of voice. Speaking calmly and clearly, and loudly enough, helps to control the general panic when things go wrong. Shouting, sarcasm or curses under the breath may help to vent your spleen but do not usually improve your assistants' performance.

Nurses value feedback and appreciate thanks for the assistance they provide, and this is an easy, and for most anaesthetists, effortless task to perform.

'Thanks for all your help today, Max. It was a great idea to try the Proseal on that lady'.

Furthermore, the provision of teaching and practical training helps to engage nurses' attention and gives them a greater understanding of the tasks that they assist with. As an example, teaching laryngoscopy to anaesthetic nurses gives them an understanding of the anatomy and the potential problems that an anaesthetist may face.

Whilst many anaesthetists may be denied the luxury of a regular highly trained anaesthetic nurse, communication can easily be improved by undertaking the steps of:

- introducing ourselves;
- assessing the capabilities of the nurse;
- giving clear instructions, ideally having written your requirements in advance;
- giving and receiving feedback during and after cases;
- addressing other colleagues by name (if you are sure you know it!) when asking for a particular task to be performed.

Handover between anaesthetists

It is interesting to reflect that anaesthetists spend far more time communicating with surgeons and nurses than they do with their peers. Aside from coffee room gossip, the most common interaction between anaesthetists is handing over patients in theatre or from a round, and informing a colleague of a problem patient on a list.

Standardized operating procedures (SOP) for use during handovers help to ensure that the essential information is transferred in an explicit, efficient manner (see Safety-critical communication—Chapter 16).

Handover of responsibility of anaesthetized patients

Handover of responsibility for ongoing anaesthesia is a practice made more common by current working patterns and the relative frequency of 'solo' anaesthetist lists or cases. Often, by their nature, such cases are emergencies, or protracted and complex cases, where quality communication is essential to maintain patient safety and anaesthetic standards. Smooth transfer of responsibility is an essential factor in maintaining patient safety and retaining surgical confidence during stressful situations.

Despite the predictable risk of adverse events attributable to poor handover practice, little has been written either on what ought to happen or indeed on what actually takes place in practice. The only national guideline we are aware of on how this communication should occur and how the necessary information should be transferred was produced by the Australian and New Zealand College of Anaesthetists (ANZCA)[14].

Despite this, it appears to be uncommon for hospitals to have local protocols for when and how handovers should be conducted and, importantly, when handover of responsibility is unacceptable. A survey from 2004 in the UK suggested that even when handover protocols were available, dissemination to trainees was poor and resulted in lack of adherence[15].

The ANZCA guidelines begin with the advice that assurance of competence of the relieving anaesthetist be ascertained before handover is considered. This presents significant issues. For example, consider the style of communication between trainees during handover. It is possible that anaesthetists may be compelled to continue cases that are beyond their perceived competence simply by the style of communication of the transferring colleague.

> '*It has been a nightmare shift. This last case has been horrendous—you're happy to take over aren't you?*'

As opposed to:

> '*It has been a nightmare shift; this last case is complicated. I'll give you all the details and I am happy to wait for the consultant before completing handover*'.

The junior trainee may or may not be well equipped to deal with the case, but in the first instance, if then asked if he/she feels confident, will almost invariably acquiesce. The second example allows room for the relieving anaesthetist to take handover and assume responsibility dependent on their perception of their capabilities.

Ensuring patient safety during handover is an obvious prerequisite, therefore relative patient stability is a must. Crisis or instability, present or imminent, is not the time to begin handover! Handover communication should be conducted under circumstances where both receiving and transferring anaesthetist can devote their attention to the process. However, almost inevitably the operating room is the likeliest site for communication; relative quiet from the rest of the theatre team should be sought.

A structured system for handover should then be used. This should be clearly supported by written information, a well-completed anaesthetic chart and, where available, a specific handover sheet. The handover should emphasize the important details whilst avoiding extraneous information. A clear concise handover supported by bullet-point-style written notes as an aide-memoire is the ideal standard.

The ANZCA guidelines provide a useful template stating that handover information should include the following:

1 Previous health status and current condition of the patient.

2 An outline of the anaesthetic technique drugs used, lines sited (gauge, quality), airway security, fluid management, untoward events, potential problems, intraoperative and post-operative plans.

3 The current surgical status and its anaesthetic implications.

4 Patient observations as recognized by the relevant national standards.
5 A check of relevant anaesthetic and monitoring devices.
6 Notification of the operating surgeon.
7 Notification of the responsible consultant anaesthetist if it is a trainee-to-trainee handover.

Most of the recommended information about anaesthetic technique, patient observations, preceding health, etc. should already be documented in the appropriate sections of anaesthetic charts. Handover sheets should then be considered as additional supplements and prompts as most essential information will be conveyed through both the anaesthetic chart and effective verbal communication. No matter how well completed charts are, spoken communication will continue to provide the 'narrative'—the unwritten 'feel' of anaesthetic experience to complement 'formal' sources of knowledge contained in the chart (see Chapter 5).

Using 'GREAT' for handover

In conjunction with the ANZCA guidelines above, the '**GREAT**' template is a useful way of structuring a handover and facilitates quality communication. A typical handover using this structure might look like the following.

Greeting, Goals

Dr Dover: '*Hi. I'm Dr Dover but please call me Han. I'm a 4th year registrar and am on for emergency theatre this morning. Are you able to hand over now—is the patient stable?*'
Dr Young: '*Yes. Things have settled now, but this is only my first month of anaesthesia and the consultant is just in the coffee room. I don't think there is too much to tell you, but maybe we should get him back in. I'll get the handover sheet*'.

It is important for both anaesthetists involved in handover to understand each other's clinical experience and capacity to take over care if this is unknown.

Rapport

Dr Dover: '*Welcome to the department. You look pretty comfortable with this case at the moment; perhaps you could give me the "heads up" before the consultant gets back from coffee*'.

Dr Dover has put the junior trainee at ease and provided him with an opportunity to make a direct contribution to the patient's care and use this as a potential teaching experience.

Evaluation, Examination, Explanation, Expectations

Dr Young: '*This 54 year old poorly controlled asthmatic… presented with an acute abdomen … and her imaging showed …. We gave her … she was a grade one intubation but on "bagging" her ventilation pressures were pretty high … salbutamol seemed to settle things. She has got a 16-gauge cannula in both hands, a 4 lumen CVC in her right internal jugular …. She's had 2 litres of … I've already arranged for Hb … a cross-match of 4 units which should be ready in half an hour. As for the surgery they've had some difficulty … I think they are planning to do a right hemi-colectomy. We had planned to wake her up; however, I have spoken to critical care and they have a bed if required*'.

This dialogue represents the principal information exchange as detailed in the ANZCA guidelines above.

Asking and Answering questions, Acknowledging and Addressing concerns

Dr Dover: *'OK, I just want to check what the post-op analgesia plan is?'*
Dr Young: *'I wish now I'd put an epidural in. I guess it might have been better for her chest. She hasn't been consented for one asleep'.*
Dr Dover: *'I notice she's got a sat probe on her nose—has there been a problem?'*
Dr Young: *'I've had to keep moving the saturation probe around to get a decent signal. Are you OK to take over? I'll let the consultant know'.*
Dr Dover: *'Hang on a moment. Is she a bit cold or under filled?'*
Dr Young: *'Errrrrrr...! I'm not sure'.*
Dr Dover: *'Well let's ask the boss....'*

This component of the '**GREAT**' template allows clarification of aspects of the handover that need expansion before taking over the care of the patient. If there are no questions the anaesthetist 'taking over' probably hasn't listened properly!

Thanks, Termination

Dr Dover: *'... well now that's all clear, I'm happy to let ICU know 20 minutes before we come round. Thanks for your help'.*

Interacting with anaesthesia trainees in theatre

Perhaps the most important interaction that occurs between anaesthetists is that which occurs during teaching. Part of becoming an anaesthetist involves the acquisition of 'anaesthetic culture'—the sense of professional identity which may be either a positive or negative one[13] (see Chapter 18).

Communicating with secretarial staff

Most anaesthetists would acknowledge that the anaesthetic secretary is the backbone or nerve centre of any department. In order to get the most out of interactions with secretarial staff here are a few key pointers—other than buying coffee and remembering Secretaries' Day! Generally speaking secretaries are masters, or, more commonly, mistresses of communication, it's their core activity! They often expect similar skill levels from anaesthetists—but sadly they are often disappointed.

Here are a few rules to help communication run smoothly:

1 If you are somewhere at variance with your planned or normal routine, let the secretaries know and ensure they have a contact number. If you don't want to be found/contacted or disturbed tell them so.

2 If you require a specific task or item completed by a certain time be specific and write it down.

'Dear Gill, please can you sign off the attached order ASAP as I need it by next Wednesday (21st)?'

Not

'FYA—urgent'

3 If you require a document copy-typed ensure your handwriting is legible (get someone else to read it!), if not, then use a Dictaphone.

4 When dictating letters avoid 'the stream of consciousness'. Think about the content and if necessary make notes before launching into a monologue. Indicate punctuation, new paragraphs and side headings. Spell unusual names and replay at least part of the tape to ensure it has recorded properly.

Written communication

In contrast to the majority of our medical colleagues, anaesthetists can get away with a bare minimum of written communication. Unless working in a Pain Clinic anaesthetists virtually never write letters and, with the exception of pain round entries in the notes, most anaesthetists tend to function at the level of 'fit & well' and 'routine post-op care' on the anaesthetic record.

The tick box format of many anaesthetic records and the computer printout that accompanies it are rapidly making the possession of a pen an optional extra for registrars! It does however behove the anaesthetist to ensure that the documents to be completed are conscientiously filled in, signed, with surname in block letters, and dated. A brief skim through any selection of anaesthetic records inevitably reveals missing data such as start time, operator or instructions for post-operative care. This is a source of great concern to the medical administration staff, quality controllers and lawyers! An audit of anaesthetic record completeness often provides useful insights into our deficiencies.

Having possibly faltered at the first hurdle of the anaesthetic record, the concept of writing to another doctor may represent a further challenge to many anaesthetists. All letters need to contain the patient's full name, date of birth and hospital ID. A heading detailing the salient problem and required action is an efficient feature for the busy GP who will not spare the time to read a two page letter about the difficult intubation.

Some departments have *pro forma* letters (see Figure 17.1) to deal with specific issues such as difficult intubation, post-dural puncture headache (PDPH), etc., and these are useful documents to generate.

Dear Dr Brown

RE: Margaret Smith
DOB: 5.11.42
MRN: 27.04.KY

Problem: *Anaphylactic reaction to Rocuronium*
Action required of GP: *Documentation in patient's case notes.*

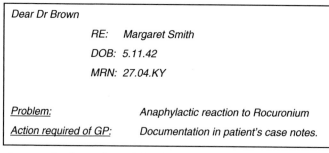

Fig. 17.1 An example of a *proforma* letter.

Key points

1. Quality communication in theatre between members of the theatre team facilitates useful interactions that are an important aspect of patient care, safety and professional job satisfaction.
2. Understanding the issues surrounding surgeons, their attitudes and behaviours, and our own, enables anaesthetists to optimize their working relationships with surgeons.
3. There is a multitude of practical ways to improve communication with colleagues.
4. Poorly written communication is a frequent source of problems, many of which are easily avoidable.

References

1 Lingard L, Reznick R, Espin S, Regehr G, DeVito I (2002). Team communication in the operating room: talk patterns, sites of tension, and implications for novices. *Acad Med*, **77**, 232–4.

2 Lingard L, Espin S, Whyte S, Regehr G, Baker GR, Reznick R et al (2004). Communication failures in the operating room: an observational classification of recurrent types and effects. *Qual Saf Health Care*, **13**, 330–4.

3 Lingard L, Espin S, Rubin C, Whyte S, Colmenares M, Baker GR et al (2005). Getting teams to talk—development and pilot implementation of a checklist to promote inter-professional communication in the OR. *Qual Saf Health Care*, **14**, 340–6.

4 Awad S, Fagan S, Bellows C, Albo D, Green-Rashad B, De la Garza M et al (2005). Bridging the communication gap in the operating room with medical team training. *Am J Surg*, **190**, 770–4.

5 Sexton J, Makary M, Tersigni AR, Pryor D, Hendrich A, Thomas EJ et al (2006). Teamwork in the operating room: frontline perspectives among hospital and operating room personnel. *Anesthesiology*, **105**, 877–84.

6 Gawande A, Zinner M, Studdert D, Brennan T (2003). Analysis of errors reported by surgeons at three teaching hospitals. *Surgery*, **133**, 614–21.

7 Reader TW, Flin R, Cuthbertson BH (2007). Communication skills and error in the intensive care unit. *Curr Opin Crit Care*, **13**, 732–6.

8 Elks KN, Riley RH (2009). A survey of anaesthetists' perspectives of communication in the operating suite. *Anaesth Intensive Care*, **37**, 108–11.

9 Flin R, Yule S, McKenzie L, Paterson-Brown S, Maran N (2006). Attitudes to teamwork and safety in the operating theatre Surgeon. *Surgeon*, **4**, 145–51.

10 Makary M, Sexton JB, Freischlag J, Holzmueller C, Millovian E, Rowen L et al (2006). Teamwork in the operating room.: teamwork in the eye of the beholder. *J Am Coll Surg*, **202**, 746–52.

11 Sexton JB, Thomas EJ, Helmreich R (2000). Error, stress and teamwork in medicine and aviation. A cross-sectional surveys. *BMJ*, **320**, 745–9.

12 Kitto S, Villaneuva E, Chesters J, Petrovic A, Waxman BP, Smith JA (2007). Surgeon's attitudes to and usage of evidence-based medicine in surgical practice: a pilot study. *ANZ J Surg*, **77**, 231–6.

13 Lingard L, Reznick R, DeVito I, Espin S (2002). Forming professional identities on the health care team: discursive constructions of the 'other' in the operating room. *Med Educ*, **36**, 728–34.

14 Australian and New Zealand College of Anaesthetists (2004). *Guidelines on the handover of responsibility during an anaesthetic.* ANZCA professional Document PS10 Available at: http://www.anzca.edu.au/resources/professional-documents/professional-standards/pdfs/PS10.PDF (Accessed 14 March 2010).

15 Horn J, Bell M, Moss E (2004). Handover of responsibility for the anaesthetised patient—opinion and practice. *Anaesthesia*, **59**, 658–63.

Chapter 18

Teaching and research

Susie Richmond, Andrew F Smith, and Suyin GM Tan

'…the sole hope of human salvation lies in teaching'.
George Bernard Shaw

'Research is the act of going up alleys to see if they are blind'.
Plutarch

What this chapter is about

This chapter is designed to give an overview of a number of specific situations in teaching and research relating to anaesthesia where communication skills may be useful. Whilst there are many others, these have been chosen because, in the authors' experience, they are often unfamiliar or poorly performed, or assumed to be part of the 'tacit' skill set that cannot be formally taught.

Giving feedback to trainees

Perhaps the most important interaction that occurs between anaesthetists is that which occurs during teaching. Communicating with trainees in order to bring about a change in knowledge, skills and attitude is probably the most sophisticated form of communication anaesthetists employ other than the context of therapeutic communication with patients. Scant attention is often paid to the unconscious way in which anaesthetics trainees learn. Anaesthesia, like surgery, is learnt, not taught. Much of the beliefs, behaviours and attitudes that trainees acquire comes implicitly as they observe and copy their mentors' actions. Part of becoming an anaesthetist involves the acquisition of 'anaesthetic culture'—the sense of professional identity which may be either a positive or a negative one[1]. When working with trainees, not only should they be taught the knowledge and skills to do the job, but, more importantly, senior anaesthetists should be modelling, and explicitly teaching them, better ways to interact with colleagues.

It is far beyond the scope of this chapter to address the issues surrounding education in anaesthesia. However, it is useful to explore one aspect of teaching—that is, feedback in order to highlight some basic principles. Everyone loves feedback—so long as it is positive! No-one likes to feel that they are being unfairly, or even fairly, criticized. So how can anaesthetists give the feedback our trainees so desperately crave? As in all communication the key lies in establishing a rapport. Most trainees spend long enough in a department to establish a reasonable relationship with at least one or two trainers. It is difficult to give feedback to a trainee whose baseline capabilities are uncertain.

'Does he always make a pig's ear out of arterial cannulation or is he just having a bad day?

Furthermore, trainees may have difficulties in accepting feedback, especially negative feedback, from someone they feel doesn't really know them. However, it is possible to give feedback to trainees, of whom you have little experience, if a structured approach is utilized. Depending on circumstance, the anaesthetist may elect to do a formalized feedback based on an entire list or a case, or may choose a more informal approach.

As in all communication, orientation to the task prior to commencing is the first step.

'OK Matt—today we are doing Dr Jessop's gynae list, I thought I'd use it as an opportunity to give you some feedback on your airway skills. How does that sound to you?

Giving feedback can occur little and often within the context of everyday communication.

'Good to see you've sutured that central line in properly'.

Although it may sometimes feel that what is being said is barn door obvious, it does convey and reinforce important learning points for trainees.

As an adjunct, a more formalized feedback may be chosen, using a structured or semi-structured form—for example, ANTS (anaesthetists' non-technical skills) or a critique approach[2,3]. Critique utilizes questions exploring the trainee's perception of the emotional content of the event, and the positive and the negative aspects of the experience—for example:

'How did you feel about putting in your first thoracic epidural?
'What did you think went well?
'What do you want to work on for next time?

The questions allow trainees to explore their emotional response to the event and to reflect on the experience as a whole. The 'strengths and weaknesses' questions give the trainer a valuable insight into how the trainee perceives the event and enables the trainer to give guidance as to how to improve future performance. Getting started with giving feedback in a conversational context will help trainees to engage with trainers and builds the confidence to move on to more structured feedback. It is important to be specific in giving both positive and negative feedback.

'You handled that difficult epidural really well. I could see you had thought carefully about positioning and had confirmed your landmarks beforehand'.

As opposed to

'That was good—I didn't think you'd get that in!'

Particularly when the trainee is having difficulties, feedback should include strategies for correction.

'I can see you're still finding your way with thoracic epidurals. Have you thought about angling the Tuohy needle a little more cephalad? We are running a new simulation course next month if you are interested'.

Choosing the best time to give feedback is a skill in itself. Ideally it should be close enough to the event to remain pertinent but also allow the trainee and trainer time for reflection and processing. If the feedback relates to a particularly difficult or traumatic event—for instance, failed intubation in an obstetric patient—it is prudent to allow a period of time to elapse in order for emotions to settle before embarking on a debrief.

As a final point, choice of location is also an important issue. Real-time feedback obviously needs to happen in the presence of patients and staff, but a more detailed dissection of performance deserves a quiet and private space, however positive the feedback or delicate the criticism.

Much of this last section has been directed at trainers giving feedback to trainees. However, it should be acknowledged that the pinnacle of trainee–trainer communication is when trainees are able to give constructive, uncensored feedback to their trainers. Few trainers feel sufficiently secure to solicit feedback on their teaching, communication and clinical skills, and the majority of trainees are inhibited by the authority gradient, a lack of experience or confidence in giving feedback, and perhaps a fear of prejudicing their career choices. Cultivating an environment where communication skills are explicitly recognized, modelled and reinforced, enhances teaching and ultimately generates the confidence both to give and to receive the feedback which is an integral part of improving practice.

Communicating for supervision

Communicating with trainees is not something that people suddenly know when they are appointed as consultants. It is a skill that develops over time and with practice. There are many opportunities, often unrealized, that can be used to help learn and develop these skills at all stages of a career[4].

Supervision skills can begin to be learned at an early point in a career. When a trainee is still being closely supervised themselves they are subconsciously watching and learning from their supervisors. When, later on in their career they start to supervise trainees they are often surprised by how much they know without being conscious of having learned it!

There are many opportunities that can be used as learning experiences—even something as mundane as giving advice over the telephone. In this situation there are educational opportunities for both parties involved—the consultant has to learn several very important concepts:

1 Accepting what the trainee on the other end of the phone tells them is true.

2 Being comfortable about giving advice over the phone without having seen and assessed the patient for themselves.

3 Knowing when to come straight into the hospital from home, without even being asked. Sometimes here the trainee may not even know they need help!

Communicating, and therefore learning, in the operating theatre is also partly done in a similar way. After the initial 'new starter' phase has passed, trainees may not be aware that they are learning while 'doing a list' with a consultant or a more senior trainee. However, all the time that the two doctors are together in the anaesthetic room and theatre there is subconscious learning going on. Communication during this 'learning' can be non-verbal as well as verbal.

During a longer case there is usually time for some more traditional teaching to occur on a one-to-one basis. This may involve an interesting aspect of the case on the table and can be expanded to a '*What if…*' scenario involving the case. This may also be an opportunity for more formal tutorial style teaching on a one-to-one basis.

Another area of communication that can occur within the operating theatre is a form of mentoring. Doing a list with a trainee can be an opportunity to get to know him or her as an individual instead of just as a trainee. The majority of trainees will probably never need any form of mentor but will still appreciate a consultant getting to know them. Equally, if consultants know a bit about their trainees, they will be in a better position to judge what is needed if rung for advice when 'on call'. To be in a position to coach or mentor a trainee it is important to know about them as an individual.

Encouraging and motivating the failing trainee

Trainees fail for many different reasons[5]. To be able to encourage and motivate a failing trainee the reason for the failing needs to be known. It may not be immediately obvious that a trainee is having difficulties—the difficulties may be clinical where it will be obvious, or could be a personal matter, where it may not be. Sometimes it is only when colleagues start to comment about unusual behaviour patterns, such as consistently being late for a shift, and someone takes the time to speak to the trainee that things are discovered. Any individual who has problems needs someone in whom they feel they can confide and would feel comfortable discussing often highly personal things with.

Encouraging and motivating trainees who are failing is not about sorting out all their problems for them. The person in whom they confide should act more as mentor. A mentor for failing trainees is someone who listens actively and with empathy to the trainees but does not draw any conclusions or form judgements, but instead helps the trainees try to find the answers for themselves. This involves listening to the stories and trying to encourage the trainees to see any blind spots they might have about themselves or their situation. A degree of insight by the failing trainee is needed for any kind of mentoring to work.

The next stage of mentoring involves helping the trainees decide what the right course of action for them is and then helping them find ways of achieving their plan. Sometimes this might involve the use of a '**SMART**' goal—this is something that is

Specific,

Measurable,

Achievable,

Realistic and and has a

Timescale appropriate for the situation (not too long).

Mentoring is not an instant fix for an individual's problems. The process can take several weeks or may take many months depending on the nature of the problem and the individual's insight into the problem. During this time it is important that trainees are supported since they can feel very vulnerable. Positive encouragement is needed regularly along with reassurance that they are *'doing OK'*. A regular informal meeting every week is useful for both parties to keep updated on how things are progressing. Some weeks will be better than others!

Sometimes a trainee has been failing for a long time. The warning signs that all is not well have not been obvious and have therefore not been noticed. In this situation the trainee is often not in a fit state to use a mentor to help, and has often moved into a state of passive acceptance of everything that is said to or about them, and everything that is done to them. Trainees in this state of mind are more in need of counselling than mentoring—they need someone to tell them what to do and generally how to sort their lives out until they are able to take control for themselves. As the situation improves and the trainees feel ready, a gentle mentoring approach can be introduced to encourage them to take some responsibility for themselves.

A failing trainee may become apparent as a result of a clinical incident that may or may not have resulted in serious harm to a patient. In this situation, a multi-pronged approach involving more than one person is needed. Someone needs to deal with the sequelae of the clinical incident and ensure it is handled properly through the correct channels. A second person needs to be there for trainees as they will need debriefing and support, both emotional and practical (see Chapter 12). Again an incident like this often reduces trainees to a passive state where they need someone to 'sort their lives out' for them.

Maintaining positivity towards a trainee is important, and any criticism needs to be positive and constructive. As a result of an incident like this there may need to be involvement with external agencies such as the medical defence organizations and the regional training committee. Any communication from these agencies needs to be shared with the trainee as soon as possible—it is important to be open and up front about everything. The trainee will trust the consultant and any advice offered, if it is felt that the consultant is 'on their side'. Apart from the consultant trying to manage a situation like this alone, there are various organizations available for trainees in these types of situations. It is important that a trainee has all the information available about these organizations and should be encouraged to at least approach them and see what they can offer or advise.

As a result of being a failing trainee, there may be a desire or a need to consider changing career path. This may involve leaving the training programme for a non-specialist position or, more seriously, giving up anaesthetics or even medicine. This is not a decision that will be reached easily, and trainees should be supported in whatever they decide, independent of the consultant's own feelings about it.

Communicating with an examiner during a viva

Vivas are sometimes viewed as the most formidable part of an exam. This is definitely so if knowledge is lacking due to poor preparation. The purpose of a viva examination is to convince the examiner that all the hard work and viva practice that the trainee has been doing has not been in vain. The best communicator in the world will still fail a viva if the necessary preparation hasn't been done.

Preparing for a viva has usually taken several months, and the stress that this fact adds can lead to a candidate performing less well than is expected and possibly failing the exam undeservedly.

There a certain rules to remember when sitting a viva:

1. Dress smartly and appropriately for the occasion.
2. Don't look like a frightened rabbit caught in car headlamps—or you will soon behave like one.
3. A pleasant smile at the examiners is a good start. Non-verbal communication is hugely important.
4. Don't look or behave in an overconfident manner.
5. Equally don't behave as if you are so scared that you can hardly utter a word—a viva is a ***spoken*** exam.
6. Answer the question that the examiner asks, not the question you would like them to have asked.
7. If you don't understand the question, say so—it is then up to the examiner to rephrase the question so you ***do*** understand what they are asking you.
8. Don't argue with the examiner as the examiner is always right!
9. Try to look as if you are enjoying yourself.
10. Don't fidget or gesticulate with your hands as you answer.
11. Speak clearly and coherently.
12. A diagram may make your point much more clearly than a garbled spoken answer.

Communicating with an editor of a journal as an author and responding to reviewers

Getting a paper accepted for publication is a long process. For a start, try to remember that, far from being the end of the process, submitting a paper is merely the start of a new round of developments. Although only the authors are credited at the top of the first page of the finished product, a published paper is very much a joint effort between the authors, the reviewers and the editor of the journal. But, in reality, the chances of publication are set much earlier than this, at the design stage of the research project. Some research papers are doomed to undergo multiple rejections simply because they report work that should never have been performed. Asking the wrong question, choosing an inappropriate methodological approach and allowing bias to creep in because of sloppy methodology are all irretrievable problems. Poor presentation of an otherwise soundly conducted study can be corrected, but it is too late to wish the study had been done differently. Much more preferable than hearing this from the journal's reviewers is asking as many people as possible for advice on the project ***before*** the work begins, rather than waiting until it is completed.

First, be realistic. This is partly about science and partly about salesmanship and, although scientific writing may be specialized, it must still conform to the same principles as any other good writing. Here then is one downfall. Trainees in anaesthesia are not expected to give anaesthetics without appropriate training and supervision, yet anaesthetists are often expected to be able to write without any special preparation or experience.

Follow the 'Instructions for authors' carefully and write clearly. Remember the importance of a first impression. Editors are usually volunteers, or, if they are paid, are often not paid much. If their work is made easier for them, so much the better. Formatting references and checking spelling and grammar are tiresome, and they might be thought unnecessary tasks, but imagine having to perform such tasks on not one but on 200 manuscripts per year. Remember that editors are only human. They want to publish the best, but they are also relieved when the painstaking and time-consuming work of preparing a manuscript for final publication is done for them by the author. This leaves them free to concentrate on the science and structure of the paper.

Assuming some decent work has been done and the paper has been written and submitted, the editor will send an acknowledgement. Some time later the editor will send a further communication—depending on the journal, this can be a few days or many months. Again, depending on the journal, this may be a brief note declining publication, or a considered response accompanied by the reviewers' comments upon which the editor's verdict is based. If the editor has sent comments, authors are advised to take a deep breath and steel themselves.

The reviewers' comments are occasionally unfair, they may appear to have misunderstood the writer, they may be unduly picky or the writer may feel they are abusing their power. However, these are unusual situations and, in any case, the editor will usually know what an individual reviewer is like and will be trying to steer a middle course through the, sometimes conflicting, comments.

Remember it is almost unheard of for a paper—any paper—to be accepted without amendment. Most accepted papers are accepted provisionally on the understanding that the author will make certain changes. Authors should try not to take this as a personal criticism—especially if it is a first attempt at writing, where a considerable intellectual and emotional investment will have been made in it. It is easy, then, to become 'precious' and possessive about the paper, and easy, too, to regard those who criticize it with the ferocity of a lioness guarding her cubs!

The most useful sets of comments not only say what is wrong with the paper, but make suggestions as to how improvements can be made. Ideally, they will be provided as a list of numbered points. The writer should then prepare a letter outlining responses to the comments and, if in agreement with a particular comment, say so and thank the reviewer. If in disagreement, then politely point out why and state the preference for leaving the text as it stands.

At this stage of the process, as at all others, it is not only courteous but also wise to highlight in the text where changes have been made, using a different colour or different fonts. Add to that the relevant page and line numbers in the response letter so that the changes can be easily identified. In time, there will be another reply from the editor. Sometimes reviewers want to see the revised version, and sometimes not. If the writer's responses are well laid out and easy to follow, it is certain the paper will be dealt with promptly. Many papers require two or even more revisions. This is not unusual, and, like the first revision, the writer should bear in mind that the comments are designed to improve the paper and protect both the author and the journal from damage to their reputations.

If the paper is rejected, the reviewers' comments on it will still be sent. This will allow the author to decide whether it is redeemable and can be submitted to another journal, or whether it is beyond hope. As stated earlier, serious faults in methodology cannot be dealt with at this stage as it is too late to conduct the study again. Editorial advice is given free and is a useful source of ideas for improvement.

Communicating with an editor of a journal as a reviewer

Journal editors rely on their reviewers for a number of reasons[6]. No editor can know his subject well enough to be an expert in all its aspects. It also takes a long time to establish a journal's reputation, and publishing hastily written papers can lose this reputation very quickly. Expert reviewers can help spot potentially embarrassing mistakes. Lastly, most manuscripts can be improved by advice. These improvements may have nothing to do with grammar or style, but may have to do with references that are missed, conclusions which are too bold or techniques which need further description[6]. However, reviewing each paper can cause delays and adds to the time it takes for a journal to handle the manuscript.

Most journals transmit the reviewers' comments direct to the author with the editor's decision. Usually, however, reviewers can also submit confidential comments to the editor, which are not relayed to the paper's author. Whether or not the reviewer's comments are seen by the author, one should be courteous and polite at all times. Constructive criticism is always welcome, but the review is not an opportunity to vent one's spleen, even if the paper is unspeakably bad.

Many journals operate an open peer review policy—that is, the reviewer's identity is revealed to the author. Although this is not universal practice, it is a good idea always to write as if it were. If opinions cannot be defended objectively, then they should not be expressed. There are some simple rules to being a reviewer:

1 It is important to be prompt when asked to review. If unable to read and comment on a manuscript within a reasonable time, the editor will need to be informed immediately to allow another reviewer to be found who can complete the review within the time frame.

2 If the editor is asking for replies to specific questions, these need to be addressed.

3 Do not recommend acceptance or rejection, unless the editor asks for this specifically.

4 Do not make too much of minor mistakes and problems. There is no need to share every preference—for instance on how results are expressed,

5 It is important to remember that even well-known departments or famous clinicians can have their names on poor quality work—the association with eminence does not guarantee that the cited authors have been part of the work or even have had the opportunity to read it.

6 Do not get in touch directly with the author during the review process. If reviewers are meant to be anonymous, they should stay anonymous.

Key points

1. Communication skills are a vital part of teaching and supervising trainees.
2. Knowing how to communicate effectively can make the difference between passing and failing a viva.
3. Critical comments to authors from journal reviewers are inevitable, and where at all possible should be considered as constructive feedback.

References

1 Lingard L, Reznick R, DeVito I, Espin S (2002). Forming professional identities on the health care team: discursive constructions of the 'other' in the operating room. *Med Educ*, **36**(8), 728–34.

2 Glavin RJ (2009). Excellence in anesthesiology: the role of nontechnical skills. *Anesthesiology*, **110**(2), 201–3.

3 Fletcher G, Flin R, McGeorge P, Glavin R, Maran N, Patey R (2003). Anaesthetists' Non-Technical Skills (ANTS): evaluation of a behavioural marker system. *Br J Anaesth*, **90**(5), 580–8.

4 Greaves D (2003). Clinical supervision. In: Greaves D, Dodds C, Kumar CM, Mets B (eds) *Clinical teaching: a guide to teaching practical anaesthesia*. pp. 13–9. Lisse: Swets and Zeitlinger.

5 Mets B (2003). Giving feedback and monitoring progress. In: Greaves D, Dodds C, Kumar CM, Mets B (eds). *Clinical teaching: a guide to teaching practical anaesthesia*. pp. 183–93. Lisse: Swets and Zeitlinger.

6 Pyke DA (1979). Referee a paper. In: *How to do it*. pp. 143–6. London: BMJ Books.

Chapter 19

Administrators

Scott W Simmons

'Not everything that counts can be counted'.
A sign in Einstein's office

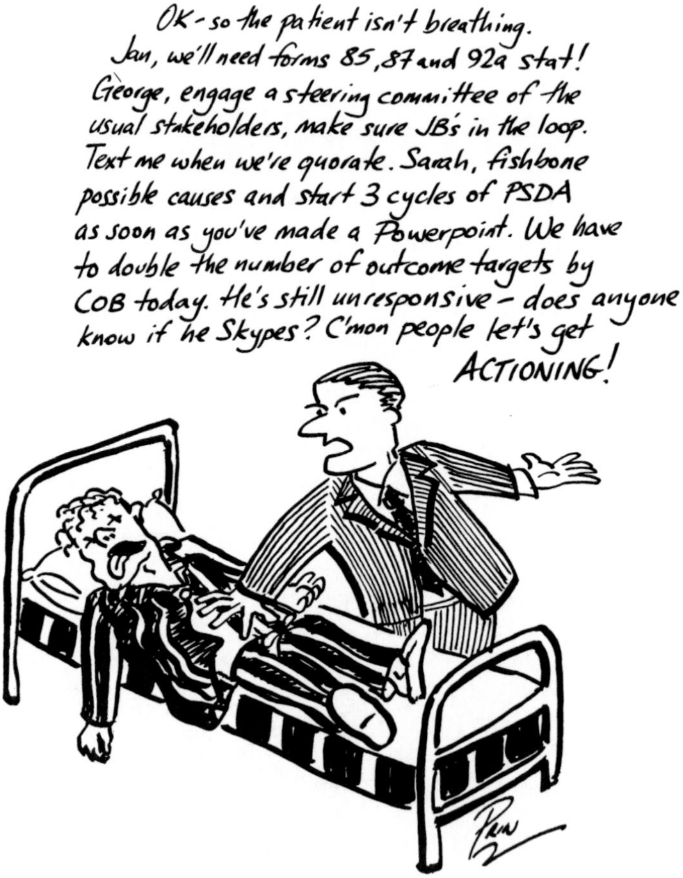
OK - so the patient isn't breathing.
Jan, we'll need forms 85, 87 and 92a stat!
George, engage a steering committee of the usual stakeholders, make sure JB's in the loop.
Text me when we're quorate. Sarah, fishbone possible causes and start 3 cycles of PSDA as soon as you've made a Powerpoint. We have to double the number of outcome targets by COB today. He's still unresponsive - does anyone know if he Skypes? C'mon people let's get ACTIONING!

What this chapter is about

Appreciating different perspectives

In our modern healthcare systems, clinicians find themselves dealing face-to-face with administrators at many different levels. Unfortunately, there often appears to be a major disconnect between the two parties, and priorities may appear to be vastly different. For the busy clinical anaesthetist who encounters this in passing, there may be transient frustration and confusion before simply getting on with the job. For the anaesthetist with a designated management role, the problem doesn't go away that easily. Both, however, will benefit from some deeper insight into the nature of these interactions to help everyone to better achieve their goals.

The '**LAURS**' concept as presented in Chapter 2 emphasizes the generic attributes of the approach to a meaningful interaction. Of particular interest in attempting to apply this framework to our dealings with administrators is the recognition that the management 'world' is exactly that—a seemingly different place that abounds with its own distinctive language, practical tools, and approaches to problem solving with which most clinicians have little familiarity. There may indeed be a sense of entering a different domain, much like the person entering the healthcare system as a patient. Hence in this chapter there is a deliberate intent to present some of these practical tools and perspectives to help better understand this other world and the people who abide there and relate it to these general principles. The results may be surprising.

A scenario

Dr Celia Roberts has recently been appointed Director of the Anaesthesia Service of a large public teaching hospital. Being an expert in her field she had conducted research, written several papers and been responsible for the teaching of specialist trainees. There is little in her chosen area of expertise that she doesn't know how to deal with. In her day-to-day work she needs to think on her feet, work independently and be

accountable for her individual actions. Where appropriate, she assumes a leadership role, giving clear and concise instructions to the team around her. Celia approaches her work with a high commitment to one-to-one interaction between herself as a skilled exponent of a specialised craft—clinical anaesthesia—and the patients who are seeking her help. She has a sense of achievement and satisfaction, engendering quiet self-confidence. When approached some four months before to step up to the role of Director of Anaesthesia, she was initially very reluctant, but eventually agreed.

Unfortunately for Celia, the combined effect of recent retirements from the department and an increasing workload related to the closure of a nearby hospital is impacting seriously on the anaesthesia service. Her colleagues have been working under considerable pressure for more than a year, and the extra case load is beginning to tell. On taking up her appointment, Celia immediately set about making a thorough analysis of the workload versus staffing levels and the potential impact on patient safety. The ultimate result was a 15-page document with references and appendices constructed in her usual analytical style, resembling a clinical research paper. The work completed, she sought a meeting with new CEO, Monika Kreutzinger, only to be told that the next available appointment was in three weeks. Despite her frustration, Celia accepts that there is no choice, and that the meeting will have to wait. Meanwhile however, with a view to keeping the ball rolling, she sends off her document via e-mail.

Monika Kreutzinger was recruited 18 months previously, when significant organizational changes were being considered by the Board of Management. Her track record as a 'mover and shaker' was well known within the health bureaucracy. However, she was quite unknown to the hospital's clinicians, and the Board felt this meant she would bring no unwanted 'baggage' at a time when some difficult and unpopular decisions would be necessary to achieve their reform agenda.

Monika has been in healthcare most of her working life, starting as a radiographer in a busy private medical imaging firm. Coming from a family with a small business background, she worked to develop management skills, acquiring several post-graduate diplomas and, ultimately, an MBA. She has natural leadership skills and has taken opportunities for advancement whenever these have arisen. As her resumé has grown, so too has her sense of achievement and satisfaction, engendering quiet self-confidence. It seemed to her a natural progression to accept the three-year contract as CEO—and its challenges—as a possible step on the ladder to even greater heights.

At the time of receiving Celia's e-mail, however, she is extremely busy, including dealing with potential strike action by laboratory staff. Also, the Minister of Health, being under parliamentary pressure over certain election promises, has generated much 'burning of the midnight oil' in the hospital executive suite, with everyone working through a swathe of ministerial briefing notes. A log of claims from an important clinical group such as the anaesthetists is the last thing Monika needs. What's more she receives between 500 and 600 e-mails per week—something of which Celia is totally unaware.

Same, same but different!

Monika and Celia are both intelligent high achievers. There are in fact many similarities between top executives and clinicians, and both will have considerable capacity for problem solving or obfuscation. A key difference is typically the individual patient perspective that the clinician usually brings to the mix, while the manager will focus more broadly. This can be interpreted by clinicians as a lack of concern or interest in individual patient welfare. While Celia has to explain to Mrs Smith that her operation has been cancelled because theatre has over-run, Monika has to face her Board of Management, the Health Minister, the media or the relatives of many Mrs Smiths repeatedly. The challenge for both parties is to appreciate each other's realities, appreciate strengths and abilities and so seek opportunities for alignment. In this way solutions can be developed that build rather than sabotage each other's priorities.

The story continues...

Three weeks have passed since the e-mail and Celia has sat in a small waiting area for 20 minutes past the appointed meeting time. She is starting to become annoyed, used as she is to having access to all areas and control over her world. Eventually she is ushered into the executive suite and, after some initial pleasantries, Monika acknowledges receipt of Celia's 'rather comprehensive' document. Whilst indicating a degree of sympathy for her position, at the end of the day no extra funding is available. Monika had also asked her Director of Medical Services to look into theatre efficiency, and his preliminary report suggested that all key performance indicators were being met. As a measure of how seriously she considered the issue, Monika had also personally done a literature search and consulted with her colleagues via the health executives' e-forum. If anything, it would appear that their hospital was relatively overstaffed by usual benchmarking standards.

Despite Celia's best attempts to draw attention to key figures in her analysis, it appeared that Monika had some counter-point that in her view was actually more significant. After a few minutes it becomes clear that the CEO just isn't 'getting it' and apparently doesn't care about the plight of her staff. With frustration and tone of voice both rising, the discussion goes off at a tangent. After another few minutes there seems to be little point in continuing and Celia leaves, having undertaken to do some more homework, and can't believe what has just transpired. With little experience of dealing with management, she had, nonetheless, felt that her request for extra staff was a 'slam dunk'. However, the CEO had not only failed to give her what, in her view, was obviously required, but in fact had left her with the perplexing and frustrating impression that somehow she was to blame for the problem and all that was needed was for her and her staff simply to work harder.

Solving the problem

Historically, 'communication' has been rather broadly defined as, 'the imparting, conveying or exchange of ideas and knowledge'[1]. This type of definition, in its simplest form, implies nothing more than data transfer from point A to point B. Expanding on this, the human resources literature, more familiar to managers than to clinicians, has emphasized the 'commonness' implied within the word, leading to a definition as 'the transmission of information and understanding through the use of common symbols'[2]. This is a more active view which requires the parties involved coming to some sort of shared position based on an exchange. Although this is entirely consistent with the principles of reflective listening, acceptance, utilization, reframing and suggestion as presented throughout this book, how can we usefully apply this to the type of interaction between Celia and Monika? What can you actually do, for example, to facilitate reflective listening, or use the language that the administrator best understands?

A useful starting place may simply be the personal insight into the nature of the difference between the doctor–patient relationship and that of the clinician and manager. This raises numerous questions that are beyond the scope of this book in relation to personal motivators, and psychological needs, etc. Simplistically, clinicians generally go to work each day to help people and are then presented with people seeking help. Does the manager, like Monika, have the same primary motivation, in this case specifically to help Celia, or is it more that Celia represents a problem amongst many others that needs to be solved?

Typically, management is about making decisions around allocation of finite resources—who gets what and who does not. There are two perspectives that have been developed in the management literature that are worth considering in this context. First, to view each interaction as a form of conflict that must be resolved. This invokes consideration of such things as the importance of the issue to both parties, and the need for an enduring relationship. Second, that the process of coming to an agreement is commonly manifested as a negotiation between two or more parties. Such negotiations have definable characteristics and agreed 'rules of engagement'.

Conflict resolution

Greenhalgh has described a conflict diagnosis model, as seen in Table 19.1, which includes seven dimensions for consideration[3]. For each dimension, there is a continuum of possible viewpoints based on the perceived ease of resolution.

Assuming both parties are interested in resolving conflict as easily as possible, application of this model aims to facilitate moving parties to the 'easy' side of the ledger by

Table 19.1 A conflict diagnosis model

Dimension	Easy to resolve	Difficult to resolve
Size of stakes	Small	Large
Issue at hand	Divisible	Matter of principle
Interdependence of parties	Positive-sum	Zero-sum
Continuity of interaction	Long-term relationship	Single transaction
Organization of the parties	Cohesive, organized	Amorphous, factionalized
Involvement of a third party	Neutral, trusted	No neutral third party available
Perceived cost or harm from conflict situation	Equal; impact or concessions balanced	Unbalanced; one party feels more harmed

first appreciating their current situation—that is, recognizing each other's reality and then attempting, where possible, to find ways of shifting the balance. There will be no discussion of content if there is not some initial link based on a joint recognition of the possibility of going somewhere. Hence, adopting this approach, and invoking some elements of reframing and suggestion, consider the following:

Celia: *'I need three extra staff which will be $500 000 and I need it now'.*
Monika: *'You must be joking, we don't have that sort of money lying around and I have no hope of meeting this year's financial targets trying to do this at such short notice'.*

This could be reframed addressing Monika's real concerns and as an issue where the stakes are not so high:

Celia: *'There will be a total additional cost but it can be spread over 3 years, and which also allows time to develop significant cost-saving strategies that will flow from my staff doing less overtime—net effect $200 000'.*

And similarly,

Celia: *'If we don't get the staff, everyone is going to leave',*

versus

Celia: *'The extra staff will enable us to implement the new day procedure service which will not only raise more revenue but meet the Board's stated strategic direction'.*

This acceptance of the administration's reality facilitates a positive-sum solution which does not rely on simply taking resources from someone else.

Negotiating with management

A number of different approaches to negotiation have been promoted. Publications vary from superficial guides offering simple advice on tactics, through to theoretical models attempting to dissect individual's behaviours by exploring underlying personality traits and value systems. For the clinician manager such as Celia, the elements that may be most relevant in this context are the personal attributes of empathy—a dominant quality of healthcare workers, and the need to develop and maintain relationships over time with different professional groups, including management. Conversely, if Monika is under substantial pressure to rein in costs and there are no other drivers for change from the management perspective, Celia's problem will not be seen as something to take on.

A typical analysis of the elements of any negotiation as presented at length by Lewicki[4] can be broken down into: preparation; determining a negotiation strategy; deciding on tactics; and relationship building. Of value at this point is to emphasize the importance of having clearly defined outcomes and boundary points for the negotiation.

Typical elements are:

- ***Target point*** —the desired outcome. This is exactly what you want, and why, and what you are prepared to do to get it. This includes not only the direct content of your objective, but also how long it takes to be achieved, the amount of time and effort involved, the total cost, etc.

- ***Resistance point***—the absolute boundary beyond which you are not prepared to go. Anyone who has been involved in a real estate auction will understand this and the importance of defining the limit before becoming carried away in the heat of the moment.
- ***Settlement range***—the interval in which there is some overlap of the resistance points of both parties, and it is here that a solution sits. Celia would like four extra staff but is prepared to work with two; Monika only has money for one extra but is prepared to allow two with certain provisos such as a review of the situation in 12 months. The key to a solution lies where these ranges overlap—that is, two extra staff. Where genuine difficulty may arise is when there is no overlap. The parties then have to work at revising resistance points.
- ***Bargaining mix***—the full range of attributes that totally defines the objective. Celia can have funding for three senior consultant staff if she is prepared to wait 12 months or she can have two senior registrars next week. What does she really want in terms of timing, skill mix, etc., and has she considered all the options?
- ***Best alternative*** to a negotiated agreement (BATNA)—this is the ultimate backstop if no solution is found.

The one-page Executive Summary

Much of day-to-day decision making depends on analysing summary information to assess a decision's impact on relevant stakeholders, only seeking greater detail in response to specific points for clarity; such detail then needs to be quickly and easily available. Anaesthetists in the midst of a busy theatre list can immediately relate to the importance of a succinct summary of the clinical problems of the next patient and the ability quickly to obtain targeted pathology results as necessary. In contrast, a lengthy dissertation presented with no sense of relevance to the issue at hand is nothing but frustrating. Managers have the same issues. The one-page Executive Summary is the direct analogy in this context. It must tell enough of the story for the senior person synthesizing the information and ultimately taking responsibility for the decisions, to get a satisfactory grasp of the salient features. It needs to list specific recommendations and should include likely outcomes if the recommendations are met or not met. Further fine detail needs to be readily accessible for reference and scrutiny.

Such an Executive Summary that Celia might have considered is presented as Figure 19.1.

Some features to be noted:

1. How the message is sent:
   a. Use the correct medium—if the CEO prefers an organizational template to be used, get a copy and use it.
   b. The one-page summary is only one page—keep cutting to make it fit.
   c. Check for spelling errors and simple typos and ensure formatting facilitates ease of reading.

St Elsewhere Hospital

St Elsewhere Hospital

BRIEFING NOTE FOR EXECUTIVE

TO: Monika Kreutzinger, Chief Executive Officer
FROM: Dr Celia Roberts, Director of Anaesthesia
RE: Anaesthesia Staffing
DATE: 8th September 2011

RECOMMENDATIONS

It is recommended that Executive:

1. Approve the creation of one new senior registrar position as part of a strategy to reduce total cost for specialist call-backs. This is projected to save $100,000 in a full year. It will be trialled for 12 months to fully assess impact.

2. Approve the creation of three new fulltime specialist positions, each for a period of 3 years, subject to appropriate personal performance review and ongoing service needs after 12 months. This supports proposed service redesigns and will reduce uncertainty and costs related to use of casual staff. Additional cost over 3 years is $200,000.

SUMMARY OF ISSUES

a. There is currently no provision for coverage of leave: staff absences are covered by ad hoc short term arrangements dependent on availability of external staff at premium rates. Significant financial and clinical risks to the organisation exist in not being able to find suitably qualified specialist anaesthetists at short notice leading to cancellation of services and case postponements.

b. The increase in clinical activity, including total after-hours case-load, and increased patient complexity has been well-documented (Attachment 1). The impact on Specialist Anaesthetists has been increased after-hours work with resultant decreased availability for in-hours service delivery, plus increased leave-taking due to fatigue and illness (Attachment 2).

c. Certainty in staff availability, enhanced cost predictability and total cost reduction can be achieved by employing additional specialist staff on a regular basis. A Senior Registrar can perform some of the duties currently undertaken by specialists and at considerably less cost. Total overtime payments, and sick leave should fall (Attachment 3).

d. As part of planning for the proposed service redesign, modelling of the Finance Dept supports the appointment of additional staff to meet projected activity targets. Break-even points can be achieved in the range of 2-4 years dependent on actual patient numbers. (Attachment 3).

ATTACHMENTS

Attachment 1 - Patient Activity by Service Type and Complexity: Data Unit, StEH.
Attachment 2 - Annual Finance Report, Dept of Anaesthesia: Finance Dept, StEH.
Attachment 3 – Supplementary Analysis, Finance Dept, StEH.

CONSULTATION AND ADVICE FROM OTHERS

1. Jack Smith, Management Accountant, Head of Service Planning, StEH.

Fig. 19.1 Executive Summary—what Celia might have done differently.

2 What is sent:

a Lead off with the specific requests that are the decision points—this is not some sort of thriller with beginning, middle and end. Making them search for what you really want is just a nuisance and creates the possibility of a perceived hidden intent.

b Include something that is likely to be agreed to—this creates the sense of joint problem solving and the opportunity for moving further forward.

c Incorporate your predetermined negotiation points—be very clear where you are in your negotiation range and avoid ambit claims as they rarely work unless you are in a very strong position.

d There must be sufficient detail to be meaningful, and 'mandatory' fields must be completed—if requests are never considered without stating the financial bottom-line then this has to be included.

e Directly identify respected others as contributors–this is then not just about me versus you.

3 Addressing their concerns:

a The language of the business world is money in financial statements and cost projections; workload is in complexity-adjusted throughput—get the finance department to translate what you want specifically into this format.

b Identify the issues that the CEO is actually worried about—it really will not go very far if the only line you have is concern for patient safety when there have been no serious patient incidents. Other issues such as the CEO's interest in developing a new clinical service could be a source of mutual gain.

c Know who the CEO answers to and what are they concerned about.

Solutions that address the concerns of Board members and politicians will strike a chord if presented genuinely and constructively.

The communication setting

The increasing use of technology for communication over direct human contact presents considerable challenges and risks for misinformation to occur (see Chapter 1). With the ease and familiarity of pushing the 'send' button, it is easy to lose sight of the distinction between data transfer from what should actually be part of a two-way process that requires the active participation of both parties. Electronic messages are particularly hazardous! Conversations via e-mail or SMS are typically short, asynchronous and lack the precision of correct spelling and grammatical rules. The parties also do not have the benefit of non-verbal cues through direct eye contact and body language—not all of the message is being sent. It is ultimately a matter of judgement as to whether the specific issue at hand is suited to a quick 'flick' of an e-mail, a phone conversation, an informal meeting over coffee or, at the extreme, a pre-arranged meeting in the CEO's office with everybody's lawyers present. Simple electronic methods such as short e-mails and text messages are best reserved for easy-to-resolve situations when the recipient is familiar with the sender's idiosyncrasies and turns of phrase. Anything on the difficult side requires face-to-face meetings, briefing documents, engagement of other stakeholders, documentation, accurate record keeping and considered opportunities for reflection.

Promoting 'win–win' as a possible solution

A zero-sum outcome is when one party wins at the other's expense. The 'pie' is a fixed size and the end result can only be arrived at by re-division of the whole. A positive-sum outcome is when the 'pie' actually gets bigger through a process of constructive development. By reframing communications in the form of potential mutual gains, there is more likely to be a perspective focusing on solving the problem rather than an emphasis on winning and losing which comes from only seeing an ever-diminishing 'pie'.

If Celia Roberts' multi-page document ends more or less with the simplistic conclusion that management should just give her more staff, with the associated additional expense, Monika will be left to make a 'Wisdom of Solomon judgement'—perhaps more anaesthesia staff but at the cost of less nursing staff.

Alternatively, Celia's proposals could include a range of possible system redesign initiatives alongside the extra staff. For example, the extra anaesthesia staff could be involved in multi-disciplinary pre-operative planning clinics, ultimately reducing total length of stay, or unplanned admissions. This may give Monika, and perhaps other stakeholders, some ideas they can then work on rather than seeing the issue simply as a matter of one group winning at another's expense.

It should also be anticipated that senior managers are not going to appreciate being backed into a corner. It is their job to ration resources and set strategic direction for a whole range of stakeholders, and they will generally seek solutions around negotiation. A take-it-or-leave-it position is likely to create an impasse. A useful guide is to apply the test of what a reasonable third party would, even hypothetically, make of your stance—that is, appreciating the 'third reality' as discussed in Chapter 2.

Recognizing the emotional components

There is always the potential for the stakes to become a matter of winning and losing, and to lose sight of the original goal. Taking a big breath and counting to ten, rather than reacting when emotions are high, will generally be beneficial. Picking up the phone or sending off a hastily constructed e-mail are quick and easy things to do and there is a great temptation to do this when wanting to vent feelings immediately. This is generally exactly what should be avoided. Very few matters require a truly instantaneous response, and it will almost always be possible to sleep on it. If you choose to respond by e-mail, draft the content but do not enter the addressee's name until you have read and re-read what you have written to avoid inadvertently sending something half-baked. Placing either too much or too little importance strikes at credibility. If possible, seek the counsel of trusted others when the stakes are high or if uncertain of the importance.

There are very few instances when any one fact will have absolute dominance over all other considerations. For every fact that Celia wheels out, Monika seems able to find another. In both cases the veracity of the facts is not what is at question but the interpretation and relative importance being placed on them by the two parties. As extensively reviewed by the members of the Harvard Negotiation Project[5], one of the major sources of failing to move forward in a conflict situation is when the two parties descend into the 'I'm right and you're wrong' debate. Energy is then increasingly expended in defending a position and attacking the other party, rather than accepting facts as facts, and coming to some agreement about their relative significance. The important insight is that the other party ***believes*** it is 'right' and has valid concerns. This is where acceptance is helpful to move forward. The task for both parties is then to repeatedly attempt to restate goals in ways that are mutually acceptable. For example, Monika's problem is commitment to the burden of recurrent expense, specifically at this point in time. Solutions from Celia that are less costly in the short term—for example, temporary appointments—enable an agreement to be reached.

There will be instances in difficult conversations when the emotional impact actually becomes the issue. A common misperception is that impact equates to intent. Hence, there is a risk that Celia will conclude that the negativity of rejection stems from a desire by Monika ***intentionally*** to cause harm. Failing to separate impact from intent will adversely affect Celia's capacity to remain objective and argue her case constructively and in a way that is meaningful to Monika. This will be influenced by numerous factors including personal values and previous experiences. Celia could well begin to think, '*...being made to wait 3 weeks for an appointment, then another 20 minutes on the day; being kept in an ante-room like being back at school and then to be told you can't even get the facts straight, is not how an intelligent professional should be treated*'.

Celia's time in conversation with Monika is then being spent wrestling with her emotional response to the situation and not on the substance of the matter. Not surprisingly Monika is also likely to begin responding emotionally. If the conversation appears to be more about emotions, personality and reactivity, it is essential to stop, recognize the subconscious response and revert back to substance as the most useful and likely strategy to sort this out.

There is an issue of self-image attached to any interaction like this. As explored at length in classic works by Alfie Kohn[6], high achievers such as Celia and Monika are typically products of reward systems which from an early age reinforce a sense of self-worth based on gold stars and public adulation. 'Failure', in the form of not getting the staff, is not only unfamiliar territory for Celia, but is likely to raise self-doubt about competency and self-esteem. This is analogous to the impact on clinicians of dealing with a major patient incident or medico-legal action. At least acknowledging that this reaction is happening is an important part of staying focused on the matter in hand.

Converting 'matters of principle' to 'matters of fiscal accountability'

Generally, issues will be broken down to a perspective based on resource allocation. Any issue that cannot be framed in terms of some form of financial bottom-line will make it difficult for the manager to relate to the criteria they have to work with. It will be easier to have a discussion which includes a financial outcome—many doctors find this conflicts with their value system. However, the patient safety initiatives in healthcare over the past two decades are examples of how 'matters of principle', which may be ignored, can become matters of fiscal accountability which get implemented. This is a major topic in its own right[7–12].

Maintaining profile and a sense of urgency

Senior managers—like anaesthetists—are time-poor and are continuously realigning job lists at short notice, depending on the priorities set from a number of competing sources. Even if the Anaesthetic Department issues are important today, it could easily seem less so tomorrow. Maintaining profile and a sense of urgency is almost expected. Senior managers have a relatively short tenure compared with most medical staff. It is usual for executives to move on after a comparatively short period. One of the major challenges identified in management thinking since the 1980s has been the emphasis on the capacity for change. There is abundant literature on concepts such as the 'learning organization' and the type of executive that is required in this environment[13]. Clinicians frequently interpret these features as signalling a lack of commitment or poor work quality. However, a manager operating in a corporate world where tenure is expected to be short, and job progression is based on results, has considerable motivation to achieve much in a relatively short time. This should be seen for what it is and put to good use where possible.

The buck stops here...

After the highly unsatisfactory meeting with Monika, Celia returns to the familiar home territory of her department, feeling some relief after the disappointment and slowly evolving anger. However, this sense of comfort quickly evaporates when two of the senior staff approach her.

'Well, when do we get the extra staff?' one of them asks.

It is at this point that the grim reality of the situation and the complexity of her new role sink in for the first time. As her colleagues' representative she is now carrying the responsibility for their quality of life in this work environment and they are clearly seeing her in a different light from when she was merely a member of the clan. In her new role she is both a part of the clan and quite separate from it.

The training and clinical life of anaesthetists is based around taking individual responsibility for one's own actions in a direct face-to-face patient encounter and then personally living with the consequences. It can be difficult to assume the role of representing others and arguing the case on their behalf.

Ultimately, the role of head of department is a leadership position. However, in communicating with staff in the department, the guidance given previously for interaction with management contains equally pertinent elements. Some aspects may require different emphases, particularly when the relationship between the head and staff will typically be more personal and enduring.

There are, for example, likely to be recurrent instances of directly working with each other, a form of close contact and interdependence unlike the relationship with upper level management. In addition, the head of department will be perceived as the one who directly makes decisions influencing the quality of both professional and personal life. Decisions that do not go in favour of the staff may well attract a degree of emotion, a sense of betrayal or even accusations of 'siding with the enemy'. The ploy of shifting responsibility to the evil warlords in management can be adopted and may be useful for a while, but will ultimately wear thin!

An alternative approach

Communicating effectively with administration is, in principle, no different from any other interpersonal interaction. Listening to Monika, appreciating and accepting her reality at least temporarily, even if Celia doesn't agree with it, will increase rapport and facilitate trust. Utilizing Monika's language will assist in any reframes necessary that might facilitate insight and promote an alignment of possible solutions.

Using 'GREAT' in the context of administration

Greeting and Goals

> **Celia:** '*Hi Monika as stated in my e-mail I want to discuss how we can ensure a safe working environment where lists can be covered by appropriately trained staff*.

Early on in the interaction it can be established what goals are of common interest. Once these are identified and recognized a solution may be more likely to be found. In the initial interaction, Celia did not present Monika with the goals of providing a safe working environment where lists can be covered by appropriately trained staff.

Rapport development

> **Celia:** '*I appreciate that you have been here for a while and I recognize that like us you are overworked and, as you say, there are considerable financial pressures. From what you say it appears there may be some difficulty meeting this year's financial targets given our request for your consideration at such short notice*'.

Listening, acceptance and utilization will be the primary tools available to the anaesthetist when communicating with administration (see Chapter 2). It is particularly important to make no assumptions about the relative importance to the other party of the matter at hand. It is perhaps not surprising then that the need for ensuring that the form of the message, the timing of it and creating an appropriate contextual frame are likely to take more effort and more time when dealing with a senior manager whose background, biases, context and preferred method of data presentation may be quite different from one's own.

Evaluation, Expectations, Explanation

> **Celia:** '*What I need is a solution to my staffing problem. Now as can be seen from the one-page exec summary, we have proposed a solution that should be able to meet our requirements regarding patient care and safety, and your requirements regarding the financial constraints*'.

It is important to accurately and succinctly identify what the negotiation's key issues are about, document discussions and meetings as soon as possible after they occur, and obtain confirmation of what was discussed, what was agreed to and what was not. Whilst busy managers and clinicians must juggle many different priorities, one should remember that people sometimes forget, or were actually talking about something else at the time.

Acknowledging and Addressing concerns, Answering questions

Celia: '*I appreciate you taking the time to research staffing in other hospitals and acknowledge your concern that we appear to be adequately staffed. However, as can be seen in the summary document this doesn't take into account long-term sick leave, unexpected retirements and the other hospital closures*'.

It is essential for Celia to acknowledge and address Monika's concerns as well as voice her own if progress is to be made. Monika could well have begun the interaction with a fairly concrete idea of how it was going to end. When it is possible for both parties to enter into reasoned debate there will be perceived opportunities for gain and hence some room to manoeuvre. In contrast, a particularly difficult situation can be created when either party portrays the issue as a matter of principle. Listening reflectively, acceptance, utilization and reframing can be particularly useful techniques to promote rapport, develop trust, and facilitate engagement even if an issue was initially flagged as something not open to debate. Acceptance on behalf of the anaesthetist at least temporarily will almost always present a way forward for logical analysis.

Tacit agreement, Thanks, Termination

Celia: '*OK so we are agreed on a plan and I'll come back to you with those figures you needed—Thanks for your time*'.

The characters of Celia and Monika are fictional stereotypes. They have been created to illustrate some of the principles underlying effective communication. The model proposed is based on defining communication between clinician and manager as a two-way interactive process leading to joint understanding. This necessarily requires understanding oneself as much as understanding the person with whom you are dealing. The practical approach proposed is one of resolving conflict using commonly identified negotiation skills, which can be readily reconciled with the '**LAURS**' of communication.

The spectrum of encounters is wide. At one extreme there are one-off issues with little or no need to consider the impact on the relationship. At the other extreme is the clinician manager representing the interests of many and aware of the need to preserve an effective relationship not only with management but with the people represented, and perhaps a number of other stakeholders such as patients!

Joint problem solving is the most successful strategic choice when both share a desire for a good outcome and an enduring relationship. Clear target points and boundaries need to be set before engaging. Considerable effort may be required to acknowledge emotional impact and adverse effects on self-worth. Although financial considerations are nearly always perceived as relevant, other factors such as feeling valued, being treated as a professional, and having concerns listened to and seen to be addressed are always important.

Key points

1. Conversations in negotiation are most productive when attention is focused on the substance of the matter and mutual goals rather than emotions.
2. Openness, honesty and engagement are the mainstays enabling effectiveness in communication and preserving the relationship base within the department and with management.
3. Ensuring that the form of the message, the timing of it, and creating an appropriate contextual frame, will take more effort and more time when dealing with a senior manager whose background, biases and preferred method of data presentation may be quite different from one's own.
4. By reframing communications in the form of potential mutual gains, there is more likely to be a perspective focusing on solving the problem rather than winning and losing.
5. Addressing the basic elements of negotiation strategy through the determination of target and resistance points, acknowledging there is a bargaining mix and continuing to work to identify the settlement range should facilitate mutual understanding and achieving goals.
6. Everyone is busy; one-page summaries and clear succinct information are always helpful.

References

1 Onions CT (1973). *The shorter Oxford English dictionary on historical principles.* 3rd edn. New York: Oxford University Press.

2 Ivancevich JM, Olekalns M, Matteson M (1997). *Organisational behaviour and management.* Sydney: McGraw Hill.

3 Greenhalgh L. (1986). Managing conflict. *Sloan Manage Rev*, Summer, 45–51.

4 Lewicki RJ, Saunders DM, Barry B (2009). *Negotiation.* 6th edn. Boston: McGraw Hill.

5 Stone D, Patton B, Heen S (1999). *Difficult conversations.* New York: Penguin Books.

6 Kohn A (1993). *Punished by rewards.* New York: Houghton Mifflin.

7 WHO Patient Safety Solutions (2008). http://www.ccforpatientsafety.org/WHO-Collaborating-Centre-for-Patient-Safety-Solutions/(Accessed 21 March 2010).

8 Martin LA, Neumann CW, Mountford J, Bisognano M, Nolan TW (2009). *Increasing efficiency and enhancing value in health care: ways to achieve savings in operating costs per year.* IHI Innovation Series white paper. Cambridge, MA: Institute for Healthcare Improvement.

9 Silow-Carroll S, Alteras T, Meyer JA (2007). *Hospital quality improvement: strategies and lessons from U.S. hospitals.* The Commonwealth Fund.

10 Haynes AB, Weiser TG, Berry WR, Lipsitz SR, Breizat AH, Dellinger EP et al (2009). A surgical safety checklist to reduce morbidity and mortality in a global population. *N Engl J Med,* **360**, 491–9.

11 Institute for Healthcare Improvement. *Improvement stories.* Cambridge, MA. http://www.ihi.org/IHI/Results/ImprovementStories/; accessed February 2010.

12 Katz MH (2010). Decreasing hospital costs while maintaining quality: can it be done? *Arch Intern Med,* **170**, 317–8.

13 Senge PM (1992). *The fifth discipline.* Sydney: Random House.

Section 5

Advanced communication techniques

Chapter 20

Hypnotic techniques

Marie-Elisabeth Faymonville, Christel J Bejenke, and Ernil Hansen

'...you may say I'm a dreamer but I'm not the only one...'.
'Imagine' John Lennon

What this chapter is about

Anxiety, fear, tension and apprehension are common emotions in patients undergoing surgery. Clinicians are becoming increasingly aware of the importance of patients' psychological reactions as well as their physical needs. For instance, surgeons now explain more to their patients than was formerly the case. The anaesthetist is therefore presented with an opportunity to use the pre-operative anaesthesia assessment as a means of fostering greater rapport and providing reassurance.

There is, of course, still much reliance upon sedative and analgesic drugs to relieve anxiety and tension prior to major anaesthesia. However, sedatives are not the only answer. Sedation can be accomplished pharmacologically, but drugs cannot re-educate patients in a way that enables them to respond more positively to their medical or surgical treatment. The challenge for anaesthetists seeking to provide optimal anaesthetic care for their patients is not only to become more expert in the latest state-of-the-art technology, but rather to acquire the skills necessary to function effectively in the role of physician healer.

Hypnosis is not a 'therapy', but a potentially valuable tool in the anaesthetist's professional armamentarium, and deserves to receive equal consideration with other tools and skills which anaesthetists acquire. Hypnotic techniques can influence communication to such a degree that the patient's entire medical experience is beneficially affected[1–5]. Anaesthetists trained in the use of hypnosis can use this approach in 'formal hypnosis' or as 'awake suggestions'.

Formal hypnosis

Hypnosis has had a cyclical history of acceptance and rejection. It has been practised in one form or another for thousands of years. However, it was not until 1828 that a scientific publication first reported its effectiveness as an anaesthetic for surgery. However, when volatile agents were introduced, the use of hypnosis as a sole anaesthesia technique died out[6].

Because of its historical association with magic, hypnosis has had to struggle to become disentangled from faith-healing methods and the occult. In a number of hospitals around the world, hypnosis is used as an adjuvant to pharmacological anaesthesia, either before or after general anesthesia[7,8]. At the same time, the fact that major surgery has been comfortably performed entirely under hypnosis overcomes some of the scepticism associated with its ancillary uses[9–11]. For most people, anaesthesia and surgery is in the realm of the unknown and is associated with numerous fears.

Since 1992, anaesthetists at the University Hospital of Liège, Belgium, have replaced traditional anaesthetic techniques—general anaesthesia or sedation—with one combining hypnosis with light conscious intravenous sedation. More than 8000 patients have comfortably undergone major head and neck or breast surgery under hypnosedation. The most important benefit of this technique is that patients maintain their consciousness, and avoid general anaesthesia.

During hypnosedation, in order to help patients better cope with pain and surgery, hypnosis is used for the therapeutic purpose of inducing a controlled state of dissociation. The surgical decision to operate under local anaesthesia and hypnosedation is dependent on the surgeon's own appreciation of feasibility, and familiarity with the technique. During the pre-operative anaesthesia interview, the patient is asked about his own motivation for this specific anaesthetic technique. Information is provided about the hypnotic state but no rehearsal is offered.

After transfer to the operating theatre, each patient is invited to choose a pleasant life experience to be 're-lived' during surgery—a 'lived in imagination' technique. A hypnotic state is then induced. After approximately 10 minutes, the patient is usually at an adequate depth of hypnosis as evidenced by slow eye movements. This psychological approach is supplemented by intravenous administration of remifentanyl, and on occasion midazolam, in order to maintain conscious sedation, provide patient comfort and optimize surgical conditions.

The induction is simple and straightforward, while at the same time quite complex, and illustrative of hypnotic phenomena involving: eye fixation; internal absorption; relaxation of the body; and increasing quietness of the mind. Patients are invited to relive previous pleasant autobiographical experiences without any suggestions for analgesia. As practice continues, confidence levels increase and the clinician begins to observe opportunities to tailor the hypnotic procedure to the particular needs of the moment by utilizing what happens around the patient. This technique provides more comfort to both patient and surgeon, better perioperative pain relief and anxiolysis, more haemodynamic stability, and faster recovery with less fatigue and pain[12–14].

What is hypnosis?

Hypnotic and imagery strategies for managing acute pain symptoms and emotional factors, associated with surgery, are described in several articles[15–17]. The construct of 'hypnosis' is used to represent both a particular state of consciousness and the technique employed to induce such a state. Like any state of consciousness, the hypnotic state is difficult to measure and objectify. In hypnosis, verbal suggestions can lead to remarkable alterations in subjective experiences. These include atypical changes in perception, memory, and some behaviours which may appear to occur without volitional control. Hypnotic suggestions do not ask subjects simply to 'imagine' the suggested state of affairs, rather the person under hypnosis is 'guided' to experience, as if in real life, circumstances which would permit responses consistent with the hypnotist's suggestions.

The scientific foundations upon which the understanding of hypnosis is based have become much firmer in the last two decades. The striking changes in perception and conscious awareness that can be achieved with hypnotic communication techniques have fascinated both researchers and clinicians. Knowledge of these neurophysiological findings will help the practising clinician to better understand how hypnosis works as an important therapeutic technique in pain management[18].

We now have an opportunity to explore activity in the brain during hypnotic pain modulation with neuroimaging techniques such as regional cerebral blood flow (rCBF), modification with positron emission tomography (PET)[19,20] and functional magnetic resonance[21]. Psychologically mediated forms of pain reduction, as shown during hypnotic procedures, modulate not only nociceptive reflexes and pain-related autonomic activity, elicited by peripheral stimulation, but also supraspinal pain control systems. Functional imaging studies have identified activation in mid-cingulate cortex area 24'a as directly mediating the changes in pain perception specific to hypnotic suggestion. Hypnosis has been found to enhance functional modulation between the mid-cingulate area 24'a, and a wide network of sensory, affective, cognitive and motor-related brain regions[22].

What is important before using hypnotic techniques?

The concept of safety should be the first priority in the context of using hypnosis for pain and anxiety management. Patients need to know that a proper medical assessment has been completed before proceeding with hypnosis. This means explaining to patients that they have access to adjunct pharmacological treatments when these are appropriate and involves helping patients to believe and feel that they are understood and cared about. Also implied is the rigorous training of the anaesthetist in these techniques.

The next essential is responsibility. Clinicians need to assist patients to assume healthy responsibility for their own health. This means that patients accept some responsibility for the choices to be made about the steps they will take, to achieve more effective pain management. It also presumes the ability to consider and weigh the potential costs and risks as opposed to the benefits of alternative courses of action, and also the willingness to make decisions and follow through with them.

Hypnosis can be utilized on its own or as an adjunct to traditional therapy. To maintain ethical standards and responsible practice, there are learned societies which offer guidelines and accreditation to clinicians[23–25]. Training in hypnosis needs actual hands-on experience to generate a wider understanding of how therapeutic communication helps the patient to overcome stressful situations.

Prerequisites for hypnosis

1. By the very nature of hypnotic procedures, the hypnosis practitioner comes to recognize the individuality of the patient.
2. Before the hypnotic induction procedure, the anaesthetist has asked about, and listened to, the patient's specific needs. Thereby, the patient feels respected and legitimately understood and cared about, and feels safe.
3. Hypnotic techniques rely on a harmonious trustful relationship. During the induction procedure, the anaesthetist uses specific communication skills to help guide a patient to put him or her into the hypnotic state. It is a cooperative construction where the hypnotist responds with verbal and non-verbal suggestions to the patient's needs.
4. To assist the patient appropriately, the practitioner of hypnosis must also accept another person's alternative reality. The practitioner's communication is adapted, by integrating the patient's words and behaviours, even if these may run counter to the practitioner's own beliefs or experiences. Patients knows what is good for them, and hypnosis can help them to be involved in their own recovery, and take an active role through the employment of these self-management skills.
5. Hypnotic communication skills allow anaesthetists to integrate patients' concerns by using and speaking the patients' language to enhance patients' strengths and abilities to cope with the situation. These techniques help anaesthetists to reframe patients' concerns into more therapeutic thoughts, perceptions or behaviours.
6. Working with patients during surgery by using hypnosis or teaching self-hypnosis techniques empowers them to be their own advocate and to play an active role during recovery.

The challenge for anaesthetists is how best to complement their general and regional anaesthesia skills to facilitate more comprehensive pain management. Anaesthetists are urged not to limit their concerns solely to biological issues but to expand their skills beyond traditional biomedical methods. They should recognize language as a primary intervention in the management of pain. Hypnotic, as well as non-hypnotic, communication skills are effectively taught, and easily learned and incorporated into routine anaesthesia practice without significantly lengthening the medical visit or radically changing the way medicine is practised[1].

Interestingly, without being aware of it, many anaesthetists actually do use 'hypnotic techniques' and 'hypnotic language'—most commonly with children[26]. For example: '*getting ready for a space-flight*'; applying an '*astronaut's mask*'—the anaesthesia mask; smelling '*that special astronaut air*'—the anaesthetic gas. We may tell stories, describe swings or carousels '*getting just a bit dizzy ... going back and forth*', or '*round and round—having so much fun ...*', taking a '*wonderful ride at Disneyland*'; watching a favourite TV programme; playing with a favourite toy or pet, etc. Because these techniques work, a basic knowledge of hypnotic concepts and principles can make anaesthetic care less haphazard, more efficient and more effective. Hypnotic concepts can help us understand more clearly why some of what we say works well, or why it doesn't. We can then develop approaches that work reliably.

Concepts of hypnosis

Hypnotic concepts and principles demonstrate the significance of nuances in language. For example, information, identical in content, can be perceived by patients as either threatening or reassuring. It all depends on how such information is formulated and transmitted—both verbally and non-verbally[1,27]. For example, if the surgeon, anaesthetist or nurse says to a patient emerging from anaesthesia, '*It's all over!*' or '*You're finished!*' These terms could be interpreted to mean 'death'.

What could one say instead?

> **Anaesthetist** (cheerfully—the tone of voice is important): '*Hello! Dr Smith has just completed your operation .... You have done very* **well** *... and you are* ***safe*** *.... Everything is taken care of ... and you will be going home soon .... You may even be hungry....*'

The latter two statements direct the patient's attention away from the emergency, from risks and fear, and instead direct focus on to something normal, healthy and mundane.

Hypnotic concepts also allow practitioners to recognize, and thereby avoid, inadvertent negative suggestions and to rectify them. The goal of this style of communicating is to empower patients, so that they experience themselves as active participants and as equal partners with their healthcare team, rather than viewing themselves as 'victims' of an illness or condition—powerless, passive recipients of incomprehensibly complex medical technology. This empowerment, in turn, can result in reduced anxiety, improved cooperation and increased patient satisfaction.

Stressed, fearful patients are highly suggestible during seemingly normal states of consciousness. Many patients even enter spontaneous trance states and exhibit trance-like phenomena such as: focused attention; amnesia; dissociation; regression to a child-like level of functioning, and so on. In this state any communication can function as a suggestion and be as powerful as those given during formal hypnotic states[27]. Inadvertent negative language can function as negative suggestions[28] and can result in unexpected and unintended detrimental effects (see Chapter 3).

However, rather than viewing suggestibility as a liability, it can instead be utilized as a therapeutic opportunity. Because patients are already in a hypnosis-like state, it is not necessary to induce hypnosis, as suggestions can simply be used as if the patient is already hypnotized.

Suggestions

'Suggestions' can be one of the most useful forms of communication in anaesthetic practice (see Chapters 3 and 4). They can be used with most adult and paediatric patients (see Chapters 9 and 10) and in most situations such as during the risk discussion when obtaining informed consent, induction of anaesthesia or emergence in the recovery room.

While various definitions exist for this term, 'suggestion' can be understood in the vernacular English usage as 'a proposal to consider a new or different view, idea or possibility'; 'to put forward for consideration'; 'to hint, imply or intimate'. There is no expectation of 'compliance', nor is the patient 'compelled' to carry out a suggestion. Instead, the patient is offered the opportunity to entertain a different, more beneficial view or perspective, to reinterpret sensations or experiences—and most patients will choose that option.

'*You are safe*' is one of the most important statements a patient can hear pre-, intra- and post-operatively.

'*Just try to relax ....*' confirms to the patient his inability to do so, and is apt to increase his sense of helplessness. In addition, '***try***' implies doubt in the possibility of success, and therefore conveys the expectation of failure (see Chapter 3).

'*You'll go under ...*' can imply drowning.

Alternatively consider: '*Anaesthesia has to do with comfort and safety: an anaesthetist, will care for you and make sure that you are safe and will watch everything very closely... while you are deeply relaxed and comfortable*'.

Managing negative suggestions

Sometimes nurses say to a patient who is just arriving in the recovery room:

> '*I'll put this "sick bowl" (emesis basin) right here so you have it, when you need it*', or '*when you get sick*', or '*call me when you have to throw up*'.

In contrast, when a patient does vomit, this can be utilized positively:

> '*Good! You're rid of that stale old stuff. Now you can feel so much better and already look forward to eating and drinking soon*' (this is an anti-nausea suggestion, see below).

Peristalsis can also be stimulated by the suggestion to listen for and hear '*the churning and gurgling*' in your belly which results in earlier resolution of post-operative ileus after intra-abdominal surgery[29].

Variations on the same theme:

> '*Do you have pain?*'
> '*Let me know when you have pain–here is the bell*'.
> '*Tell me when you start hurting ...*'

To patients this can mean

> '*I **will** have pain—these people know; after all, they are experts*'.
> Instead: '*Let me know how I can make you more comfortable. There are so many ways we can do that: would you like ....?*'
> For example, after a mastectomy: '*Let me put a pillow under your arm. That will help relax the muscles in your chest .... and feel so much better ....*'

The anaesthetist's communication, designed to reduce the severity of any expected post-operative pain and nausea, can include:

> '*Wouldn't it be nice ... if it would be a whole lot different for you **this** time ... and quite a bit **easier** than you might have thought?*'

Case study

When asked how a patient expected to feel after her hysterectomy, she responded, '*My doctor says I'll feel like I've been run over by a truck!*'

> **Anaesthetist:** '*Would you mind feeling better than that?*'
> **Patient:** '*You mean ... like being run over by a small truck?*'
> **Anaesthetist:** '*Better than that?*'
> **Patient:** '*By a car?*'
> **Anaesthetist:** '*Better than that?*'
> **Patient:** '*Maybe ... a small car?*'
> **Anaesthetist:** '*Better than that?*'
> **Patient:** '*You mean ... a ... motorcycle?*'
> **Anaesthetist**: '*Better than that?*'
> **Patient** (after thinking for a while): '*Aaaah ... a ... bicycle?*'
> **Anaesthetist:** '*Would you mind **not** feeling like being run over by **anything**, ... just feeling some pressure underneath your bandages ... and maybe some cramps ... like when you have a period .... and things like that?*'
> **Patient:** '*Hmm ...*'

After the operation, when asked how she felt, the patient said '*I feel like I've been run over by a bicycle*' and laughed! She did not suffer the expected (and suggested!) severe post-operative pain, but instead—to her surgeon's amazement—experienced minimal discomfort and recovered more rapidly than expected. This 'intervention' took less than one minute of suggestions as part of the anaesthetist's communication.

This style of communicating is empowering, because it gives the patient ***choices*** and ***control.*** No suggestions were given as to how the patient should, could or might feel. The anaesthetist simply utilized the patient's own creativity. The choice of feeling like '*having been run over by a bicycle*', rather than by a truck, was entirely hers.

Apart from improvements in patient cooperation and being proactive even when complications arise, there are reduced demands on carers, earlier discharge from hospital, and earlier resumption of gainful work resulting in cost savings[30]. Most importantly, this type of communication can lead to a therapeutic alliance that enhances the physician–patient relationship.

Awake craniotomy without sedation

An extreme example of hypnotically based communication skills is the use of these techniques with patients having an awake craniotomy. A tumour in the vicinity of the eloquent area or motor areas of the brain may make it necessary to have the patient awake during surgery for neurological testing. This usually is achieved by an awake–sleep–awake technique where the patient receives anaesthesia or analgesia–sedation with or without controlled ventilation[31]. Besides pain there are a number of stress factors affecting patients such as: the noises and vibration of drilling and milling the skull for craniotomy; suctioning of blood; and the knowledge of having someone working inside the brain. Pain can be managed effectively by regional anaesthesia in the form of a scalp block. At the University of Regensburg, Germany, the effects of stress are mitigated by the use of 'therapeutic communication' based on an understanding of hypnosis[27,32,33], without formal induction of hypnosis.

During the pre-operative visit, rapport is established and the patient's own resources and coping strategies are evaluated by questions about family, profession, accommodation, pets, garden, favourite holiday destinations, hobbies, sport activities, experience with relaxation techniques, and preferred place of rest and recreation. One or more of these activities can be utilized later as the patient's 'safe place'.

To seed the option of reframing stimuli, an anecdote is told.

> *'A patient visits his dentist, who declares that he will have to drill. He asks "What is your hobby?" "Motorcycling". "Where?" "California". "OK, so you can close your eyes and go biking, on Highway No.1". The dentist does his work, and finally asks "How was it?" "Well, OK. But it was great, when you really turned up the revs. Brrhmm, brrhmm!"'*

The patient in this example has reinterpreted the drilling by the dentist as the revving up of the motorbike in his 'lived in imagination'.

With only this minimal preparation, one patient, who had a 'lived in imagination' experience of 'mountain hiking' during awake craniotomy at the time of drilling of b holes into the skull, said: '*There's a helicopter—taking me away*'—a wonderful interpretation for the noise and incidentally a metaphor for being saved. These examples illustrate that patients have the best images, resources and coping strategies, if we give them the opportunity to use these resources. Patients benefit from anaesthetic guidance and the avoidance of sedative drugs.

Assurance is given by placing a hand on the shoulder:

> *'This is the hand of medicine on your shoulder, representing all our experience and knowledge, all the technology and drugs we have available for you, all the good things we can do for you. This hand of medicine will stay with you—even when I take it away—to accompany you all the time, until you have safely come through this therapeutic procedure, with the results that you have been looking for'.*

Motivation is increased by explaining that although all drugs are kept on standby and can be used, from mild sedation to deep anaesthesia, they will only be used if necessary, since the fewer of these used, the better the testing will turn out, and the more successful the surgery.

Control is given by saying,

> '*Whenever you want something to change, just let us know. We are with you all the time, and we can always do something helpful for you*'.

After establishing an IV line, an arterial canula, Foley catheter and after careful positioning, the patient is guided by the anaesthetist to dissociate from the immediate environment and to internally generate one of his 'safe places': '*We don't need you right now. You might as well go ….*'

The dissociation to the safe place can be deepened with questions to the different senses:

> '*How does it feel, the sun on the skin, the ground beneath the feet? Is there a smell in the air? What colours are around? Can you hear birds, or the wind?*'

The noises in the operating room can be ***utilized*** and ***reframed***. The suction: '*Maybe there is water running somewhere*'. Rattle of instruments: '*There might be birds singing, or branches breaking. Just watch, with an open and interested mind, what comes up*'.

Non-verbal support is given by hand-holding. This helps to detect any tension. A hand on the shoulder is not only a monitor of respiration but also a tool for deepening and slowing down of breaths—by delayed pressure during expiration and delayed release with inspiration. It is not necessary or even helpful to talk to the patient all the time. As long as he is calm and relaxed there is no need to interfere. But as soon as his facial expression indicates concern or discomfort, he moves, his respiration or heart rate goes up, he opens his eyes to look around, then is the time to bring him back to his safe place. Actually, this intervention can be delayed a little, and if he closes his eyes again this indicates that he has checked for himself that he is more comfortable there.

As in Qigong or Pranayama, breathing can be used both for calming and relaxing, and as a basis for metaphors.

> '*With every breath in, you can take up fresh air and oxygen that is so essential for all the cells of the body—and with every breath out, get rid of all the used air and waste of cellular metabolism … and breathe in the good oxygen… and you may want to hold and keep it for a while—and along with expiration let it flow through your body all the way down to your toes—and take up fresh air and all the good things that can help you now—and blow away with expiration the used air and all the things that are not useful for you now or disturb you—to have the lungs ready for another deep breath to take up calmness and confidence—and exhale all stress—and take up strength and healing power…*'.

These words are spoken to the rhythm of breathing, slower and slower.

The prominent role of the theatre environment as a major negative suggestion became obvious in one patient, who was fine throughout his awake craniotomy, until, at the end of surgery, he developed a vaso-vagal reaction without reporting pain. What had happened? The lights were switched back on in the OR after microscopy. The neuropsychologist responsible for neurological testing said good-bye. The patient opened his eyes to look around and noticed a monitor showing the closure of his dura mater. The neurosurgeon let him see a rivet used for closure of the craniotomy, the patient became aware of the theatre environment and then developed hypotension—systolic blood pressure 70 mmHg—bradycardia—heart rate of 35/min—and cold sweating.

This example demonstrates to anaesthetists that what is familiar to them may be most disturbing to the patient. All that this patient needed was to be taken back to the 'walk in the woods' he had been on during the procedure.

While arousal from trance usually is expected from any disturbance, actually such events can be utilized to deepen the trance and dissociation. It is effective to point out that disturbance is not a fact, but it is the patient's and the doctor's misconception and expectation that noise has to disturb relaxation.

> '*And whenever you feel more than you want to, you can go deeper and deeper into that wonderful, calm experience of nature—and rest. Any sensation, any noise you experience can be a signal for you that everything is proceeding well here, and that you can relax and have a good time, like going for a walk or swimming after you have given your car to the garage*'.

The author (EH) has performed more than 30 awake craniotomies and more than 30 electrode placements for deep-brain stimulation in Parkinsonian patients in the above manner, with minimal or no additional analgesic, and without any sedation, and to a high level of patient satisfaction. Initially pre-emptive propofol and remifentanil were given prior to incision and craniotomy, with concomitant haemodynamic instabilities and desaturation. Subsequently, with the safety of having these tools on standby—to encourage anaesthetists to try to use less medication—it became apparent that with proper therapeutic communication, sedative medication was not required.

It may be equally true that in many cases of regional anaesthesia sedation is given for the anaesthetist's benefit rather than that of the patient. The feeling of being abandoned cannot be treated by sedation. So the question arises whether our patients should be treated under regional anaesthesia but with more effective communication. Therapeutic communication is bidirectional. We can help patients utilize their own resources, life experiences and coping strategies for pain and stress, thereby releasing them from prescribed passivity. From hypnotherapy one can learn to watch and listen to the patient and personalize therapy. Much can be learned from patients on how to improve their treatment.

Hypnotic communication relies on indirection to guide patients' associations. On one level common everyday phenomena can be spoken about, while on another suggestions are indirectly interspersed about controlling discomfort. One of the anaesthetist's key tasks is to elicit ideodynamic effects, whereby associations drive behaviour. Such multi-level communication can generate more desirable behaviour through the patient's own initiative.

Hypnosis is not a therapy in itself. Integration and application of hypnotic communication into a core therapeutic armamentarium will make sense to experienced clinicians who are willing to think creatively with each new individual patient.

Key points

1. Anaesthetists will benefit from a change in attitudes and receptiveness by using different communication skills.
2. Be aware of inadvertent negative suggestions—'innocent remarks'.
3. Information and choices are empowering.
4. '*You are safe*' is important for patients to hear.
5. The therapeutic alliance is of utmost importance.
6. Anaesthetists will benefit from a solid grounding in the principles and practices of hypnosis, and an understanding of how to integrate these into their own practice.
7. Hypnotic communication permits anaesthetists to work more effectively with a wider range of patients.

References

1 Bejenke CJ (1996). Preparation of patients for stressful medical interventions: some very simple approaches. In: Peter B, Trenkle FC, Kinzel C, Duffner A, Iost-Peter A (eds) *Munich lectures on hypnosis and psychotherapy. Hypnosis International Monographs* **2**, 27–36.

2 Lambert SA (1996). The effects of hypnosis/guided imagery on the postoperative course of children. *J Dev Behav Pediatr*, **17**, 307–10.

3 Lang E, Berbaum K, Faintuch S, Hatsiopoulou O, Halsey N, Li X et al. (2006). Adjunctive self-hypnotic relaxation for outpatient medical procedures: a prospective randomized trial with women undergoing large core breast biopsy. *Pain*, **126**, 155–64.

4 Enqvist B, von Konow L, Bystedt H (1996). Stress reduction, preoperative hypnosis and perioperative suggestion in maxillo-facial surgery: somatic responses and recovery. *Hypnosis*, **23**, 76–82.

5 Ginandes CS, Brooks P, Sando W, Jones C, Aker J (2002). Can medical hypnosis accelerate post-surgical wound healing? Results of a clinical trial. *Am J Clin Hypn*, **45**, 333–51.

6 Elliotson J (1843). *Zoist. Numerous cases of surgical operations without pain in the mesmeric state.* Philadelphia, http://books.google.com.au/books?id=XZ5xJq7qovMC&pg=PA241&lpg=PA241&dq=elliotson+1843&source=bl&ots=2T-jFYo4-I&sig=LoZjxulazuzHdP7NyVe5v5b6jL0&hl=en&ei=FeScS-3BEZCIswOCysm_Aw&sa=X&oi=book_result&ct=result&resnum=1&ved=0CAYQ6AEwAA#v=onepage&q=elliotson%201843&f=false (Accessed 15 March 2010).

7 Enqvist B, Bjorkllund C, Engman M, Jakobsson J (1997). Preoperative hypnosis reduces postoperative vomiting after surgery of the breasts. A prospective, randomized and blinded study. *Acta Anaesthesiol Scand*, **41**, 1028–32.

8 Montgomery GH, Weltz CR, Seltz M, Bovbjerg DH (2002). Brief presurgery hypnosis reduces distress and pain in excisional breast biopsy patients. *Int J Clin Exp Hypn*, **50**, 17–32.

9 Minalyka EE, Whanger AD (1959). Tonsillectomies under hypnosis: report of cases. *Am J Clin Hypn*, **2**, 87–9.

10 Rausch V (1980). Cholecystectomy with self-hypnosis. *Am J Clin Hypn*, **22**,124–9.

11 Steinberg S (1965). Hypnoanesthesia—a case report in a 90-year-old patient. *Am J Clin Hypn*, **7**, 355.

12 Faymonville ME, Mambourg PH, Joris J, Vrijens B, Fissette J, Albert A et al (1997). Psychological approaches during conscious sedation. Hypnosis versus stress reducing strategies. A prospective randomized study. *Pain*, **73**, 361–7.

13 Faymonville ME, Meurisse M, Fissette J (1999). Hypnosedation: a valuable alternative to traditional anaesthetic techniques. *Acta Chir Belg*, **99**, 141–6.

14 Defechereux T, Degauque C, Fumal I, Faymonville ME, Joris J, Hamoir E et al (2000). L'hypnosédation, un nouveau mode d'anesthésie pour la chirurgie endocrinienne cervicale. Etude prospective randomisée. *Ann Chir*, **125**, 539–46.

15 Lang EV, Benotsch EG, Fick LJ, Lutgendorf S, Berbaum ML, Berbaum KS et al (2000). Adjunctive non-pharmacological analgesia for invasive medical procedures: a randomized trial. *Lancet*, **355**, 1486–90.

16 Montgomery GH, David D, Winkel G, Siverstein JH, Bovbjerg DH (2002). The effectiveness of adjunctive hypnosis with surgical patients: a meta-analysis. *Anesth Analg*, **94**, 1639–45.

17 Wobst AKH (2007). Hypnosis and surgery: past, present and future. *Anesth Analg*, **104**, 1199–208.

18 Vanhaudenhuyse A, Boly M, Laureys S, Faymonville ME (2009). Neuro-physiological correlates of hypnotic analgesia. *Contemp Hypn*, **26**, 15–23.

19 Faymonville ME, Laureys S, Degueldre C, Del Fiore G, Luxen A, Franck G et al (2000). Neural mechanisms of antinociceptive effects of hypnosis. *Anesthesiology*, **92**, 1257–67.

20 Faymonville ME, Roediger L, Del Fiore G, Degueldre C, Phillips C, Lamy M et al (2003). Increased cerebral functional connectivity underlying the antinociceptive effects of hypnosis. *Cogn Brain Res*, **17**, 255–62.

21 Vanhaudenhuyse A, Boly M, Balteau E, Schnakers C, Moonen G, Luxen A et al (2009). Pain and non-pain processing during hypnosis: a thalium-YAG event-related fMRI study. *Neuroimage*, **47**, 1047–54.

22 Faymonville ME, Vogt B, Maquet P, Laureys S (2009). Hypnosis and cingulate-mediated mechanisms of analgesia. In: Vogt B (ed.) *Cingulate neurobiology and disease*. pp. 381–400. Oxford: Oxford University Press.

23 Yapko MD (2010). *The art and science of clinical hypnosis: why it enhances treatment so well. Overview*. http://www.sash.asn.au (Accessed 2 February 2010).

24 Code of Conduct of the American Society of Clinical Hypnosis. http://www.asch.net (Accessed March 12 2010).

25 Ethical Guidelines of the European Society of Hypnosis. http://www.esh-hypnosis.eu/ (Accessed March 16, 2010).

26 Bejenke CJ (1993). Hypnosis for surgical interventions, including an historical review. *Hypnos: Swedish J Hypn Psychother Psychosm Med*, **17**, 214–20.

27 Bejenke CJ (1996). Painful medical procedures. In: Barber J (ed.) *Hypnosis and suggestion in the treatment of pain. A clinical guide*. pp. 209–66. New York: WW Norton.

28 Bejenke CJ (1990). Operating room equipment: useful hypnotic induction aids in anesthesiology. In: Van Dyck R, Spinhoven Ph, Van der Does AJW, Van Rood YR, De Moor W (eds.) *Hypnosis: current theory, research, and practice*. pp. 199–205. Amsterdam, The Netherlands: V.U. University Press.

29 Disbrow E, Bennett H, Owings J (1993). Effect of preoperative suggestion on postoperative gastrointestinal motility. *West J Med*, **158**, 488–92.

30 Lang EV, Rosen MP (2002). Cost analysis of adjunct hypnosis with sedation during outpatient interventional radiologic procedures. *Radiology*, **222**, 375–82.

31 Piccioni F, Fanzio M (2008). Management of anesthesia in awake craniotomy. *Minerva Anestesiol*, **74**, 393–408.

32 Jacobs DT (1991). *Patient communication for first responders and EMS personnel.* Brady: Englewood Cliffs, NJ.

33 Cheek DB (1994). *Hypnosis: the application of ideomotor techniques.* Boston: Allyn and Bacon.

Index